IFMBE Proceedings

D1806684

Volume 74

The IFMBE Proceedings Book Series is an official publication of *the International Federation for Medical and Biological Engineering* (IFMBE). The series gathers the proceedings of various international conferences, which are either organized or endorsed by the Federation. Books published in this series report on cutting-edge findings and provide an informative survey on the most challenging topics and advances in the fields of medicine, biology, clinical engineering, and biophysics.

The series aims at disseminating high quality scientific information, encouraging both basic and applied research, and promoting world-wide collaboration between researchers and practitioners in the field of Medical and Biological Engineering.

Topics include, but are not limited to:

- Diagnostic Imaging, Image Processing, Biomedical Signal Processing
- Modeling and Simulation, Biomechanics
- Biomaterials, Cellular and Tissue Engineering
- Information and Communication in Medicine, Telemedicine and e-Health
- Instrumentation and Clinical Engineering
- Surgery, Minimal Invasive Interventions, Endoscopy and Image Guided Therapy
- Audiology, Ophthalmology, Emergency and Dental Medicine Applications
- Radiology, Radiation Oncology and Biological Effects of Radiation

IFMBE proceedings are indexed by SCOPUS and EI Compendex. They are also submitted for ISI proceedings indexing.

Proposals can be submitted by contacting the Springer responsible editor shown on the series webpage (see "Contacts"), or by getting in touch with the series editor Ratko Magjarevic.

More information about this series at http://www.springer.com/series/7403

Kang-Ping Lin · Ratko Magjarevic ·
Paulo de Carvalho
Editors

Future Trends in Biomedical and Health Informatics and Cybersecurity in Medical Devices

Proceedings of the International
Conference on Biomedical and Health
Informatics, ICBHI 2019, 17–20 April, 2019,
Taipei, Taiwan

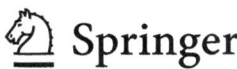 Springer

Editors
Kang-Ping Lin
Department of Electrical Engineering
Chung Yuan Christian University
Taoyuan, Taiwan

Ratko Magjarevic
Faculty of Electrical Engineering
and Computing
University of Zagreb
Zagreb, Croatia

Paulo de Carvalho
Department of Informatics Engineering
University of Coimbra
Coimbra, Portugal

ISSN 1680-0737   ISSN 1433-9277   (electronic)
IFMBE Proceedings
ISBN 978-3-030-30635-9   ISBN 978-3-030-30636-6   (eBook)
https://doi.org/10.1007/978-3-030-30636-6

This Springer imprint is published by the registered company Springer Nature Switzerland AG
The registered company address is: Gewerbestrasse 11, 6330 Cham, Switzerland

Preface

The Technology Translation Center for Medical Device, Chung Yuan Christian University, Taiwan, and IFMBE WG on Health Informatics and eHealth organized the ICBHI 2019 in Taipei, held on April 17–20, 2019. The ICBHI 2019 was one of the most important scientific events initiated from the IFMBE Working Group on Health Informatics and eHealth, gathering together expertise from biomedical, technological, and health information fields. The goals of the conference focused on future trends in Biomedical and Health Informatics & Cybersecurity in Medical Device.

Biomedical information and health informatics is a rapidly growing field that brings healthcare system into a new era with innovative medical devices, eHealth, mHealth, and personalized health (pHealth) technologies. The developments may involve the following areas

- Medical devices, medical imaging, and biosignal processing
- Biomedical informatics
- Cybersecurity and healthcare Information
- AI in medical image
- Biodata management and analytics
- Advanced mHealth-inspired applications
- User interaction systems and data/information exchange
- Applied connected health and integrated care systems
- Personalized health systems
- Preventive and multimorbid disease management tools
- Patient safety and efficient public health systems
- Biomedical informatics and technology education

By incorporating from data to effective information, ICBHI 2019 was expected to integrate the achievements of the above various topics and provide a new development mechanism for biomedical information and bioinformatics to fulfill health care, patient safety, and medical quality. In addition, the conference was expected to obtain in-depth biological data through a variety of ICT technologies for assisting healthcare system and facilitating growth of biomedical knowledge.

The conference focused on the link and integration of information of medical devices, specifically topics related to bio-information security and cybersecurity, which have gradually expanded to various personalized medical devices. With respect to cloud computing applications, the development of artificial intelligence and deep learning in biological signal processing and medical image processing was also important topic of the conference. "Data Sharing" experts were invited to share current open data topics and its future trends, which was a highlighted feature of the conference. In addition to topics related to biomedical engineering (BME), medical physics (MP) experts were also invited to present current status of image information and possible future integration of BME and MP. Young Investigator Competition, Student Paper Competition, and Scientific Challenge were also held at the conference with the Student Paper Competition being jointly organized with IFMBE Asia-Pacific Activity Working Group which was another special feature of the conference.

The editors would like to sincerely appreciate all the members of Organization Committee, Scientific Advisory Committee, and the IFMBE Officers for their time and effort in preparing this conference. The experts contributed valuable expertise and young researchers presented innovative findings enriched the content of the conference and broadened our horizon. The Technology Translation Center for Medical Device, Chung Yuan Christian University, Taiwan, and IFMBE WG had given a considerable amount of time and effort to organize this conference, along with the assistance from Taiwanese Society of Biomedical Engineering and Chinese Society of Medical Physics, Taipei. In addition, without the support and sponsor from the Ministry of Science and Technology and the National Health Research Institutes, Taiwan, and without the Springer Nature's publication of the IFMBE proceedings, the ICBHI 2019 conference wouldn't have been completed with such success. The editors are also grateful to the dedicated efforts of the Local Organizing Committee members and their supporters for carefully preparing and operating the conference. The editors would also like to specially thank all the team members from Technology Translation Center for Medical Device, Chung Yuan Christian University, for their dedication to the event.

Kang-Ping Lin
Ratko Magjarevic
Paulo de Carvalho

Organization

Conference Chairperson

Kang-Ping Lin   Chung Yuan Christian University, Taiwan

Conference Co-chair

Ratko Magjarević   University of Zagreb, Croatia

Honorary Chairs

Feng-Huei Lin   Institute of Biomed Eng & Nanomed.,
                                    National Health Research Institutes, Taiwan
Jaw-Lin Wang   National Taiwan University, Taiwan

Conference Secretary

Yung-Hsin Chen   Technology Translation Center for Medical
                                    Device, Chung Yuan Christian University,
                                    Taiwan
Julia Pei-shu Tsai   Technology Translation Center for Medical
                                    Device, Chung Yuan Christian University,
                                    Taiwan

IFMBE Officers

Shankar Krishnan (President)	Boston, USA
Ratko Magjarević (Vice President)	University of Zagreb, Croatia
James Goh (Past President)	National University of Singapore, Singapore
Kang-Ping Lin (Secretary-General)	Chung Yuan Christian University, Taiwan
Marc Nyssen (Treasure)	Vrije Universiteit Brussel, Belgium

IFMBE WG on Health Informatics and eHealth

Chair

Paulo De Carvalho

Co-chair

Ratko Magjarevic

Advisor

Yuan-Ting Zhang

Members

Shankar Krishnan
Marc Nyssen
Nitish Thakor
Bruce Wheeler
May Wang
Nicos Maglaveras
Esteban Pino
Kang Ping Lin
Maurício Cagy
Erik Bresch

Organization Committee

James C. H. Goh (Chair)	National University of Singapore, Singapore
Shaou-Gang Miaou (Co-chair)	Chung Yuan Christian University, Taiwan
Virginia Laura Ballarín	Universidad Nacional de Mar del Plata, Argentina

Eric Laciar Leber   Universidad Nacional de San Juan, Argentina
Nicos Maglaveras   Aristotelian University, Greece
Leandro Pecchia   University of Warwick, UK
Madan Rehani   Duke University, USA
Magdalena Stoeva   Medical University of Plovdiv, Bulgaria
Yung-Nien Sun   National Cheng Kung University, Taiwan
Slavik Tabakov   King's College London, UK
Hua-Nong Ting   University of Malaya, Malaysia
Guang-Zhi Wang   Tsinghua University, China
Suiren Wan   Southeast University, China

Scientific Advisory Committee

Shankar M. Krishnan (Chair)   Wentworth Institute of Technology, USA
Pai-Chi Li (Co-chair)   National Taiwan University, Taiwan
María Teresa Arredondo   Universidad Politécnica de Madrid, Spain
Cholid Badri   University of Indonesia, Indonesia
Virginia Laura Ballarín   Universidad Nacional de Mar del Plata,
                                Argentina
Eva Bezak   University of South Australia, Australia
Enkhjargal Biziya   Mongolian University of Science
                                and Technology, Mongolia
Paulo Carvalho   University of Coimbra, Portugal
Martha Zequera Diaz   Pontifical Javeriana University, Colombia
Yu-bo Fan   Beihang University, China
Bin He   University of Minnesota, USA
Ernesto Iadanza   University of Florence, Italy
Andrew Laine   Columbia University, USA
Hong-En Liao   Tsinghua University, China
Toh Siew Lok   National University of Singapore, Singapore
Dong Ming   Tianjin University, China
Xiao-Chuan Pan   The University of Chicago, USA
Esteban Pino   Universidad de Concepción, Chile
Marius N. Roman   Technical University of Cluj-Napoca, Romania
Ichiro Sakuma   The University of Tokyo, Japan
Nitish Thakor   National University of Singapore, Singapore
Virginia Tsapaki   Konstantopoulio General Hospital, Greece
Bruce Wheeler   University of Florida, USA
Luis Miguel Zamudio   Instituto Politecnico Nacional, Mexico
Yuan-Ting Zhang   City University of Hong Kong, Hong Kong
Yong-Ping Zheng   The Hong Kong Polytechnic University, China

Local Organizing Committee

Cheng-Yuan Chang	Chung Yuan Christian University, Taiwan
Chih-Chung Huang	National Cheng Kung University, Taiwan
Ching-Fen Jiang	I-Shou University, Taiwan
Wen-Chen Lin	Chung Yuan Christian University, Taiwan
Guang-Hwa Shiue	Chung Yuan Christian University, Taiwan
Hsiang-Ho Chen	Taipei Medical University, Taiwan
Pai-Chi Li	National Taiwan University, Taiwan
Shaou-Gang Miaou	Chung Yuan Christian University, Taiwan
Shih-Tsang Tang	Ming Chuan University, Taiwan
Tsai-Chi Kuo	Chung Yuan Christian University, Taiwan
Yao-Jen Chang	Chung Yuan Christian University, Taiwan
Ying-Hui Lai	National Yang Ming University, Taiwan
Yuan-Hsiang Chang	Chung Yuan Christian University, Taiwan
Yu-fang Chiu	Chung Yuan Christian University, Taiwan
Yuh-Show Tsai	Chung Yuan Christian University, Taiwan
Yung-Nien Sun	National Cheng Kung University, Taiwan

Contents

Artificial Intelligence (AI) for Dental Intraoral Film Mounting   1
Meng-Chi Chen, Cheng-Hsueh Chen, and Mu-Hsiung Chen

Exploring the Possibilities to Characterize the Soft Tissue
Using Acoustic Emission Waveforms   9
Yashbir Singh, Wei-Chih Hu, Alfredo Illanes, and Michael Friebe

Real-Time Intelligent Healthcare Monitoring and Diagnosis System
Through Deep Learning and Segmented Analysis 15
Edward B. Panganiban, Wen-Yaw Chung, Wei-Chieh Tai,
Arnold C. Paglinawan, Jheng-Siang Lai, Ren-Wei Cheng,
Ming-Kai Chang, and Po-Hsuan Chang

The Prolonged Effect on Respiratory Sinus Arrhythmia Response
of Individual with Internet Gaming Disorder
via Breathing Exercise 26
Hong-Ming Ji and Tzu-Chien Hsiao

Automatic Liver and Spleen Segmentation with CT Images
Using Multi-channel U-net Deep Learning Approach 33
Ting-Yu Su and Yu-Hua Fang

Classification of Breast Cancer Malignancy Using Machine
Learning Mechanisms in TensorFlow and Keras 42
Yuan-Hsiang Chang and Chi-Yu Chung

A New Numerical Simulation Process for Footwear Slip
Resistance Analysis. 50
Shu-Yu Jhou, Wei-Chun Hsu, and Ching-Chi Hsu

A Numerical Study of Different Hallux Valgus Treatments Using
Three-Dimensional Human Musculoskeletal Lower
Extremity Models 57
Kuan-Ting Huang, Kao-Shang Shih, and Ching-Chi Hsu

**Point-of-Care Testing System of Uric Acid for the Prevention
from Urolithiasis Recurrence**   63
Lin-Chen Yen, Cheanyeh Cheng, Wen-Yaw Chung, and Vincent Tsai

**A Transcutaneous High-Efficiency Battery Charging System
with a Small Temperature Increase for Implantable Medical
Devices Based on the Taguchi Method**   72
De-Fu Jhang, Szu-Ying Kao, Kuan-Ting Lee, and Chiung-Cheng Chuang

**Using Bi-planar X-Ray Images to Reconstruct the Spine Structure
by the Convolution Neural Network**   80
Chih-Chia Chen and Yu-Hua Fang

**Biomechanical Analysis of Pullout Strength of Spinal Pedicle
Screws with Full Insertion and Back-Out Using Finite
Element Method**   86
Yu-You Chen, Chian-Yun Hsu, Kao-Shang Shih, and Ching-Chi Hsu

**A Free-Hand System of the High-Frequency Single Element
Ultrasound Transducer for Skin Imaging**   91
Wei-Ting Zhang, Yin-Chih Lin, Wei-Hao Chen, Chia-Wei Yang,
and Hui-Hua Kenny Chiang

**Ultrasonography Classification of Obstructive Sleep Apnea (OSA)
Through Dynamic Tongue Base Motion Tracking and Tongue
Area Measurements**   100
Cyrel Ontimare Manlises, Jeng-Wen Chen, and Chih-Chung Huang

**A Novel Multi-direction Adjustment Strategy for Reducing Ghost
Artifact in Body Tomosynthesis**   108
Yu-Ching Ni, Chia-Yu Lin, Chia-Hao Chang, Fan-Pin Tseng,
Sheng-Pin Tseng, and Keh-Shih Chuang

Blood Pressure Variation Trend Analysis Based on Model Study   115
Pei-Ying Chen, Hao-Jen Ting, Mei-Fen Chen, Wen-Chen Lin,
and Kang-Ping Lin

**Raman Spectroscopic Urine Crystal Detection and Clinical
Significance Study on Urolithiasis Management**   122
Chih-Hao Wang, Jing-Xiang Zeng, Pin-Chuan Chen,
and Hui-Hua Kenny Chiang

**A Real Time Fall Detection System Using Tri-Axial Accelerometer
and Clinometer Based on Smart Phones**   129
Yi-Sheng Su and Shih-Hsiung Twu

**Automatic Classification of Lymph Node Metastasis
in Non-Small-Cell Lung Cancer (NSCLC) Patient
on F-18-FDG PET/CT**   138
Tsu-Chi Cheng, Nan-Tsing Chiu, and Yu-Hua Fang

Feasibility Study of Developing a Brain-Dedicated SPECT Scanner . . . 143
Hsin-Chin Liang, Yu-Ching Ni, and Hsiang-Ning Wu

**Development of Urine Conductivity Sensing System
for Measurement and Data Collection** 148
Roozbeh Falah Ramezani, Abdul Hadi Nograles, Wen-Yaw Chung,
Jennifer Dela Cruz, Kuan-Hua Li, Chean-Yeh Cheng, and Vincent Tsai

**Spectrogram and Deep Neural Network Analysis in Detecting
Paroxysmal Atrial Fibrillation with Bottleneck Layers
and Cross Entropy Approach** 156
Edward B. Panganiban, Wen-Yaw Chung, and Arnold C. Paglinawan

**3D Fluorescence Tomography Combined with Ultrasound
Imaging System in Small Animal Study** 166
Shih-Po Su and Hui-Hua Kenny Chiang

**Main Barriers and Needs to Support Clinical Cancer Research
via Health Informatics** 174
Laura Lopez-Perez, Silvana Canevari, Leandro Pecchia,
Maria Teresa Arredondo, Lisa Licitra, and Giuseppe Fico

**Stability Evaluation of a Tissue Oxygen Saturation
Measurement System** 183
Shao-Hung Lu, Tieh-Cheng Fu, Wei-Cheng Lu, Po-Hung Chang,
Kang-Ping Lin, and Cheng-Lun Tsai

**Liquid Phantom for Calibrating Tissue Oxygen
Saturation Measurement** 191
Po-Hung Chang, Shao-Hung Lu, Tieh-Cheng Fu, Kang-Ping Lin,
and Cheng-Lun Tsai

**Instantaneous Respiratory Phase Response of Individual
with Internet Gaming Disorder During Watching Game Video** 198
Hong-Ming Ji and Tzu-Chien Hsiao

Photoplethysmographic Signals Measured at the Nose 204
Pin-Lu Li, Shao-Hung Lu, Kang-Ping Lin, and Cheng-Lun Tsai

**Correlation Between Time-Domain Features of Electrohysterogram
Data of Pregnant Women and Gestational Age** 212
Chomkansak Hemthanon and Suparerk Janjarasjitt

A Study of Speech Phase in Dysarthria Voice Conversion System 219
Ko-Chiang Chen, Ji-Yan Han, Sin-Hua Jhang, and Ying-Hui Lai

Toward the Precision Medicine for a Psychiatric Disorder: Light Therapy for Major Depressive Disorder with Neuroimaging Validation 227
Fan-pei Gloria Yang, Wei-cheng Chao, Sung-wei Chen, Ernie Du, Chi-chin Yang, Li-chi Su, and Mu-tao Chu

Integrated RFID Aperture and Washing Chamber Shielding Design for Real-Time Cleaning Performance Monitoring in Healthcare Laundry System 235
Kampol Woradit, Setta Sassananan, Sasithorn Boonjun, and Amaraporn Boonpratatong

Manual Wheelchair Propulsion and Joint Power Transmission Efficiency for Diagnosis of Upper-Limb Overuse 243
Supanat Sakunwitunthai, Worapol Aramrussameekul, and Amaraporn Boonpratatong

Individual Margins of Instantaneous Dynamic Stability: Verification in Elderly with Mobility and Balance Tests 252
Pattranit Kitiratchai, Waranya Mongkholhatthi, Sugunya Wongbuangam, and Amaraporn Boonpratatong

Cyber-Physical Secure VLC Applications 260
Noriharu Miyaho, Noriko Konno, Takamasa Shimada, Kana Egawa, Kosuke Watai, Kotaro Murase, and Atsuya Yokoi

Empirical Modeling of Photopolymerization for Oxygen-Mediated Anti-cancer 268
Kuo-Ti Chen, Jui-Teng Lin, and Hsia-Wei Liu

Investigating the Use of Wearables for Monitoring Circadian Rhythms: A Feasibility Study 275
Rossana Castaldo, Marta Prati, Luis Montesinos, Vishwesh Kulkarni, Micheal Chappell, Helen Byrne, Pasquale Innominato, Stephen Hughes, and Leandro Pecchia

Quantitative Reduction in the Dynamic Endothelial Function on Foot Microcirculation in Patients with Diabetes Mellitus 281
Jia-Jung Wang, Xuan-Hao Su, G. Hung, Hsin-Yen He, and Wei-Kung Tseng

Promises and Challenges in the Use of Wearable Sensors and Nonlinear Signal Analysis for Balance and Fall Risk Assessment in Older Adults 288
Luis Montesinos, Rossana Castaldo, and Leandro Pecchia

Arrhythmia Detection Using Curve Fitting and Machine Learning 296
Po-Chuan Chiu, Han-Chien Cheng, and Shu-Nung Yao

**Combining Multi-classifier with CNN in Detection
and Classification of Breast Calcification** 304
Kuan-Chun Chen, Chiun-Li Chin, Ni-Chuan Chung, and Chin-Luen Hsu

**Evaluation of Left Ventricular Ejection Fraction Obtained from
^{201}Tl Myocardial Perfusion Scan by CZT Cardiac Camera** 312
Hsiao-Ling Chiang, Chien-Hsin Ting, Cheng-Pe Chang, Bang-Hung Yang,
Jyh-Shyan Leu, Chi-Long Juang, and Wen-Sheng Huang

**Cardiopulmonary Resuscitation Support Using Accelerometer
Signals from the Carotid** 320
Diogo Jesus, Paulo Carvalho, Jens Muehlsteff, and Ricardo Couceiro

**Input Clinical Parameters for Cardiac Heart Failure
Characterization Using Machine Learning** 328
Ernesto Iadanza and Camilla Chilleri

**An Investigation on Phase Characteristics of Galvanic Coupling
Human Body Communication** 335
Weikun Chen, Wenzhu Liu, Ivana Čuljak, Xingguang Chen, Haibo Zheng,
Yueming Gao, Željka Lučev Vasić, Mario Cifrek, and Min Du

Noise Reduction for Continuous Positive Airway Pressure Machine . . . 342
Cheng-Yuan Chang, Sen M. Kuo, and Xiu-Wei Liu

**Dysphonia Measurements Detection Using CQT's
and MFCC's Methods** 349
Mario Lopez-Rodríguez, Mireya Sarai García-Vázquez,
Luis Miguel Zamudio-Fuentes, and Alejandro Ramírez-Acosta

**Quantification of Systolic Time Intervals Using Continuous Wavelet
Transform of Electrocardiogram and Phonocardiogram Signals** 356
Suparerk Janjarasjitt

PEP and LVET Detection from PCG and ECG 363
Yi-Fang Yang, Yu-Sheng Chou, and Jia-Yin Wang

**To Determinate PEP and LVET Through Analyzing LPC
of Heart Sounds** 371
Jin-Hao Ou, Ming-Hao Yang, Ming-Hsien Yu, and Wen-Chien Chen

**Improvement of Environment and Camera Setting on Extraction
of Heart Rate Using Eulerian Video Magnification** 381
Bo-Yu Huang and Chi-Lun Lin

Deep Learning Method to Detect Plaques in IVOCT Images 389
Grigorios-Aris Cheimariotis, Maria Riga, Konstantinos Toutouzas,
Dimitris Tousoulis, Aggelos Katsaggelos, and Nikolaos Maglaveras

Fall Risk Assessment in Older Adults with Diabetic
Peripheral Neuropathy 396
Jhonathan Sora Cárdenas, Martha Zequera Díaz,
and Francisco Calderón Bocanegra

COP Analysis in Type 2 Diabetics with Peripheral Diabetic
Neuropathy 405
Daissy Carola Toloza, Martha Zequera, and Gustavo Castro

Comparison of Human Fall Acceleration Signals Among
Different Datasets 413
Goran Šeketa, Lovro Pavlaković, Sara Žulj, Dominik Džaja,
Igor Lacković, and Ratko Magjarević

Handling Missing Data in CGM Records 420
Sara Zulj, Paulo Carvalho, Rogerio Ribeiro, and Ratko Magjarevic

Based on DICOM RT Structure and Multiple Loss Function
Deep Learning Algorithm in Organ Segmentation of Head
and Neck Image 428
Ya-Ju Hsieh, Hsien-Chun Tseng, Chiun-Li Chin, Yu-Hsiang Shao,
and Ting-Yu Tsai

Author Index 437

Artificial Intelligence (AI) for Dental Intraoral Film Mounting

Meng-Chi Chen[1], Cheng-Hsueh Chen[2], and Mu-Hsiung Chen[3]($\boxtimes$)

[1] Taipei Chang Gung Memorial Hospital Dental Department,
Taipei Association of Radiological Technologists, Taipei, Taiwan
[2] Tungs' General Hospital Dental Department,
Taichung Association of Radiological Technologists, Taichung, Taiwan
[3] Department of Dentistry, National Taiwan University Hospital,
Taipei Association of Radiological Technologists,
No. 1, Changde Street, Zhongzheng District, Taipei, Taiwan
hsiung@ntuh.gov.tw

Abstract. Until today, In the daily work of dental radiologists, the flipping and identification of the intraoral x-ray images must be controlled by humans. No software or artificial design software can be improved, which causes the radiologist to take time and flip the teeth and put them into the correct tooth area. Therefore, under the increasing workload, how to shorten the time spent by the radiologist in handling is particularly important. In this study, through the Convolutional Neural Network (CNN) architecture in Deep Learning, the most commonly used intraoral films (Periapical, Horizontal Bite Wing, Vertical BiteWing) were inverted and identified to show the tooth area, and 16 tooth positions were designed for AI identification and learning; a total of 15,752 dental x-ray films (including original images, inverted 90°, 180° and 270° each 3938) for AI training. Therefore, in this study, 328 tests were performed after AI training (testing 1. tooth position recognition 2. flipping 90°, 180°, 270° image recognition each time), the recognition success rate is: 1. tooth position identification the success rate was 97.56%. 2. The average success rate of flip image recognition was 97.56%. Therefore, there is a great relationship between the number of AI learning images and the classification of image features and the success rate of recognition. In this study, the AI has been linked to the browser, and it can be used for teaching and research in the industry, research reference, etc., and is expected to be used clinically to reduce the workload of dental radiologists and dentists.

Keywords: Intraoral x-ray images identification · Artificial Intelligence · Deep Learning · Convolutional Neural Network

1 Introduction

In the daily work of the dental radiologist, there is a step in which the outside world is ignorant and must be manipulated manually. This is the flipping and identification of the intraoral film. In recent years, dental medicine has made rapid progress, but whether it is a software package or a software designed by hand. It can't be improved, it takes a

© Springer Nature Switzerland AG 2020
K.-P. Lin et al. (Eds.): ICBHI 2019, IFMBE Proceedings 74, pp. 1–8, 2020.
https://doi.org/10.1007/978-3-030-30636-6_1

lot of time for the radiologist to flip the teeth and put the images into the correct tooth area. Under the increasing workload, there seems to be a need for improvement.

In 2018, Artificial Intelligence has been covered in newspapers and media. If AI can be applied to this problem, it will undoubtedly reduce manpower and time waste, and may even surpass human recognition and reduce medical care caused by flipping photo errors. Negligence; this research will also link AI and browser, and the future can be used for teaching and research in the industry and academia.

Based on the aforementioned motivations, the research purpose of this study is twofold:

1. Through the AI, the most frequently photographed intraoral films (Periapical, Horizontal Bite Wing (BW), Vertical BiteWing (VBW)) for adults will be identified and inverted to show the tooth position area. In the future, we hope to cooperate with the software manufacturers to add the data of the research results to the existing ones. In software, let the software be more integrated.
2. The development of AI software can also be used by researchers in the dental field in the future to expand its functions, such as dental diagnosis, disease, etc., so that AI can help humans solve more problems.

2   Methods

First, hardware and images, CPU: Intel Xeon Processor E5-2650, DRAM: 16 GB, GPU: GTX-1060 6G. Software: Python, CNN, ResNet-34 model in TensorFlow. Image data: Database: 3938 films (jpg) and test strips: 328 films (jpg.); intraoral films are: 1. Dental CR#2 (about 1700*1200 pixels); 2. Dental DR#2 (1200*825 pixels).

Second, write the AI software to the computer and design 16 tooth positions (Periapical 10, Bite Wing 2, Vertical Bitewing 4); the image data is divided into original image 0°, flipped 90°, 180° and 270° each of 3938 films and start AI learning. (e.g. Table 1)

Table 1. Dental position setting

Teeth area	Intraoral film direction	* Selection criteria
Upper and Lower teeth 2–2	Straight	Image contains upper and lower center incisors and lateral incisors
Upper and Lower teeth 3–5	Straight	The image includes upper and lower canines, first permolars, and second premolars
Upper and Lower teeth 6–8	Horizontal	The image contains the upper and lower first molars, the second molars, and the third molars (wisdom teeth)
BW Left side and Right side	Horizontal	The image includes upper and lower first permolars, second permolars, first molars, and second molars
VBW Left and Right front	Straight	The image contains the upper and lower first permolars and the second permolars
VBW Left and Right behind	Straight	The image contains the upper and lower first molars and the second molars

* Images that cannot be clearly classified are not used

Third, the test image is divided into original image 0°, inverted 90°, 180°, 270° each 328, into the browser, test the tooth recognition and flip recognition success rate. (e.g. Table 2)

3 Results

The accuracy of the identified AI in the tooth area was 97.56%; the accuracy of the inverted image recognition was also 97.56% (Table 2). Therefore, it can be known from the research that the AI does not misjudge the direction of the image when performing image interpretation, but the image that is flipped will be wrong when the original image is misjudge.

At the same time, this experiment also found that the following factors affect AI identification:

1. **Number of database images:** In this experiment, the data of each tooth position area is about 100–400, which is slightly insufficient. It is recommended that a single tooth area needs at least 500–1000 images, which will have a good recognition rate; but in the end, there will be limits. There will still be a slight error rate. (e.g. Figs. 1, 2, 3 and 4)
2. **Special image:** Due to the limited number of people in this experiment, we chose to increase the conventional intraoral images as a database, and less training special images. Therefore, AI will be weaker for signs, implants, and missing teeth, thus reducing the recognition rate. (e.g. Figs. 5, 6)
3. **The image classification is correct:** Because each tooth in the mouth is closely connected with the teeth, some images will have blurred spaces in both teeth, which will affect the AI interpretation, resulting in a decrease in the recognition rate. (e.g. Fig. 7)
4. **Test image quantity and classification:** The more the number of test images, the slowly increasing the error rate will cause the recognition rate to decrease. If the test image is not classified, the recognition rate will decrease. (e.g. Fig. 8)
5. **To avoid affecting the correct rate, the test group must be separated:** In order to meet the number of IRB application studies, the study set the medical record number from 1 to 8 for the database image, a total of 280 people; the first 9 of the medical record number is the test group image, a total of 20 people, no confusion.

Table 2. Identification rate statistics

Teeth area	AI learning the number of films	Number of test films	Number of errors	0° correct rate(%)	90° correct rate(%)	180° correct rate(%)	270° correct rate(%)
18–16	222	17	0	100	100	100	100
15–13	396	43	2	95.35	95.35	95.35	95.35
12–22	374	32	2	93.75	93.75	93.75	93.75
23–25	404	41	0	100	100	100	100
26–28	245	20	0	100	100	100	100
46–48	259	15	0	100	100	100	100
45–43	391	31	0	100	100	100	100
42–32	283	26	3	88.5	88.5	88.5	88.5
33–35	372	28	0	100	100	100	100
36–38	244	17	0	100	100	100	100
BW Right side	167	9	0	100	100	100	100
BW Left side	167	10	0	100	100	100	100
VBW Right front	106	9	0	100	100	100	100
VBW Right behind	102	11	1	90.91	90.91	90.91	90.91
VBW Left front	104	10	0	100	100	100	100
VBW Left behind	102	9	0	100	100	100	100
Total	3938	328	8	*97.56	97.56	97.56	97.56

*Correct rate: (328–8)/328 = 97.56%

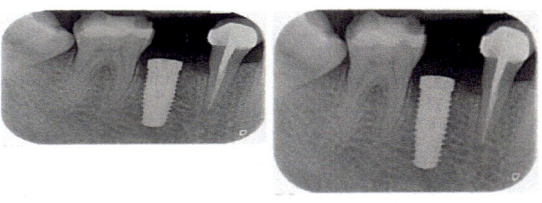

46~48,機率 0.99995

Fig. 1. The left picture shows the implant image of the "46–48" tooth position area, and the AI is accurately identified.

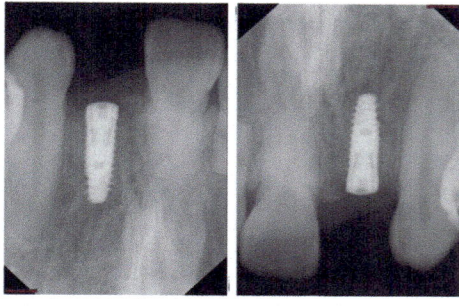

12~22，機率0.99999

Fig. 2. The picture on the left is "12–22 180° flipping the image", the AI is flipped correctly and identification.

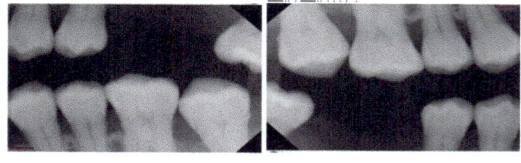

右BW（1Q.4Q），機率1.0

Fig. 3. The picture on the left is "BW right side 180° flipping the image", the AI is correctly flipped and identification.

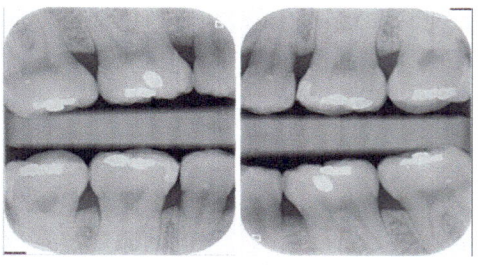

左後VBW（2Q.3Q），機率0.99999

Fig. 4. The picture on the left is "VBW left behind 180° flip image", high difficulty, AI correct flip and identification.

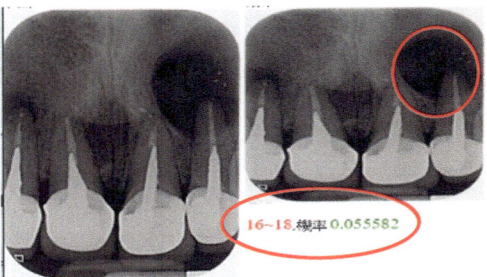

Fig. 5. The left picture shows the "12–22" tooth position area, which failed due to symptom identification, and the probability of 0.055 means that almost no such image has been studied.

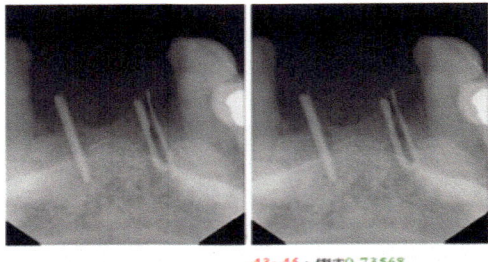

Fig. 6. The left picture shows the positioning of the implants in the "32–42" tooth position. Because the image training is less, the AI is misjudged as "43–45".

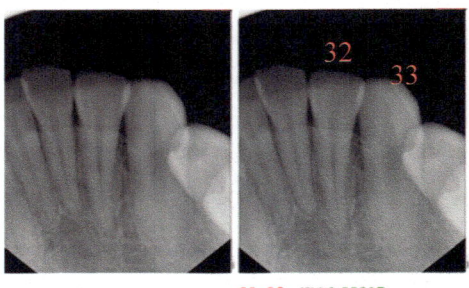

Fig. 7. The picture on the left is the "32–42" tooth position area, but the 32 and 33 are too close in the image. Therefore, when classifying the image of the database, the image is classified as "33–35", which leads to AI misjudgment.

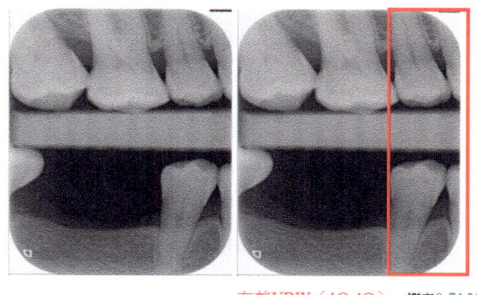

右前VBW（1Q.4Q），機率0.71506

Fig. 8. The picture on the left is "right behind VBW", because the test image contains the second premolars, which causes the AI to be mistakenly judged as the "right front VBW", so it is not recommended to include the controversial image in the test.

4   Conclusion

This experiment is an important step for clinical dental image recognition. In the future, it can not only be added to children's dentistry, oral surgery, oral pathology, craniofacial correction or even intra-oral images of various medical centers, and is combined into a complete database. It can also work with a dentist to identify and assist in the diagnosis of dental images and find a symptom that is difficult to be observed with eyes. In the future, as long as the amount of AI learning database is sufficient, there is a chance to surpass human identification.

Conflict of Interest. The authors have not conflicts of interest.

Compliance with Ethical Standards
   1. **Conflict of interest** The authors declare that they have no conflict of interest
   2. **Statistics and biometry** No complex statistical methods were necessary for this paper.
   3. **Informed Consent** This study belongs to the case review study without patient consent.
   4. **Ethical approval Institutional** Review Board approval was obtained.

References

Yang, J., Xie, Y., Liu, L., Xia, B., Cao, Z., Guo, C.: Automated dental image analysis by deep learning on small dataset. In: 2018 IEEE 42nd Annual Computer Software and Applications Conference (COMPSAC), pp. 492–497 (2018)

Fei, L., Junran, Z., Hao, Y.: Research progress of medical image recognition based on deep learning. Chin. J. Biomed. Eng. **37**(1), 86–94 (2018)

Eun, H., Kim, C.: Oriented tooth localization for periapical dental X-ray Images via convolutional neural network. In: 2016 Asia-Pacific Signal and Information Processing Association Annual Summit and Conference (APSIPA), pp. 1–7 (2016)

Shiyuan, L., Yi, X.: Challenges and opportunities of deep learning artificial intelligence in medical imaging. Chin. J. Radiol. **51**(12), 899–901 (2017)

Dong, X.: A brief discussion on the related technologies of deep learning in image medicine. In: 2017 Health Guide, vol. 44, p. 229 (2017)

Dong, X.: Three basic technologies of artificial intelligence in medical treatment. In: 2017 Health Guide, vol. 44, p. 171 (2017)

Dong, X.: The attempt of deep learning in image medical processing. In: 2017 Health Guide, vol. 44, p. 55 (2017)

Yu, Y-J.: Machine learning for dental image analysis. Eprint arXiv:1611.09958

Exploring the Possibilities to Characterize the Soft Tissue Using Acoustic Emission Waveforms

Yashbir Singh[1]([⊠]), Wei-Chih Hu[1], Alfredo Illanes[2],
and Michael Friebe[2]

[1] Department of Biomedical Engineering,
Chung Yuan Christian University, Zhongli, Taiwan
Yashbir143@gmail.com, weichihhu@cycu.edu.tw
[2] Electrical Engineering and Information Technologies,
Otto-Von-Guericke-University, Rötgerstraße 9, Magdeburg, Germany
{alfredo.illanes,michael.friebe}@ovgu.de

Abstract. Minimal invasive device insertion into the soft tissue is a very important medical approach that is helpful for local drug delivery, biopsy, regional anesthesia, blood sampling, and radiofrequency ablation. These methods need to introduce the MID inside the body for exploring the tissue texture pattern. We propose a novel approach by acquiring acoustic emission data from the proximal end of the MID for the tissue using phase angle, power spectral to identify the texture. By performing these signal processing approach to the soft tissue, the pattern of the tissue can be understood. The result shows a new study to obtain soft tissue texture information.

Keywords: Minimal invasive device · Acoustic emission · Tissue texture · Non-invasive sensors

1 Introduction

Nowadays, physicians are facing the problem to determine the abnormal tissue such as ovarian cyst or tumor in the body, which is very challenging. Numerous recent clinical practices are involved in soft tissue treatment and some local therapies. Advanced technologies are used in the laparoscopic surgery that allows finding the accurate information of the soft tissue characteristics [1].

There are many devices available in the market such as biopsy needle, catheter and guidewire for regional anesthesia, and brachytherapy which considered as a medical interventional device (MID). These applications, needle and catheters have to penetrate into the soft tissue to find the texture information of the soft tissue. The effectiveness of the diagnosis is depended on the accuracy of the penetration of the device into the soft tissue. Medical studies have revealed that misplacement of the needle insertion into the soft tissue will be a problematic [2, 3]. Nowadays, through the MID insertion procedure has become a very significant way to evaluate the texture of the tissue because a variety of pathological conditions in humans directly or indirectly involve remodeling or regenerating the collagenous framework in tissue. Accurate placement of MID is very important because biopsy of an unintended tissue region can effect in misdiagnosis.

© Springer Nature Switzerland AG 2020
K.-P. Lin et al. (Eds.): ICBHI 2019, IFMBE Proceedings 74, pp. 9–14, 2020.
https://doi.org/10.1007/978-3-030-30636-6_2

Many studies suggest that the inappropriate MID insertion can be caused by many factors like tissue in homogeneity, tissue anisotropy, anatomical obstructions. A MID has assumed as the rigid rod and the soft tissue has elasticity property to deform under the external forces and to release stored energy to drive the function of other tissues. MID penetration method is divided into pre-puncture, puncture and post-puncture phases. Soft tissue deformation happens at the pre-puncture and post puncture phases [4–6]. There are numerous irregular gaps inside the tissue and the tissue is simply compressible under the external loads. When MID goes into the soft tissue leads to the volume change with its deformation. This volume change of the tissue can be used to measure the deformation. Tissue deformation includes three cases which are the displacement of the tissue, comparative sliding of multilayer soft tissue and motions of the organs. usually, soft tissue contains three layers which are skin, muscle, and fat. The inhomogeneous characteristic sallow the adjective layers to slide with each other under the asymmetrical forces [7]. The connection between needle deflection and needle geometry are discussed [8]. In general, when a tensile event happens, the sides of the deformation move away from each other, and consequently, a few energy transmits in the waveforms which means acoustic emission waveform emitted by a tensile event.

However, it is very hard to calculate the changed volume of soft tissue but we are trying to get some information about the tissue texture. The impact of the research presented in this paper lies in its contribution to extract the texture comparison information of the soft tissue using the audio signal.

2   Method

In this research, we setup the experiment for MID which was an 18G 200 mm length biopsy needle with the needle core (ITP, Germany), placed inside a flushed 1.9 F micro catheter of 1.5 m length were implemented. A gelatin phantom was filled with different fruits such as grape, persimmon, breast and, liver of chicken to perform the analysis (Fig. 1). We attached a microphone to the proximal end of the needle to the soft tissue (Gelatine phantom filled with fruits) using testing machine (Zwicki, Zwick GmbH & Co. KG, Ulm).

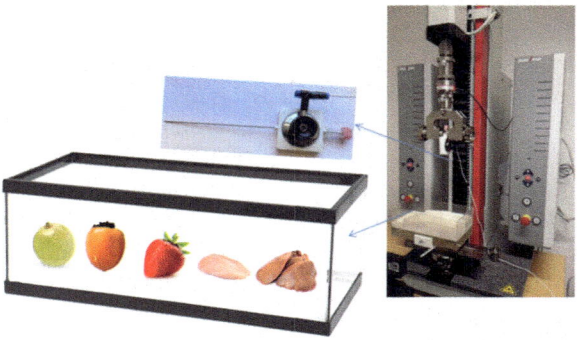

Fig. 1. Experiment setup (Illanes et al. 2018)

Penetration velocity rate of the needle was 3 mm/s, recorded 80 audio signals in WAV format with a sampling frequency of 44672 Hz because it is very common sampling frequency in the digital audio system. Insertion of the needle timing and exit timing were observed. We performed the filtration process to obtain the filtered audio signal from the raw audio signal (Fig. 2). In this study, we focused on the signal processing to find the texture of the tissue using the audio signal. We used the biopsy needle to get the match in the different structures of tissue. The experimental tissues were persimmon, grape, breast and liver of chicken with different texture of the tissue. Since It is very important to implement a signal processing approach to get more hidden information which is not possible by naked eyes.

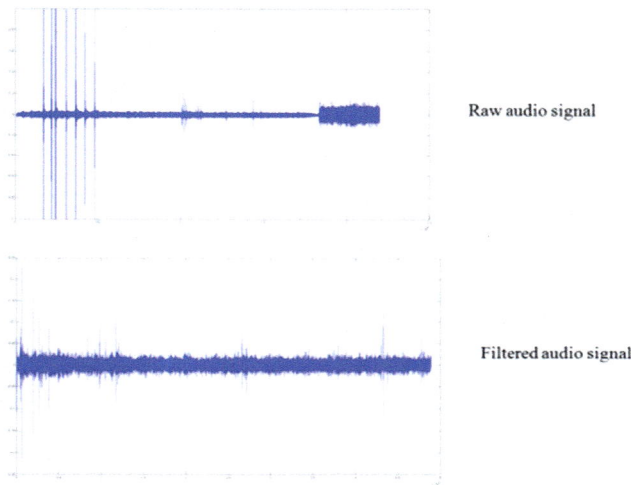

Fig. 2. Original and filtered audio signal

The *Matlab R2015b* is used to perform signal processing for the audio signal analysis. The algorithm used on filtered audio signal for the digital analysis of amplitude, frequency, phase angle pattern detection among the tissue successfully [9–11]. Finally, we performed cross-correlation to determine inter-observer and intra-observer variability. The objective of this research is to evaluate tissue texture when the needle passes into dissimilar tissue structures.

3 Results

In this section, we observed more friction dynamics in the breast and liver of chicken at the time of needle penetration rather than fruits, obtained different elasticities of tissue structures which is different patterns of the soft tissue. We particular made the block on the graph where is the more different peaks variation clearly differentiate from other tissue (Fig. 3). Numerous research suggests the muscle tissue is composed out of different fibre strands and fruit tissue have different. These kind of alignment will lead to a directed light distribution with the fibre direction in the piece of tissue. After performing the power spectral, phase angle among the tissues. Power spectral graph represents the difference among the tissue which is shown in the graph (Fig. 3). Though, frequency distribution is important for human perception. These kinds of information may be acquired by computation power spectrum.

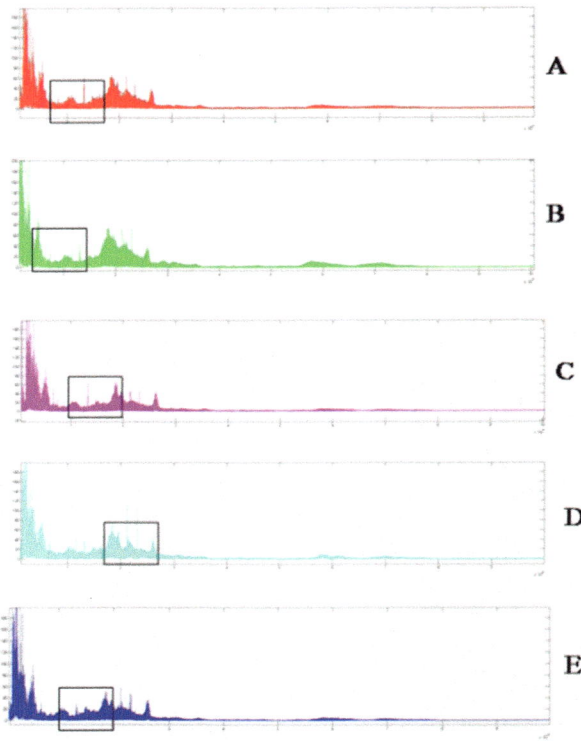

Fig. 3. Power spectral analysis of the various tissues.

Phase angel graph is also representing the difference among the tissues, we have shown in the graph (Fig. 4). In the graph, we have made the block where is the dense area which is fibre that also differentiate the tissue pattern to each other. The phase angle ($p(\alpha, \varphi', \theta')$) of the soft tissues have strong deviations at the incident of penetration and scattering angles (φ', θ'). MID insertion is directed into fibre direction that can propagate to get the inside organization of the tissue. We compared all results of the soft tissue texture pattern. Our comparison reveals differences among the soft tissues that can be seen pattern consistency of the data.

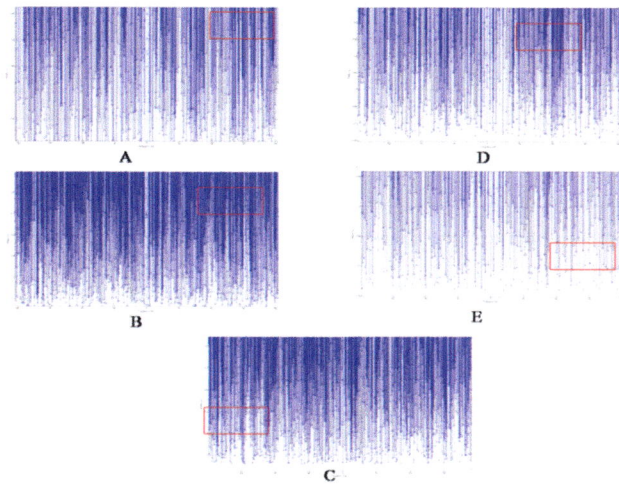

Fig. 4. Phase angle of the different tissues.

Finally, we performed the cross-correlation to get the pattern among the tissue which is shown in the graph as well (Fig. 5). Here, we have shown the graph only a few signal patterns for the representation purpose. Upper and lower part of the graph peaks are different that shows the variability of the signal at different points (Fig. 5). We obtained the angle variation that strongly dependent on the incident direction.

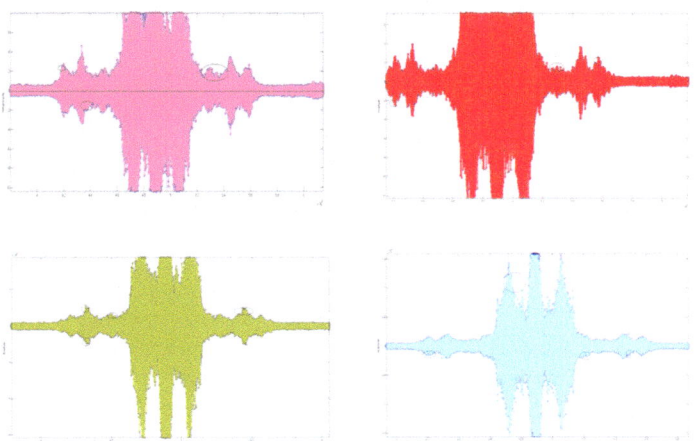

Fig. 5. Cross correlation among the tissues

This study shows an interesting approach to get fruitful information between the MID and tissue. This experiment was performed in a laboratory controlled physiological environment. We strongly believe that this research would play a very significant role in medical science.

4 Conclusions

This research suggests that it is a novel method to extract the helpful information of the Medical interventional device. We used advanced signal processing algorithms to get the in-homogeneities and elasticity properties of that tissues and obtained the texture difference in between. As we know, In the clinical world where digital pathology is becoming more popular, automatic classification could be a very helpful tool for the pathologist. and it could provide a new direction to the medical science.

Acknowledgment. This work was supported by Deutscher Akademischer Austauschdienst (DAAD), Germany. We thank to INKA research (OVGU, Magdeburg, Germany) Group for the cooperation.

Conflict of Interest. We have no conflicts of interest relationship with any companies or commercial organizations.

References

1. Horgan, S., Vanuno, D.: Robots in laparoscopic surgery. J. Laparoendosc. Adv. Surg. Tech. **11**(6), 415–419 (2001)
2. Abolhassani, N., Patel, R.: Deflection of a flexible needle during insertion into soft tissue. In: Engineering in Medicine and Biology Society, 2006. EMBS 2006. 28th Annual International Conference of the IEEE, pp. 3858–3861. IEEE (2006)
3. Illanes, A., Boese, A., Maldonado, I., Pashazadeh, A., Schaufler, A., Navab, N., Friebe, M.: Novel clinical device tracking and tissue event characterization using proximally placed audio signal acquisition and processing. Sci. Rep. **8**(1), 12070 (2018)
4. van Gerwen, D.J., Dankelman, J., van den Dobbelsteen, J.J.: Needle–tissue interaction forces–A survey of experimental data. Med. Eng. Phys. **34**(6), 665–680 (2012)
5. Dedong, G.A.O., Yong, L.E.I., Bin, Y.A.O.: Analysis of Dynamic Tissue Deformation during Needle Insertion into Soft Tissue. IFAC Proc. Volumes **46**(5), 684–691 (2013)
6. Mostaço-Guidolin, L.B., Ko, A.C.T., Wang, F., Xiang, B., Hewko, M., Tian, G., Sowa, M.G.: Collagen morphology and texture analysis: from statistics to classification. Sci. Rep. **3**, 2190 (2013)
7. Lee, H.K., Chung, J., Chang, S.I., Yoon, E.: Real-time measurement of the three-axis contact force distribution using a flexible capacitive polymer tactile sensor. J. Micromech. Microeng. **21**(3), 035010 (2011)
8. Okamura, A.M., Simone, C., O'leary, M.D.: Force modeling for needle insertion into soft tissue. IEEE Trans. Biomed. Eng. **51**(10), 1707–1716 (2004)
9. Boedeker, K.L., McNitt-Gray, M.F.: Application of the noise power spectrum in modern diagnostic MDCT: part II. noise power spectra and signal to noise. Phys. Med. Biol. **52**(14), 4047 (2007)
10. Kienle, A., Forster, F.K., Hibst, R.: Influence of the phase function on determination of the optical properties of biological tissue by spatially resolved reflectance. Opt. Lett. **26**(20), 1571–1573 (2001)
11. Cheong, W.F., Prahl, S.A., Welch, A.J.: A review of the optical properties of biological tissues. IEEE J. Quantum Electron. **26**(12), 2166–2185 (1990)

Real-Time Intelligent Healthcare Monitoring and Diagnosis System Through Deep Learning and Segmented Analysis

Edward B. Panganiban[1,2,3]([⊠]), Wen-Yaw Chung[1], Wei-Chieh Tai[1], Arnold C. Paglinawan[2], Jheng-Siang Lai[1], Ren-Wei Cheng[1], Ming-Kai Chang[1], and Po-Hsuan Chang[1]

[1] Department of Electronic Engineering, Chung-Yuan Christian University, Chung-Li, Taoyuan city, Taiwan, R.O.C.
[2] School of Electrical Electronics and Computer Engineering, Mapua University, Muralla street, Intramuros, Manila, Philippines
[3] College of Computing Studies, Information and Communication Technology, Isabela State University, Echague, Isabela, Philippines
ebpanganiban@isu.edu.ph

Abstract. Medical facilities and technologies have been greatly improved through the application of biosensors, healthcare systems, health diagnosis and disease prevention technologies. However, wireless transmission and deep learning neural network are essential applications and new methods in biomedical engineering nowadays. Hence, authors established a new real-time and intelligent healthcare system that will help the physician's diagnosis over the patient's condition and will have a great contribution to medical research. Physiological conditions can be monitored and primary diagnosis will be determined which will help people primarily for personal health care. This paper focused on the collection, transmission, and analysis of physiological signals captured from biosensors with the application of deep learning and segmented analysis for the prediction of heart diseases. Biosensors employed were non-invasive composed of infrared body temperature sensor (MLX90614), heart rate and blood oxygen sensor (MAX30100) and ECG sensor (AD8232). This research used these biosensors to collect signals integrated with Arduino UNO as a central module to process and analyze those signals. ESP8266 Wi-Fi microchip was used to transmit digitized result signals to the database for deep learning analysis. The first segment of deep learning analysis is the Long-Short Term Memory (LSTM) network applied for the temperature, heart rate and arterial oxygen saturation prediction. A rolled training technique was used to provide accurate predictions in this segment. The second segment used was the Convolutional Neural Network (CNN), which comprises three hidden layers to analyze the ECG signals from the image datasets. Deep learning tools used were the powerful python language, python based Anaconda, Google's TensorFlow and open source neural network library Keras. The algorithm was used for evaluation using the available MIT-BIH ECG database from Physionet databases which attained 99.05% accuracy and arrived at only 4.96% loss rate after 30 training steps. The implementation of the system is comprised of physiological parameter sensing system, the wireless transmission system and the deep neural network prediction system. User interfaces were also developed such as

© Springer Nature Switzerland AG 2020
K.-P. Lin et al. (Eds.): ICBHI 2019, IFMBE Proceedings 74, pp. 15–25, 2020.
https://doi.org/10.1007/978-3-030-30636-6_3

the LCD display which shows values of body temperature, heart rate and arterial oxygen saturation level. Web page and app were created to allow users or doctors for visual presentations of the results of analysis. The webpage contains information about the system, deep learning networks used, biosensors and the historical graph of about the patient's body temperature, heart rate and oxygen saturation. It also indicates the normal ranges of the physiological parameters.

Keywords: Physiological signals · Biosensors · Deep learning · CNN · LSTM

1 Introduction

Through the advancement of medical technology, the remote monitoring of physiological parameters has been possible for use in society [1, 2]. The wireless transmission and deep learning methods provide medical staff the medical information then analyze these through conditional deep learning with segmented reasoning [3]. According to ranking of global population deaths in 2016 as shown in Fig. 1, heart disease is the top cause of death in the world. The world population density is gradually increasing and the impact of an aging society and the urban-rural gap becomes larger which led to widespread disparity in social medical resources.

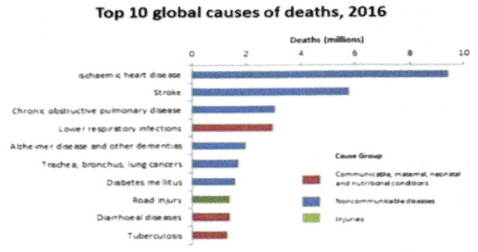

Fig. 1. Ranking of global population deaths in 2016

Even today, many social health policies and health insurance premiums are proposed, but these does not ultimately solve the most fundamental problems. This paper can help ease some problems encountered with the people in the uneven medical distribution area through an intelligent monitoring and diagnosis system [4, 5]. Detected values and signals are transmitted back to the database for deep learning analysis. It can diagnose the possible causes so that people in the uneven medical distribution area can detect the physiological condition first and then go to the hospital for further treatment.

2 Materials and Methods

2.1 Concept

This paper has the concept as shown in Fig. 2. Users or patients use biological sensors to detect physiological parameters for heart disease and vital signs like body temperature, pulse rate and oxygen saturation level. The values from these sensors are then fed into interfaces so that information can be understood by the users. Wireless transmission is used to send the gathered data to the database. Simultaneously, the microcontroller utilized deep learning analysis and segmentation reasoning to predict the outcome and the possible causes. Finally, the results and data are displayed in the user interface. Medical practitioner like the doctor or nurse validates and confirms if the results are reliable.

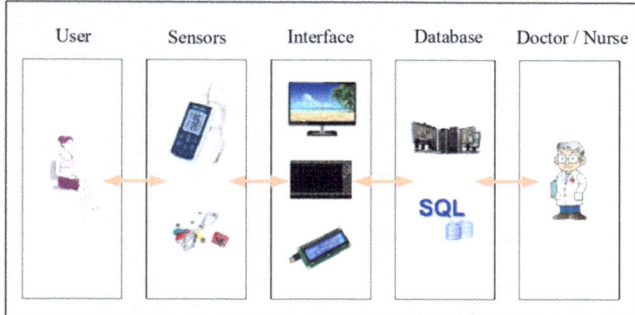

Fig. 2. Concept

2.2 System Architecture

The system architecture of this research is divided into three parts, physiological parameters sensors system, wireless transmission system and the deep learning prediction system. The system comprises of body temperature (MLX90614), ECG (AD8232), heart rate and blood oxygen sensors to collect the signals of the measured physiological parameters of the body. Figure 3 show the system architecture which explains how the system works. Both heart rate and blood oxygen values are gathered by only one sensor (MAX30100). Analog-to-Digital Converter is also employed for conversion of signal. Inter-Integrated Circuit (I2C) communication is the built-in feature of the microcontroller (Arduino UNO) to send the data to be displayed on LCD. The data were sent to the database through wireless transmission.

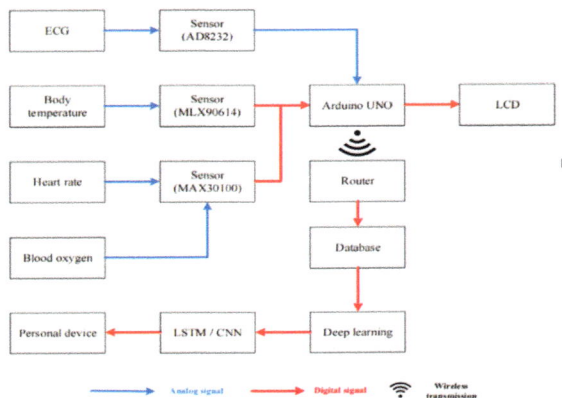

Fig. 3. System architecture

These data were processed in a deep learning technique using Long Short-Term Memory (LSTM) for the purposes of prediction of next occurrence and Convolutional Neural Network (CNN) to analyze the electrocardiogram (ECG) images. The prediction result is then shown on the user interface.

2.3   System Components

2.3.1   Temperature sensor

The body temperature sensor is a tiny electronic component that people can measure human body temperature. The researchers use MLX90614 because of its accuracy than can reach up to 0.02 °C. This is an infrared temperature sensor that is small in size, cost is low and easy to use.

2.3.2   Heart rate and blood oxygen sensors

For human, heart rate and blood oxygen are one of the physiological parameters that most directly affect heart disease. The researchers utilized the Integrated Circuit (IC) MAX30100, which is an integrated pulse oximetry and heart rate monitor sensor. It is a combination of two light emitting diodes (LEDs), a photo detector, optimized optics and low-noise analog signal processing that can detect both heart rate and blood oxygen saturation level. Its principle is the optical measurement of changes in blood flow in blood vessels called photoplethysmography (PPG).

2.3.3   ECG sensor

ECG is the best way to measure and diagnose abnormal heart rhythms [6]. AD8232 is a portable ECG sensor and a fully integrated single-lead ECG front end for biopotential signal acquisition. It can extract, amplify and filter small biopotential signals like ECG even with a presence of noisy conditions. The sensors output can be monitored using the serial monitor or can be sent directly to the cloud with the help of a microcontroller.

2.3.4   Inter-Integrated circuit (I2C) communication protocol

I2C (Inter-Integrated Circuit) is a two-wire transmission protocol which uses two bidirectional open-drain call SDA (serial data) and SCL (serial clock). This protocol is used for LCD interface compatibility and data transmission (Fig 4).

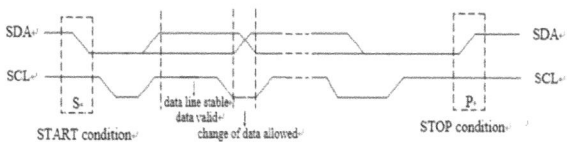

Fig. 4. Data transmission protocol

2.3.5   Microcontroller

The Arduino UNO type of microcontroller is used in the system. This is a single-chip microcontroller in processing development environment and serves as a central system in analyzing data signals. The system also used this due to its I2C communication protocol feature to transfer data.

2.3.6   Wireless transmission

Wireless transmission technology transmits information in space like Wi-FI is what the system used in transferring data. The researchers chose Wi-Fi chip ESP8266 to transmit digitized signals to the database for deep learning analysis because of its low price and reliability. It has also convenient application development, abundant learning resources, flexible design and enhanced function. On the other hand, the system also used Bluetooth technology to transport ECG data because of its large property. The HC-05 is the Bluetooth which has a low price and easy to operate. It has a master-slave feature for easy use. It is also a serial port for transport wireless serial connection setup.

2.3.7   Database

The data uploaded were temperature, heart rate, blood oxygen and ECG. The ECG need is the image type for the CNN deep learning, while other physiological parameters uploaded were in value type. The MySQL database management tool is used which is based on PHP for Internet compatibility.

2.3.8   Deep learning architectures

The deep learning involved in this paper is to perform multi-level function operations and machine learning for meanings expressed by data such as pictures, sounds, and numbers. Deep learning is an algorithm based on representational learning of data in machine learning [7, 8].

2.4   LSTM network

A recurrent neural network (RNN) consist of LSTM units are LSTM network. This network has the feature that the current output of a sequence is associated with the previous output. It means that the network memorizes the previous output message and applies it to the calculation of the current output. It is composed of forget gate, input gate and output gate [9]. This network is the first segment of deep learning analysis which is applied for the temperature, heart rate and arterial oxygen saturation estimation. The forget gate performs filtering out the previous data if there is new input data, input gate determines whether the new input data should be added to the LSTM network while output gate determines whether the current data will be added to the output.

The architecture of temperature deep learning using the LSTM algorithm is shown in Fig. 5. The body temperature values from the sensor are the input data and converts its property into CSV file for normalization using python. Analysis of data defines the weight of each gate to get the prediction model. Then it builds a model to let the machine train itself. The final deep learning model is then established through comparison of prediction versus the training model. The correct model is the finalized based from the comparison.

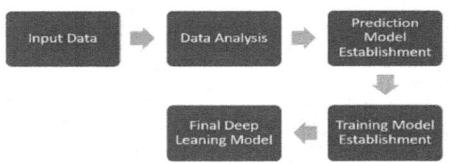

Fig. 5. Temperature deep learning architecture

2.5   Convolutional Neural Network

The second segment of this research is the Convolutional Neural Network (CNN) to analyze the ECG signals from the image datasets [10, 11]. Its functions is a feed forward neural network consisting three convolutional hidden layers associated with weights and pooling layers and a fully connected layer at the last stage.

2.5.1   Deep Learning Development Tools

For this research to become attainable, it used several deep learning development tools like the powerful python programming language, python based Anaconda, Google's TensorFlow and open source neural network Keras library. Python is a high-level programming language was used to analyze signals from sensors and also performs smooth learning. It supports open source framework like TensorFLow from Google. Anaconda is the platform used for python distribution for scientific computing established in this research. Data flow diagram based from TensorFlow with the aid of Keras library was done for quick analysis of the signals acquired from sensors [8].

3   Results and Discussion

3.1   Temperature Deep Learning Results

3.1.1   Smooth Training

The temperature datasets were loaded into the database and underwent neural network model and allowed access to the data of the memory cell of the LSTM network. The body temperature smoothing training chart in figure is the result of the smooth training of temperature values. Based from the figure, it is explained that for more than 300 times of training, the temperature difference only if from − 0.2 to 0.4 unit of temperature. The training model has a quite good result, however, smooth prediction can only take its average values and cannot predict the next occurrence (Fig 6).

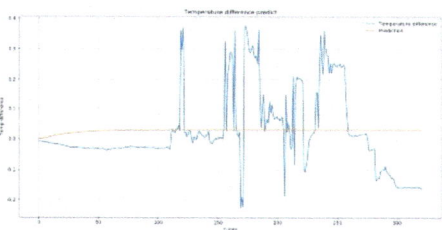

Fig. 6. Body temperature smoothing training chart

3.1.2   Rolling Training

There are two type of analysis done for temperature rolling training in this paper. These are body temperature rolling training and body temperature difference rolling training which are presented in Figs. 7 and 8 respectively. The horizontal axis denotes the number of training times. From these figures, it can be seen that there is not much difference between the datasets and the predicted values. The temperature difference is also not large. Hence, the correct training result is quite high and it can be validated that the weights and the LSTM model are correct. From those results, the researchers concluded that rolling prediction is more accurate for body temperature prediction.

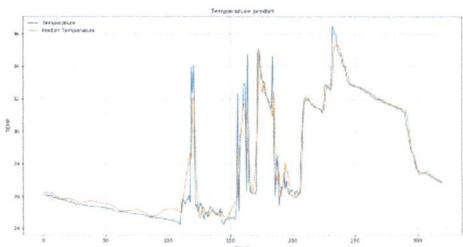

Fig. 7. Body temperature rolling training chart

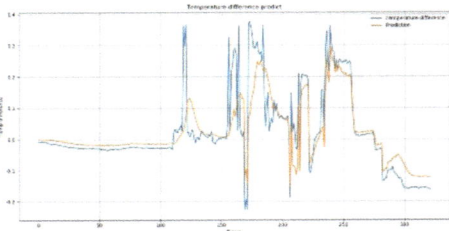

Fig. 8. Body temperature difference rolling training chart

3.1.3   ECG Deep Learning Results

In the deep learning of ECG, the ECG signal is analyzed by the CNN for the characteristics of its images through its pattern. The ECG signal used by the researchers are acquired from MIT-BIH datasets from physionet.org databank. Through the application of CNN deep learning, the training model was able to classify diseases specifically in heart. Figure 9 illustrates the architecture of the deep learning system for ECG signals. ECG input signals are fed into CNN for deep learning process. It contains of three convolutional layers comprising of hidden and pooling layers and a final fully connected layer. Each convolutional layers contain eigenvalue filter and rectified linear units (ReLu) activation functions. The first layer in each data has 64 features and has size of 3×3, second layer with 128 features and has 3×3 size while the last layer has 256 features with 3×3 size. It was then compressed to a 2×2 in length and width to become flat. Finally, the fully connected layer act as a classifier. If the training model has high accuracy, then final model is determined then stored for the implementation stage.

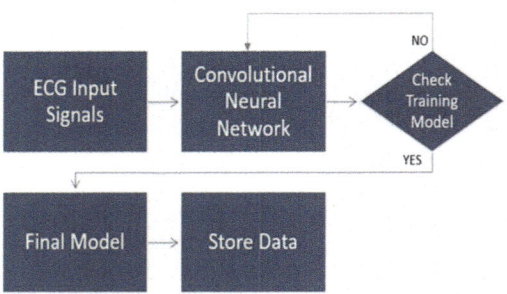

Fig. 9. ECG deep learning system architecture

3.1.4   ECG Training

MIT-BIH database are divided into four categories, namely normal, arrhythmia, noisy and other abnormalities. In the four groups, the training data has 6048 sets of data, and the validation group has 1513 sets. The method used to determine the type of ECG signal is mainly to analyze whether the user is healthy through identifying the RR interval of the ECG signal. In addition, the RR interval can also calculate the user's heart rhythm. The results of the test are established in each training generation, wherein the data loss rate and the accuracy rate are determined. In the experiment, the researchers trained 30 generations. The summary of the tests are presented in Table 1. It can be seen that after 30 training generations, the loss rate went down to 4.96% and its accuracy attained 99.05%.

Table 1. Training result

Generation	Loss rate	Accuracy rate
1	54.01%	75.96%
5	20.13%	96.71%
10	12.00%	97.66%
15	9.31%	98.03%
20	7.49%	98.31%
25	6.16%	98.77%
30	4.96%	99.05%

3.2   User Interface System

User interface is developed for better understanding of the users in the system. LCD display, APP and website are the types of interfaces the researchers have established.

3.2.1   LCD display

This allows the user to see instantly the physiological parameters about their health status obtained by sensors attached to their body. The temperature, heart rate and blood oxygen saturation level are displayed on LCD.

3.2.2   Website

The website is composed of home and inner pages. Homepage shows the background of the system and its process involved. Inner pages shows the various data gathered from sensors. The interface of the website is built using HTML, CSS, JavaScript and Lua as illustrated in Fig. 10.

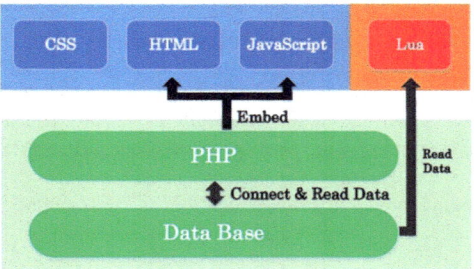

Fig. 10. Website architecture

3.2.3   Mobile APP

Java Eclipse is used to design the ECG user interface APP. It can display ECG and heart rate values as well as it can save previous measured records. Bluetooth HC-05 was used to transmit ECG signals for easier transmission protocol and ECG interface.

4   Conclusion

The CNN algorithm used using the available MIT-BIH ECG database from Physionet databases obtained 99.05% accuracy and 4.96% loss rate after 30 training generations. Whereas, in LSTM algorithm, the rolling training prediction technique is identified to be more accurate than smooth training body temperature values. The main innovation involved in this paper is the new algorithm established which composed of physiological parameter sensing system, the wireless transmission system and deep neural network prediction system. Its functionalities were tested and validated to attain its desired performance. User interfaces displayed values of body temperature, heart rate and arterial oxygen saturation level that allow users like doctors or other medical staff for visual presentations and validation of results. Overall, the researchers came up with a simple and yet reliable real-time intelligent healthcare monitoring and diagnosis system through deep learning and segmented analysis.

Acknowledgment. The authors would like to thank Chung Yuan Christian University for allowing the researchers use the Mixed-Mode IC laboratory in the Department of Electronic Engineering which made this paper possible and attained its objectives.

Conflict of Interest. The authors declare no conflict of interest.

References

1. Baba, E., Hammouch, A.: A health remote monitoring application based on wireless body area networks, pp. 1–4. IEEE (2018)
2. Kaur, A., Jasuja, A.: Cost effective remote health monitoring system based on IoT using arduino UNO. Adv. Comput. Sci. Inf. Technol. **4**, 80–84 (2017)
3. Deng, L., Yu, D.: Deep learning: methods and applications (2013). https://doi.org/10.1561/2000000039
4. Shinjo, D., Aramaki, T.: Geographic distribution of healthcare resources, healthcare service provision, and patient flow in Japan: a cross sectional study. Soc. Sci. Med. **75**, 1954–1963 (2012)
5. Wilson, N., Coopuer, I., De Vries, E., Reid, S., Fish, T., Marais, B.: A Critical review of interventions to redress the inequitable distribution of healthcare professionals to rural and remote areas. Int. Electron. J. Rural Remote Heath Res. Educ. Pract. Policy **9**(1060), 1–21 (2009)
6. Gacek, A.: ECG signal processing, classification and interpretation. Springer, vol. 1, no. 289 (2015)

7. Parsa, M., Panda, P., Sen, S., Roy, K.: Staged inference using conditional deep learning for energy efficient real - time smart diagnosis, pp. 78–81. IEEE (2017)
8. Khan, U.M., Kabir, Z., Hassan, S.A., Ahmed, S.H.: A deep learning framework using passive WiFi sensing for respiration monitoring. In: 2017 IEEE Global Communications Conference GLOBECOM 2017 – Proceedings, pp. 1–6 (2018)
9. Lipton, Z.C., Kale, D.C., Elkan, C., Wetzel, R.: Learning to diagnose with LSTM recurrent neural networks, pp. 1–18 (2015)
10. Acharya, U.R., Fujita, H., Oh, S.L., Hagiwara, Y., Tan, J.H., Adam, M.: Application of deep convolutional neural network for automated detection of myocardial infarction using ECG signals. Inf. Sci. **415–416**, 190–198 (2017)
11. Lu, L., Zheng, Y., Carneiro, G., Yang, L.: Deep learning and convolutional neural networks for medical image computing (2017). https://doi.org/10.1007/978-3-319-42999-1

The Prolonged Effect on Respiratory Sinus Arrhythmia Response of Individual with Internet Gaming Disorder via Breathing Exercise

Hong-Ming Ji[1] and Tzu-Chien Hsiao[2,3(✉)]

[1] Institute of Computer Science and Engineering, College of Computer Science, National Chiao Tung University, 1001 University Road, Hsinchu, Taiwan
[2] Department of Computer Science, College of Computer Science, National Chiao Tung University, Hsinchu, Taiwan
[3] Institute of Biomedical Engineering, College of Electrical and Computer Engineering, National Chiao Tung University, Hsinchu, Taiwan
labview@cs.nctu.edu.tw

Abstract. Students playing Internet game become a daily activity in campus life. They usually struggle for fun and stay at audio-visual stimuli of Internet games for a long period of time. Some players hardly controlling the impulses of game engagement despite negative consequences can be described as a term of Internet gaming disorder (IGD). They always perform a psychological property, called tolerance symptom, for increasing the amounts of playing time to achieve satisfaction. Studies found that breathing exercise can alleviate IGD symptoms because breathing can facilitate the psychophysiological regulation. Few studies, moreover, observed the effect of breathing exercise on tolerance response of IGD symptom. This study explores the prolonged effect on respiratory sinus arrhythmia (RSA) of individuals with IGD from rest to watching game videos as stimuli through abdominal breathing (AB) training. 7 persons of high-risk IGD (HIGD) and 17 persons of low-risk IGD (LIGD) were recruited. The results showed that both of HIGD and LIGD presented an increasing RSA value with AB training from rest to stimuli. In contrast to those with LIGD, those with HIGD showed higher RSA value during negative stimuli. Our findings suggested that AB training can be a potential method to reduce psychophysiological responses of persons with HIGD during game-related cue stimuli, negative game especially. It may provide researchers insight into the effect of breathing exercises on psychophysiology responses of persons with IGD and further develop related application, such as alleviative method. A further study could investigate the effect on autonomic nervous system activities for a long-period AB training.

Keywords: Internet gaming disorder · Tolerance symptom · Respiratory sinus arrhythmia · Abdominal breathing

© Springer Nature Switzerland AG 2020
K.-P. Lin et al. (Eds.): ICBHI 2019, IFMBE Proceedings 74, pp. 26–32, 2020.
https://doi.org/10.1007/978-3-030-30636-6_4

1 Introduction

With development of game industry, the population of game players is gradually increased in recent years. The population of game players increased 1.04% from 2003 to 2010 in Taiwan [1] and 0.24% from 2014 to 2020 in the US (The Statistics Portal) [2]. In the population, some players cannot control their game use, and overuse causes them to risk relationship, education, or work performance. American psychiatric association noticed the severity and included Internet gaming disorder (IGD) into the Diagnostic and Statistical Manual of Mental Disorders fifth edition (DSM-5) in 2013 [3]. The World Health Organization announced gaming disorder as a mental disease in the International Statistical Classification of Diseases 11th Revision in 2018 [4].

Persons with IGD show tolerance symptom, who spend a lot of time on games, and they need to increase the amounts of time playing games to achieve satisfaction [3]. Researchers consider that the tolerance symptom is an important psychological property of IGD. Petry et al. proposed that tolerance symptom not only denotes increasing amounts of time but also denotes increasing games' excitement and powerful software or hardware [5]. King et al. pointed out that the motivations of increasing time on game were playing more complicated, difficult, or consuming games [6]. The aforementioned studies mainly focused on observing cognition and behavior of persons with IGD.

Persons with IGD stay at dynamically visual and acoustical stimuli for a long period of time, and they control their psychophysiological responses during stimuli. Breathing can control psychological responses (e.g. emotion) and physiological responses (e.g. autonomic nervous system (ANS)) [7]. Breathing responses may be an important index to explore psychophysiological mechanism of persons with IGD under tolerance symptom. Chang et al. noted that persons with problematic Internet use & excessive online game increased breathing rate during playing game [8]. Kim et al. also agreed that persons with IGD increased breathing rate during watching game video [9]. Moreover, breathing can affect the rhythmic oscillation in heart period, also called respiratory sinus arrhythmia (RSA). RSA can link with emotion regulation [10]. RSA as an index is adopted to investigate breathing and emotional responses of persons with IGD. The severity of IGD is associated with high RSA withdrawal during solving family problems [11]. The RSA value of persons with high-risk Internet addiction (HIA) was lower than those of persons with low-risk Internet addiction (LIA) [12]. The empirical studies [8, 9] suggested that persons with IGD showed higher sympathetic nervous system (SNS) activity during game stimuli, and the empirical studies [11, 12] indicated that persons with IGD felt more displeasure and less parasympathetic nervous system (PNS) activity.

In recent years, breathing exercise has been used to assist psychotherapies with alleviating psychological symptoms of IGD and relaxing emotions [13, 14]. Breathing exercises may be a potential method to affect psychophysiological responses of persons with IGD under tolerance symptom. However, few studies observed the effect of breathing exercises on psychophysiological responses of persons with IGD for longer period of time. In this study, our purpose was to investigate that breathing exercises affected RSA of individuals with high-risk IGD (HIGD) and low-risk IGD (LIGD) from rest to watching game videos. We expected that our finding in this study can provide researchers to design appropriate breathing exercises to prevent and treat IGD symptoms.

2   Material and Method

Participants in this study were 32 subjects (28 males and 4 females, 20–33 years old), who were recruited from National Chiao Tung University (NCTU), Taiwan. All participants signed informed consent document. To assess the IGD and Internet addiction, we adopted IGD questionnaire (IGDQ, 9 items, 2-point Likert scale from 0 (no) to 1 (yes)) [3] and Chen Internet addiction scale (CIAS, 26 items, 4-point Likert scale from 1 (stronger disagreement) to 4 (stronger agreement)) [15], respectively. We selected video of League of Legends (video1) and Resident Evil (video2) as game-related cues to stimuli participants, and the two games were popular with students on the NCTU campus. We used self-assessment manikin (SAM, 9-point Likert scale from 1 to 9) [16] to assess participant's emotional valence (ranging from unpleasant to pleasant feeling) and emotional arousal (ranging from peace to extreme stronger).

In experimental procedure (Fig. 1), we asked each participant to fill out IGDQ and CIAS, and then subject was asked to use iso-volume maneuver (IVM) method to do abdominal breathing (AB) training (10 min) [17]. After recovery (3 min), subject completed two trials. Each trial was contained rest (6 min), watching game video as stimuli (6 min), and filling out SAM. We measured subject's electrocardiography signals (ECG, Best-C, three disposable pregelled Ag/AgCl spot electrodes) during rest and stimuli.

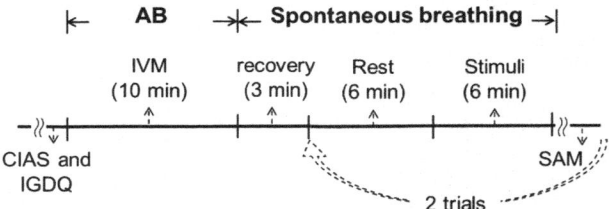

Fig. 1. The experimental procedure.

The sampling rate of ECG was 1000 Hz. We adopted auto power spectrum method to calculate frequency domain information of ECG, including low frequency bend (LF, 0.04–0.15 Hz, as measure of SNS and PNS activities) and high frequency bend (HF, 0.15–0.4 Hz, as measure of PNS activities). After that, we calculated RSA ($HF/(LF + HF)$). All signal processing were executed in LabVIEW environment (v.2016, NI Corp., Austin, USA).

3   Result

We considered that if Internet users are IGD, they must be Internet addiction. Based on the IGDQ and CIAS scores, we separated subjects into 7 HIGD (IGDQ score $\geq$ 5 and CIAS score $\geq$ 64) and 17 LIGD (IGDQ score < 5 and CIAS score < 64) people. Table 1 shows demographic information and statistical result (mean $\pm$ SD) of SAM rating after watching video1 and video2 for individuals with HIGD and LIGD. Based on the valence rating, video1 and video2 were represented positive stimuli (valence rating > 5) and negative stimuli (valence rating < 5). The valence and arousal rating of individuals with HIGD were higher than those of individuals with LIGD, except arousal after video2.

Figure 2 displays the box plot of RAS of individuals with HIGD and LIGD during rest (rest1 and rest2) and watching game videos (video1 and video2). The RSA values of individuals with HIGD and LIGD during watching game video were higher than that during rest. There are statistical significant differences ($p < 0.05$) between RSA value during rest and RSA value during watching videos, except during watching video1 for individuals with HIGD. Comparing to individuals with LIGD, the RSA value of individuals with HIGD during rest1 and rest2 were lower. The RSA value of individuals with HIGD during watching video2 was higher than those of individuals with LIGD. But there are no statistical significant differences between the RSA value of individuals with HIGD and those of individuals with LIGD.

Table 1. Demographic information and statistical result (mean ± SD) of SAM rating for individuals with HIGD and LIGD. M: males; F: females.

	HIGD (6 M, 1 F)	LIGD (13 M, 4 F)
Age	21.57 ± 0.98	22.53 ± 3.04
video1 valence	6.29 ± 0.76	5.59 ± 1.33
video1 arousal	4.71 ± 2.50	3.18 ± 2.35
video2 valence	4.14 ± 1.77	3.65 ± 1.22
video2 arousal	5.29 ± 1.98	5.59 ± 1.77

*Statistically significant differences ($p < 0.05$) according to a Mann-Whitney U test.

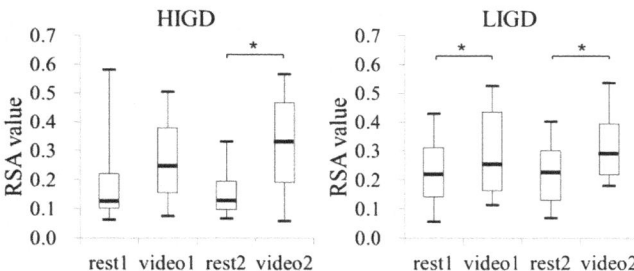

Fig. 2. The box plot of RSA of individuals with HIGD and LIGD during rest and watching game video. Statistically significant differences (*$p < 0.05$) according to a Wilcoxon signed-rank test.

4 Discussion

We investigated breathing exercise as regulation method that affect RSA responses of individuals with IGD during rest and watching game videos. We compared the difference between the RSA value during rest and that during watching game video; and the difference between the RSA value of individuals with HIGD and those of individuals with LIGD.

We found that the RSA value of individuals with HIGD and LIGD with AB training was increased from rest to positive or negative game stimuli. Coyne et al. proposed the positive correlation between the severity of IGD and high RSA withdrawal during solving family problems [11]. Compared with during rest, those of persons with HIA and LIA showed higher RSA value during positive emotion stimuli but lower RSA value, during negative emotion stimuli [12]. Compare our finding with the empirical study [11, 12], and we inferred that AB training mainly affected the psychophysiological responses of individuals with HIGD and LIGD during negative game stimuli. Deep and slow breathing was used to alleviate stress and anxiety [7]. Therefore, we suggested that AB training may effectively decrease unpleasant feeling and increase PNS activity of individuals with HIGD and LIGD during negative game cue stimuli.

In contrast to individuals with LIGD, the RSA value of individuals with HIGD during rest was lower, but the RSA value was higher, during watching negative game. Hsieh and Hsiao proposed that the RSA value of persons with HIA during rest and positive or negative emotion stimuli was lower than those of persons with LIA [12]. Persons with problematic Internet users & excessive online gaming showed lower HF and higher LF/HF value than those of control groups during rest and playing game [8]. This partially consistency may be that individuals with IGD were inexperienced in AB during rest, and they need to spend time on training AB. AB training affected reducing the psychophysiological responses of individuals with HIGD during watching negative game compared with those of individuals with LIGD. Doing deep and slow breathing can transfer unpleasant feeling to calm or temporarily disappear for patients with panic disorder [18]. We suggested that AB training may affect more PNS activity and positive feeling of individuals with HIGD during watching negative game compared with those of individuals with LIGD.

This study has two limitations. First, due to small the number of subjects, there were no statistically significant difference in RSA value between individuals with HIGD and LIGD. Second, due to only observing 6 min physiological responses, we lacked information to investigate the effect on RSA value of individuals of HIGD for a long-period AB training, such as one day later or one week later. Nevertheless, we investigate the effect of AB training on RSA of individuals of HIGD under tolerance symptom. In this study, AB training can be a potential method to regulate psychophysiological responses of individuals with IGD during game-related cue stimuli, negative game especially. We provide researchers to understand the effect on physiological responses of individuals with IGD toward breathing exercises. Our finding would promote researchers to design appropriate breathing exercises to prevent and treat IGD symptoms.

5 Conclusions

In this study, AB training as way of psychophysiological relaxation was used to investigate the effect on the RSA value of individuals with HIGD and LIGD from rest to watching game video. Individuals with HIGD and LIGD increased RSA value from rest to watching game videos. Compared with individuals with LIGD, individuals with HIGD exhibited higher RSA value during watching negative game. We inferred that AB training can be a potential way to influence psychophysiological responses of individuals of HIGD and LIGD during game-related cue stimuli, negative game especially. Our finding may provide researchers insight into the effect on psychophysiology responses via AB training and develop related application. In near future, we would like to collect more sample size and investigate the effect on ANS activities for a long-period AB training.

Acknowledgment. This study was fully supported by the Taiwan Ministry of Science and Technology (MOST 105-2221-E-009-159, MOST 105-2634-E-009-003, and MOST 107-2221-E-009-153), and was approved by the REC for Human Subject Protection, NCTU, Taiwan (NCTU-REC-104-046).

Conflict of Interest. The authors declare that they have no conflict of interest.

References

1. Chang, T.-S., Ku, C.-Y., Fu, H.-P.: Grey theory analysis of online population and online game industry revenue in Taiwan. Technol. Forecast. Soc. Change **80**, 175–185 (2013)
2. The statistics portal at. https://www.statista.com/statistics/521822/number-of-online-console-gamers-in-the-us/
3. American Psychiatric Association: Diagnostic and statistical manual of mental disorders, 5th (DSM-5). VA, American Psychiatric Association Press Inc, Arlington (2013)
4. Rumpf, H.J., Achab, S., Billieux, J., et al.: Including gaming disorder in ICD-11: the need to do so from a clinical and public health perspective. J Behav. Addict. **7**, 556–561 (2018)
5. Petry, N.M., Rehbein, F., Gentile, D.A., et al.: An international consensus for assessing internet gaming disorder using the new DSM-5 approach. Addiction **109**(9), 1399–1466 (2014)
6. King, D.L., Herd, M.C.E., Delfabbro, P.H.: Tolerance in Internet gaming disorder: a need for increasing gaming time or something else? J Behav. Addict. **6**(4), 525–533 (2017)
7. Brown, R.P., Gerbarg, P.L.: Sudarshan Kriya yogic breathing in the treatment of stress, anxiety, and depression: part I—neurophysiologic model. J. Altern. Complement. Med. **11**(1), 189–201 (2005)
8. Chang, J.-S., Kim, E.-Y., Jung, D., et al.: Altered cardiorespiratory coupling in young male adults with excessive online gaming. Biol. Psychol. **110**, 159–166 (2015)
9. Kim, H., Ha, J., Chang, W.-D., et al.: Detection of craving for gaming in adolescents with Internet gaming disorder using multimodal biosignals. Sensors **18**(1), 102 (2018)
10. Overbeek, T.J.M., van Boxtel, A., Westerink, J.H.D.M.: Respiratory sinus arrhythmia responses to induced emotional states: effects of RSA indices, emotion induction method, age, and sex. Biol. Psychol. **91**(1), 128–141 (2012)

11. Coyne, S.M., Dyer, W.J., Densley, R., et al.: Physiological indicators of pathologic video game use in adolescence. J. Adolesc. Health **56**(3), 307–313 (2015)

12. Hsieh, D.-L., Hsiao, T.-C.: Respiratory sinus arrhythmia reactivity of internet addiction addicts in negative and positive emotional states using film clips stimulation. Biomed. Eng. OnLine **15**, 69 (2016)

13. Li, W., Garland, E.L., O'Brien, J.E., et al.: Mindfulness-oriented recovery enhancement for video game addiction in emerging adults: preliminary findings from case reports. Int. J. Ment. Health Addict. **16**, 928–945 (2017)

14. Torres-Rodríguez, A., Griffiths, M.D.: The treatment of Internet gaming disorder: a brief overview of the PIPATIC program. Int. J. Ment. Health Addiction **16**, 1000–1015 (2018)

15. Chen, S.-H., Weng, L.-J., Su, Y.-J., et al.: Development of a Chinese internet addiction scale and its psychometric study. Chin. J. Psychol. **45**, 279–294 (2003)

16. Lang, P.J.: Behavioral treatment and bio-behavioral assessment: computer applications. In: Sidowski, J.B., Johnson, J.H, Williams, T.A. (eds.) Technology in Mental Health Care Delivery Systems, pp. 119–137 (1980)

17. Chen, Y.-C., Hsiao, T.-C.: Abdominal breathing by using an intelligent tutoring system. In: 2015 IFMBE Proceedings 6th European Conference of the IFMBE, vol. 45, pp. 419–422 (2015)

18. Meuret, A.E., Wilhelm, F.H., Ritz, T., et al.: Breathing training for treating panic disorder useful intervention or impediment? Behav. Modif. **27**(5), 731–754 (2003)

Automatic Liver and Spleen Segmentation with CT Images Using Multi-channel U-net Deep Learning Approach

Ting-Yu Su[✉] and Yu-Hua Fang

Department of Biomedical Engineering, National Cheng Kung University,
Tainan, Taiwan
C840131840125@gmail.com

Abstract. The detection and evaluation of the shape of liver from abdominal computed tomography (CT) images are fundamental tasks in computer-assisted liver surgery planning such as radiation therapy. The contour of spleen is also a significant factor highly related to liver diseases. However, automatic and accurate liver segmentation still remains many challenges to be solve, such as ambiguous boundaries, heterogeneous appearances and highly varied shapes of the liver and spleen. To address these difficulties, we developed an automatic segmentation model based on multi-channel U-net network. Some preprocessing steps were done to elevate the performance first. Also, an approximate liver and spleen map was generated by calculating the gradient of CT images. The area which have high possibility to be liver and spleen would be select as the training set to make sure the balance of data. Then, a deep learning U-net structure was applied for the processed training data. Finally, some post-processing methods, which include k-means clustering and morphology algorithms, would be applied in our protocol. The results indicated that a high structure similarity index (SSIM) and dice score coefficient of liver and spleen segmentation model can be achieved, which were 0.9731 and 0.9508 respectively, demonstrating the potential clinical applicability of the proposed approach.

Keywords: Liver segmentation · Deep learning ·
Computed tomography images · Gradient map · k-means clustering

1 Introduction

Nowadays, deep learning algorithm, in particular convolutional neural networks, have enormously attracted the attention on many fields and have outstanding performance in many researches. On that basis, the applications, which includes image classification, object detection, segmentation, registration and other task, have already become a widespread trend, especially for medical imaging.

In clinical, there are several kinds of advanced scanning technologies of medical imaging such as computed tomography, positron emission tomography, magnetic resonance imaging and ultrasound, which lead to the diversified procedures on diagnosis of the specific disease or region of interested. The appearance of deep learning

K.-P. Lin et al. (Eds.): ICBHI 2019, IFMBE Proceedings 74, pp. 33–41, 2020.
https://doi.org/10.1007/978-3-030-30636-6_5

method provides a possible universe solution for each imaging application under the rules which is similar and simple.

Although many challenges have not been adequately tackled yet, several high-profile successes of deep learning in medical imaging are proposed such as the work by Esteva et al. [1] and Gulshan et al. [2] in the fields of dermatology and ophthalmology, both of which showed that it is possible to outperform medical experts in certain tasks.

One particularly salient example of these medical applications is the automatic segmentation of CT images, which have went viral recently. Because of the thorny difficulties caused by the large shape and size variations of anatomy between patients and the diversified styles of pathologic tissue, automated segmentation of medical images is still challenging even for a well-trained specialist.

Furthermore, the low contrast to surrounding tissues in CT images is still a problem. Conventional approaches for segmentation are statistical shape models [3, 4] and techniques that relative to image registration. Fusion of Multi-atlas label [5–7] has been widely applied in clinical research and practice. Moreover, approaches that combine multi-atlas registration algorithm and machine learning have been proposed [8, 9]. Nevertheless, the complex shape variations between patients have also made it difficult for registration-based methods to perform adequately for very non-rigid organs, especially for abdominal organs.

Today, many successful deep learning methods [8, 10–15] are being adapted to segmentation tasks in medical imaging. Most of them are based on a purely deep learning model that allows the extraction of features to be calculated and transmitted under the simple and profound rules without any anthropogenic intervention and hand-craft features.

In clinical routine, an accurate liver or spleen segmentation is of paramount importance for liver disease diagnosis and liver surgical planning system such as radiation therapy. General speaking, manual segmentation is a monotonous and time-consuming procedure. The observer variability will also come at a cost of reduction of diagnosis sensitivity, especially for the conspicuous structures and sections. And that is the reason why an automatic computer-aided detection (CAD) system is needed just as Eugenio Alberdi et al. mentioned [16], but it still have many troubles need to be overcome, such as the ambiguity between liver parenchyma and surrounding tissue, the variation of liver among different patients and the similarity gray level values of boundary.

In this paper, we presented an automatic liver parenchyma segmentation algorithm that combines deep-learning method and clustering algorithm and achieved a higher structure similarity than manual segmentation result.

2   Experimental Data and Proposed Methods

The dataset we acquired is the 3D Image Reconstruction for Comparison of Algorithm Database (3D-IRCADb) [17], which includes 20 sets of anonymized medical images of patients and the manual segmentation of the various structures of interest performed by clinical experts and the whole protocol consists of three phases including preprocessing step, training step and post-processing step.

The first stage is the preprocessing step, in which Hounsfield unit windowing is applied in the range of specific thresholds decided by the Otsu's method to exclude the irrelevant parts of organ. Meanwhile, an approximate shape of liver and spleen is evaluated preliminarily to serve as the target sample of automatic selection of slice by calculating the gradient map of CT volume and morphology algorithm. The area having high possibility of liver and spleen would be selected as the training set according to the proportion of liver to the whole volume. Then follows the separation step, where the size of each CT slice is separated into several small patches from size of [512, 512] to [128, 128], due to the lack of GPU memory in training step. To form a collective achievement of CT slice and to take more information into consider, the data of upper and lower slice is also involved in each specific patch and become a multi-channel data format with dimension [batch_size, 128, 128, 3 or 5]. Additionally, the 3D CT data is also considered as training input, which form a 5D tensor stack with size [batch_size, 128, 128, 3, 1], finally (Fig. 1).

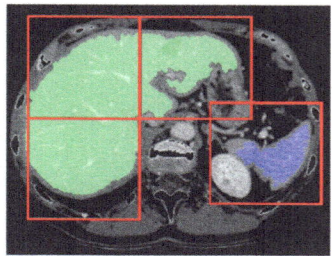

Fig. 1. The approximate shape of liver and spleen calculated by automatic segmentation algorithm. The green and blue area will be serve as the sampling criteria of the ensuring deep learning network.

The next step, perhaps the most critical step, is about the model training. The U-net deep learning structure is adopted for the segmentation of both liver and spleen. The U-net model comprises 3×3 convolutional layers followed by ReLU activation function ($3 \times 3 \times 3$ in 3D U-net), 2×2 max pooling layers ($2 \times 2 \times 2$ in 3D U-net), 2×2 up-sampling layers ($2 \times 2 \times 2$ in 3D U-net) and concatenate layers, attaching the former layer to later layer. Also, dilated convolution, which enable the enlargement of perception of each neuron unit, is applied to the deep learning model for the purpose of performance enhancement. In another way, the deep learning network of multi-channel U-net structure with dense block is also developed to elevate the accuracy, which is a deformation of U-net structure intertwined with the concept of dense network. Compared to normal U-net structure, dense network shows strong relationship between each two layers and the penalty function of network can pass through every afore-layers in the back forward stage directly (Figs. 2 and 3).

It is absolutely imperative to deal with the unbalance data as multi-classes exist, which implies that the available area of different labels are discrepant. This application indicates that the percentage of liver and spleen area in whole CT volume is substantially imbalance so that the sample of patches with specific label will be different, which may

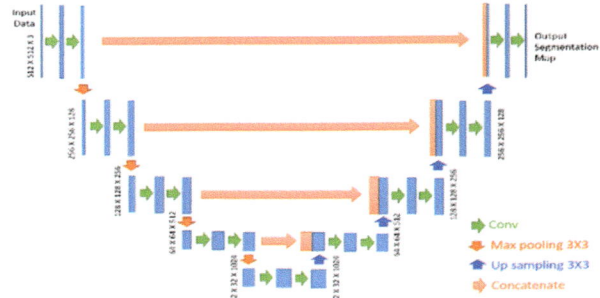

Fig. 2. The U-net deep learning structure.

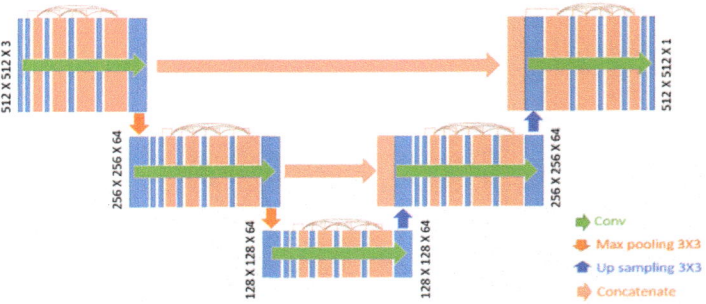

Fig. 3. The dense U-net deep learning structure.

cause the reduction of detection sensitivity of the model. That is the reason why the dice coefficient, generalizing dice coefficient and tversky score are applied as the loss function. The usage of these loss function can improve this situation and also achieve an extremely awesome performance. Note that all loss functions are analyzed under a binary classification formulation (label vs background), and the multi-label information is saved in an extend dimension in our protocol. Let R be the reference gold standard with voxel values r_n, and P be the predicted probabilistic output for the foreground label over N image elements p_n, and the background class probability be $1 - P$.

The dice coefficient is used to evaluate the segmentation performance when a gold standard or ground truth is available, comparing the similarity between prediction output and ground truth. Proposed in Milletari et al. [18] as a loss function, the 2-class discrimination of the dice loss can be expressed as

$$\text{Dice score} = 1 - \frac{\sum_{n=1}^{N} p_n r_n + \varepsilon}{\sum_{n=1}^{N} p_n + r_n + \varepsilon} - \frac{\sum_{n=1}^{N} (1 - p_n)(1 - r_n) + \varepsilon}{\sum_{n=1}^{N} 2 - p_n - r_n + \varepsilon}$$

The ε term is used to ensure the numerical item not be 0 as R and P empty.

And generalizing dice coefficient loss, proposed by Crum et al. [19], is customed to deal with the multi-label segmentation with merely a single score. The formulation of the loss function has been listed elsewise [19].

Also, Tversky similarity index, proposed by Salehi et al. [20], is adopted as the loss function in our protocol. Unlike the dice score, which take the false negative and false positive as the same weighting, Tversky index weighs false negative more than false positive in training step for unbalanced data, where detecting small region is crucial. The Tversky index is defined as:

$$T(\alpha, \beta) = \frac{\sum_{n=1}^{N} r_n p_n}{\sum_{n=1}^{N} r_n p_n + \alpha \sum_{n=1}^{N} r_n (1 - p_n) + \beta \sum_{n=1}^{N} (1 - r_n) p_n},$$

where α and β is the weighting that control the magnitude of penalties for false positive and false negative. It is significant that in the case $\alpha = \beta = 0.5$, the Tversky index simplifies to have the similar performance as the dice coefficient do.

Besides, the batch size of network is set as 64 and the loss function is minimized using the stochastic gradient descent (SGD) and Adam optimizer. The learning rate is set to $1e - 5$. The model is trained using 90% and cross validated using the remaining 10% of subjects.

The final stage is the post-processing step, where k-means clustering and morphology method are applied on segmentation output to decide the position of liver and spleen and small fragments that are not belong to our target are also removed. The whole training procedures are implemented using Keras on GeForce GTX1080 cards.

3   Result

In this part, we discuss the performance of two kinds of protocol. And the performance is evaluated by three parameters, which include dice score coefficient, (SSIM) and (PSNR). The SSIM and PSNR formula are listed below.

$$SSIM = \frac{(2\mu_r\mu_p + c_1)(2\sigma_{rp} + c_2)}{(\mu_r^2 + \mu_p^2 + c_1)(\sigma_r^2 + \sigma_p^2 + c_1)}$$

The μ and σ are the average and variation of both reference and predicted maps. And C1 and C2 are two variables to stabilize the division of weak dominator.

$$PSNR = 20 * log_{10}\left(\frac{MAX}{\sqrt{MSE}}\right), MSE = \frac{1}{N}\sum_{n=0}^{N} (r_n - p_n)^2,$$

where *MAX* is the maximum possible pixel value of the image.

In the first protocol, an automatic segmentation of liver is done by deep learning algorithm. And the spleen segmentation, afterwards, is applied on the data without liver and derive the result individually. The segmentation models of liver and spleen are independent. Here, we apply three kinds of deep learning models based on U-net structure, which include the combination of different model setting between multi-channel and 3D in input size and the approval of dilated convolution. We take dice score as loss function and apply Adam optimizer on these models.

Table 1. The comparison of liver segmentation model

Liver model-setting		Dice score	SSIM	PSNR
Multi-channel	U-net	0.950	0.974	22.284
Multi-channel	Dilated U-net	0.936	0.970	21.523
Multi-channel	Dense U-net	0.921	0.964	20.684

Table 2. The comparison of spleen segmentation model

Spleen model-setting		Dice score	SSIM	PSNR
Multi-channel	U-net	0.896	0.985	24.548
Multi-channel	Dilated U-net	0.905	0.987	25.101
Multi-channel	Dense U-net	0.955	0.991	28.609

For the second protocol, segmentation of liver and spleen are applied simultaneously by multi-label organization of data. In this protocol, we manage to handle the unbalance data by utilizing two kinds of loss functions including tversky index and generalizing dice coefficient. Discrepant optimizers are also used to enhance the performance (Tables 3 and 4).

Table 3. The comparison between different models. The loss function of these models are Tversky index.

Liver & spleen model setting		Dice score	SSIM	PSNR
U-net	Adam	0.867	0.920	15.620
Dilated U-net	Adam	0.840	0.922	15.429
U-net	SGD	0.860	0.945	17.021

Table 4. The comparison between different models. The loss function of these models are generalizing dice coefficient.

Liver & spleen model setting		Dice score	SSIM	PSNR
U-net	Adam	0.819	0.924	14.839
Dilated U-net	Adam	0.795	0.914	11.829
U-net	SGD	0.803	0.939	16.127

4   Discussion

In the result of first protocol, we listed 6 models in Table 1, and all of the results showed that the performance achievement of dice score are over 90%. In the liver segmentation part, the best model is the U-net model with multi-channel input data, dice score loss function and Adam optimizer. The deformations seem to have little improvement on it. In terms of spleen segmentation, however, it worked while a dense U-net was applied. The accuracy of dense U-net surpassed the counterpart of merely U-net, allowing an alternative choice for this application.

Here comes the result of the second protocol in Table 2. We tried 10 kinds of model above. Through these models, tversky loss function expressed an outstanding characteristic to deal with the unbalance data. The highest dice score of the model with tversky loss function is about 86%. There is no prominent difference between multi-channel and 3D input data. But the Adam optimizer seems to have better performance than SGD optimizer.

Comparing the two protocols mentioned before, the result elucidates that the performance of first protocol outperform the counterpart of second protocol. However, one of the reasons why we attempt to make use of the second protocol is to avoid the prerequisite that spleen segmentation needs to be done on the data without the liver. Without this condition, a tremendously steep accuracy will occur on automatic spleen segmentation and the area with highly false positive rate will be the liver parenchyma. Another reason is that the training time of the second protocol is considerably shorter than the first protocol to segment both liver and spleen. Although the accuracy of the second protocol did not surmount the first one, it also provided an alternative which is clinically acceptable and time-saving.

5   Conclusion

Although automatic liver segmentation using traditional algorithm is challenging because of the reasons aforementioned, deep learning algorithm provides a new solution to overcome these problems, which can have profound clinical implications for radiologist. Also, the flexible acquirement of data and changeability of model are the reasons that attract enormous attention. On this basis, our approach represents a clinically acceptable diagnostic accuracy and potential clinical applicability.

Conflict of Interest. The authors declare that they have no conflict of interest.

References

1. Esteva, A., Kuprel, B., Novoa, R.A., Ko, J., Swetter, S.M., Blau, H.M., Thrun, S.: Dermatologist-level classification of skin cancer with deep neural networks. Nature **542**, 115–118 (2017). https://doi.org/10.1038/nature21056

2. Gulshan, V., Peng, L., Coram, M., Stumpe, M.C., Wu, D., Narayanaswamy, A., Venugopalan, S., Widner, K., Madams, T., Cuadros, J., Kim, R., Raman, R., Nelson, P. C., Mega, J.L., Webster, D.R.: Development and validation of a deep learning algorithm for detection of diabetic retinopathy in retinal fundus photographs. J. Am. Medd. Assoc. **316**, 2402–2410 (2016). https://doi.org/10.1001/jama.2016.17216

3. Cerrolaza, J.J., Reyes, M., Summers, R.M., Gonzalez-Ballester, M.A., Linguraru, M.G.: Automatic multi-resolution shape modeling of multi-organ structures. Med. Image Anal. **25** (1), 11–21 (2015)

4. Okada, T., Linguraru, M.G., Hori, M., Summers, R.M., Tomiyama, N., Sato, Y.: Abdominal multi-organ segmentation from CT images using conditional shape location and unsupervised intensity priors. Med. Image Anal. **26**(1), 118 (2015)

5. Rohlfing, T., Brandt, R., Menzel, R., Maurer, C.R.: Evaluation of atlas selection strategies for atlas-based image segmentation with application to confocal microscopy images of bee brains. NeuroImage **21**(4), 1428–1442 (2004)

6. Wang, H., Pouch, A., Takebe, M., Jackson, B., Gorman, J., Gorman, R., Yushkevich, P.A.: Multi-atlas segmentation with robust label transfer and label fusion. In: Information processing in medical imaging: proceedings of the Conference on Information Processing in Medical Imaging, vol. 23, p. 548, NIH Public Access (2013)

7. Iglesias, J.E., Sabuncu, M.R.: Multi-atlas segmentation of biomedical images: a survey. Med. Image Anal. **24**(1), 205–219 (2015)

8. Tong, T., Wolz, R., Wang, Z., Gao, Q., Misawa, K., Fujiwara, M., Mori, K., Hajnal, J.V., Rueckert, D.: Discriminative dictionary learning for abdominal multi-organ segmentation. Med. Image Anal. **23**(1), 92104 (2015)

9. Oda, M., Shimizu, N., Karasawa, K., Nimura, Y., Kitasaka, T., Misawa, K., Fujiwara, M., Rueckert, D., Mori, K.: Regression forest-based atlas localization and direction specific atlas generation for pancreas segmentation. In: International Conference on Medical Image Computing and Computer-Assisted Intervention, pp. 556–563. Springer (2016)

10. Kamnitsas, K., Ledig, C., Newcombe, V.F., Simpson, J.P., Kane, A.D., Menon, D.K., Rueckert, D., Glocker, B.: Efficient multi-scale 3D CNN with fully connected CRF for accurate brain lesion segmentation. Med. Image Anal. **36**, 6178 (2017)

11. Zhou, X., Ito, T., Takayama, R., Wang, S., Hara, T., Fujita, H.: Three dimensional CT image segmentation by combining 2D fully convolutional network with 3D majority voting. In: International Workshop on Large-Scale Annotation of Biomedical Data and Expert Label Synthesis, pp. 111–120. Springer (2016)

12. Milletari, F., Navab, N., Ahmadi, S.-A.: V-Net: fully convolutional neural networks for volumetric medical image segmentation. In: 2016 Fourth International Conference on in 3D Vision (3DV), pp. 565–571. IEEE (2016)

13. Roth, H.R., Lu, L., Farag, A., Shin, H.-C., Liu, J., Turkbey, E.B., Summers, R.M.: DeepOrgan: multi-level deep convolutional networks for automated pancreas segmentation. In: International Conference on Medical Image Computing and Computer-Assisted Intervention, pp. 556–564. Springer (2015)

14. Zhou, Y., Xie, L., Shen, W., Fishman, E., Yuille, A.: Pancreas segmentation in abdominal CT scan: A coarse-to-fine approach. arXiv preprint arXiv:1612.08230 (2016)

15. Christ, P.F., Elshaer, M.E.A., Ettlinger, F., Tatavarty, S., Bickel, M., Bilic, P., Rempfler, M., Armbruster, M., Hofmann, F., Danastasi, M., et al.: Automatic liver and lesion segmentation in CT using cascaded fully convolutional neural networks and 3D conditional random fields. In: MICCAI, pp. 415–423. Springer (2016)

16. Alberdi, E., Povyakalo, A.A., Strigini, L., Ayton, P.: Computer aided detection: risks and benefits for radiologists' decisions. In: Handbook of Medical Image Perception and Techniques, pp. 1–26 (2009)

17. Li, C., Wang, X.: A likelihood and local constraint level set model for liver tumor segmentation from CT volumes. IEEE Trans. Biomed. Eng. **60**, 2967–2977 (2013)
18. Milletari, F., Navab, N., Ahmadi, S.A.: V-Net: fully convolutional neural networks for volumetric medical image segmentation. In: 2016 Fourth International Conference on 3D Vision (3DV), pp. 565–571. IEEE (2016)
19. Crum, W., Camara, O., Hill, D.: Generalized overlap measures for evaluation and validation in medical image analysis. IEEE TMI **25**(11), 1451–1461 (2006)
20. Salehi, S.S.M., Erdogmus, D., Gholipour, A.: Tversky loss function for image segmentation using 3D fully convolutional deep networks

Classification of Breast Cancer Malignancy Using Machine Learning Mechanisms in TensorFlow and Keras

Yuan-Hsiang Chang[(✉)] and Chi-Yu Chung

Department of Information and Computer Engineering,
Chung Yuan Christian University, 200 Chung Pei Road,
Chung Li, Taiwan, R.O.C.
changyh@ice.cycu.edu.tw

Abstract. Classification of breast cancer malignancy using digital mammograms remains a difficult task in breast cancer diagnosis and plays a key role in early detection of breast cancer. Inspired by rapid progress in the field of artificial intelligence, we explored several machine learning mechanisms, i.e., *Support Vector Machine* (SVM), *Logistic Regression*, *Decision Tree*, *Random Forest*, and *Deep Neural Network* (DNN) given in TensorFlow and Keras deep learning frameworks, and used Python programming to predict if a patient case is malignant or benign. This retrospective study was based on the *Breast Cancer Wisconsin (Diagnostic) Data Set* that contains a set of 30 features, e.g., radius mean, texture mean, perimeter mean, etc., previously extracted from digital mammograms. In addition, breast cancer diagnosis results were provided as the gold standard for training and testing of the machine learning mechanisms. Based on verification results on the test set, the five machine learning mechanisms achieved the *sensitivity* of 94.4%, 94.4%, 91.9%, 90.8%, 98.5%, and the *specificity* of 92.7%, 90.5%, 92.3%, 94.6%, 91.1%, respectively. In conclusion, our machine learning mechanisms achieved competitive performance results with the state-of-art techniques presented by other researchers and may provide useful *second opinion* to radiologists in breast cancer diagnosis.

Keywords: Breast cancer diagnosis · Deep learning · Machine learning · TensorFlow

1 Introduction

Recently, the American Cancer Society published the Global Cancer Statistics report [1], which evaluated 36 cancers in 185 countries. Morbidity and mortality are estimated to have approximately 18.1 million new cancer cases and 9.6 million cancer deaths worldwide in 2018. Among the most commonly diagnosed cancer, breast cancer is one of the leading cause of cancer in women, accounting for 11.6%. Fortunately, with the progress of medical treatment, if breast cancer can be detected early and treated in time, the cure rate is very high.

Lately, the field of *Machine Learning* (ML) and *Artificial Intelligence* (AI) has been greatly improved and advanced. In addition, computer hardware has been developed with high parallelism and speed. This has also led to the invention of deep learning

© Springer Nature Switzerland AG 2020
K.-P. Lin et al. (Eds.): ICBHI 2019, IFMBE Proceedings 74, pp. 42–49, 2020.
https://doi.org/10.1007/978-3-030-30636-6_6

techniques, which has set off the revolution of AI techniques. Inspired by the rapid progress in the field of AI, this article explores the conventional machine learning techniques such as *Support Vector Machine*, *Logistic Regression*, *Decision Tree*, and *Random Forest*, as well as the emerging techniques such as *Deep Neural Network* (DNN) in TensorFlow and Keras for the classification of breast cancer malignancy.

Cotes and Vapnik [2] proposed the *Support Vector Machine* (SVM) algorithm, and improved the method in 1995, which made the SVM popular for pattern classification. Boser et al. [3] presented a training algorithm that maximizes the margin between training patterns and the technique is applicable to a wide variety of the classification functions such as the radial basis functions, etc. In addition, *Logistic Regression* is a machine learning method based on linear regression, but is applied with the logistic sigmoid function for pattern classification.

The *Decision Tree* algorithm was originally proposed by Breiman [4] for pattern classification. Unlike many other statistical procedures, the algorithm can be used to regress continuous data. Further, Breiman [5] generalized the concept and presented the *Random Forests* algorithm, which is a combination of decision tree predictors for multi-dimensional patterns.

The concept of *Artificial Neural Networks* (ANNs) was based on the mathematical model originally proposed by McCulloch and Pitts [6]. However, the method encountered some technical difficulties and was quiet for many years. In recent decade, based on the ImageNet Image Recognition Competition, the *Convolutional Neural Network* (CNN) architecture built by Hinton's student Alex, namely AlexNet, was trained with multiple GPUs for object classification [7]. The performance results won the championship with a big lead than the second place using conventional techniques. Inspired by this research work, deep learning techniques has attracted great interest of many researchers lately. Many innovative and advanced AI techniques for various applications, e.g., speech recognition, computer vision, etc., are under ongoing development with great success.

2 Materials and Methods

In this study, the *Breast Cancer Wisconsin (Diagnostic) Data Set* released by the University of Wisconsin [8] was used. The data set includes 569 patient cases with suspicious breast tissue regions. The patient case information includes ID numbers and breast cancer diagnosis results, i.e., M = malignant, and B = benign. Among which, each case was previous analyzed and a set of 30 features, e.g., radius mean, texture mean, perimeter mean, etc., were previously extracted using digital mammograms.

The machine learning architectures for the classification of breast cancer malignancy is shown in Fig. 1. We compared and analyzed the results of the four conventional machine learning methods, i.e., *SVM, Logistic Regression, Decision Tree*, and *Random Forests*, as well as the emerging techniques, i.e., *Deep Neural Network* (DNN) given in TensorFlow and Keras. The technical approaches are described herein.

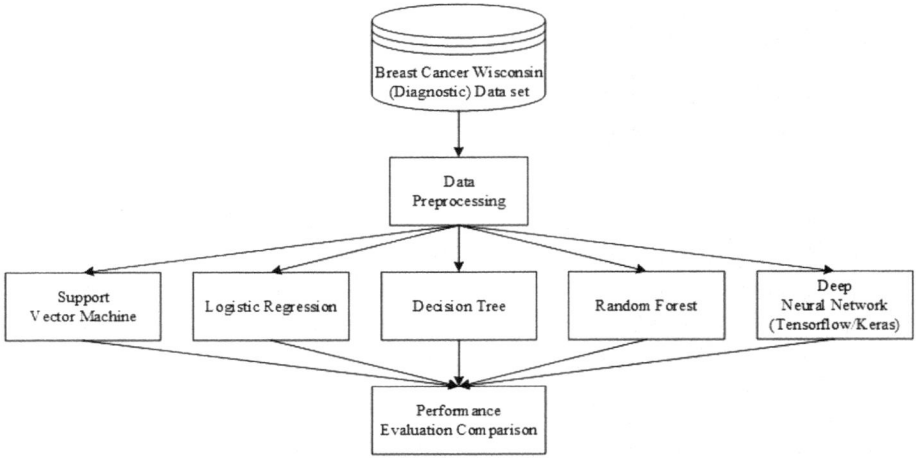

Fig. 1. Machine learning mechanisms for the classification of breast cancer malignancy.

2.1 Preprocessing

To facilitate the training and testing of the machine learning techniques, the data were first organized using preprocessing, after which the data are divided into two independent sets, namely the training set and the test set. In practice, we divided the data according to the type of breast cancer diagnosis, within which the number of benign and malign cases are balanced.

The flow chart of the preprocessing is given in Fig. 2. After preprocessing, 80% of benign and 80% of malignant cases are used as the training set, and the remaining 20% are used as the test set. Prior to the training or testing, the feature data are shuffled such that patient cases are given in random order to the machine learning techniques. Then, all the labeled data, M = malignant, and B = benign, are used for supervised learning in all machine learning techniques.

In addition, because the original feature data cover a wide range of distribution, the preprocessing is to perform data normalization on all the feature data such that accuracy of machine learning techniques can be improved. This step can also speed up the convergence of the machine learning techniques. In practice, the *min-max normalization* is used.

2.2 Support Vector Machine

The objective of the *Support Vector Machine* (SVM) is to maximize the margin by looking for an optimal separating hyperplane that is then used to classify the data [2].

Because the data set features of this study are multidimensional, the use of kernel functions is needed. This study uses the *Gaussian Radial Basis Function* (RBF) kernel [9] function, which is defined as follows:

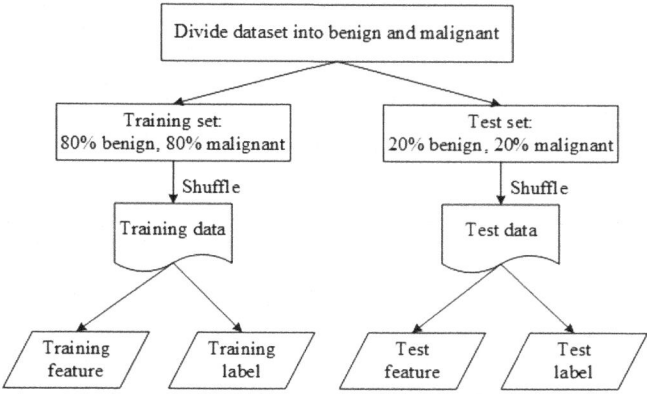

Fig. 2. Flow chart of preprocessing.

$$K(x, x') = exp\left(-\frac{\|x - x'\|^2}{2\sigma^2}\right) \qquad (1)$$

After applying the Taylor expansion, it is possible to map the feature vectors to higher-dimensional space, and then find an optimal separating hyperplane in the high-dimensional space such that feature data can be classified.

2.3   Logistic Regression

Logistic Regression (LR) can be regarded as a single-layer neural network. The idea is based on linear regression which map the input feature data to the output in the range of 0 to 1 using the sigmoid function as follows:

$$g(z) = \frac{1}{1 + e^{-z}} \qquad (2)$$

The output represents the probability that the input feature data belongs to the category 1 is defined as follows:

$$z = \theta_0 + \theta_1 x_1 + \theta_2 x_2 + \cdots + \theta_n x_n = \theta^T x \qquad (3)$$

$$g(z) = g(\theta^T x) = \frac{1}{1 + e^{-\theta^T x}} \qquad (4)$$

In this study, the loss function of the Logistic Regression, namely the *Cross Entropy* [10], is used.

2.4   Decision Tree

The objective of the *Decision Tree* (DT) algorithm is to produce a *Classification and Regression Tree* (CART) that divides the input data into two sub-data classes using the Gini impurity [5] defined as follows:

$$I_G(t) = 1 - \sum_{i=1}^{n} p(i|t)^2 \tag{5}$$

where n is the number of classes, and $p(i|t)$ is the conditional probability of the feature data given the class t.

The algorithm is implemented recursively until convergence, i.e., all the feature data are classified in the same class and no longer change. The resulting Gini impurity is a number between 0 and 1.

2.5   Random Forests

The *Random Forest* (RF) algorithm is based on the multiple decision trees algorithm [11]. The concept is to use the Bootstrapping method to randomly select n training samples from the training data, and extract a total of m times to train m decision trees. For each single decision tree model, each split is based on the Gini impurity, and at the end, each decision tree is used for voting to obtain the classification result.

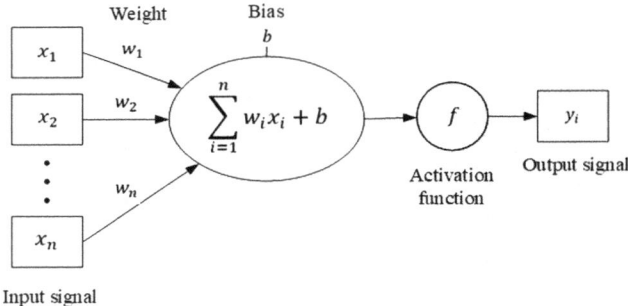

Fig. 3. Simple artificial neuron model simulating biological neurons.

2.6   Deep Neural Network

A neural network is a method of realizing artificial intelligence. It simulates the operation of biological brain cells to achieve the effect of pattern classification. A simple artificial neuron model is given in Fig. 3.

The formula for the neuron model is defined as follows:

$$y = f\left(\sum_{i=1}^{n} w_i x_i + b\right) \tag{6}$$

where w_i is the weights and b is the bias. The function f is called the activation function. We chose to use the following function, known as the *Rectified Linear Unit* (ReLu) function:

$$f(x) = max(x, 0) \tag{7}$$

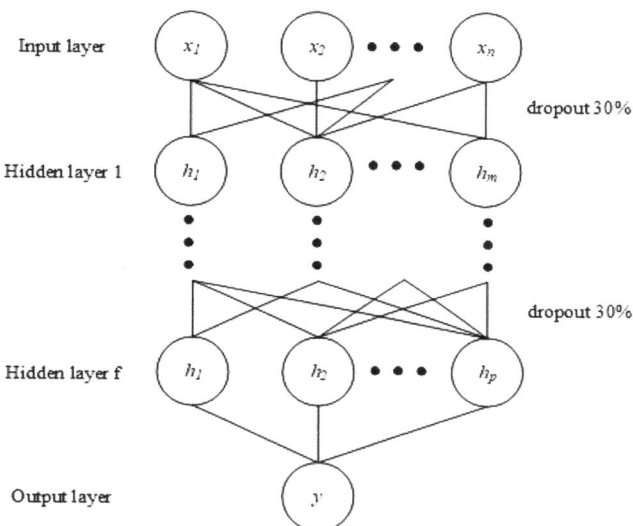

Fig. 4. Architecture of the deep neural network.

Table 1. Confusion matrix of prediction results

Predicted	Actual	
	Positive	Negative
Positive	True Positive (*TP*)	False Positive (*FP*)
Negative	False Negative (*FN*)	True Negative (*TN*)

The *Deep Neural Network* (DNN) is an interconnecting network of neurons as shown in Fig. 4. The DNN contains one input layer, hidden layers, and output layer.

Performance evaluation of machine learning mechanisms are based on a standard evaluation tool known as the ROC analysis [12]. Prediction results are presented using the confusion matrix, as shown in Table 1.

In particular, we evaluated the *sensitivity* and *specificity* as follows:

$$Sensitivity = \frac{TP}{TP+FN}, Specificity = \frac{TN}{FP+TN} \tag{8}$$

3   Results

The computer hardware is Intel (R) Core (TM) i5-6600 CPU 3.30 GHz, and 16 GB memory on Microsoft Windows 10. The GTX 1080Ti 11G graphic card is used for training and testing. The system software development tools are Microsoft Visual Studio and Python programming, with TensorFlow 1.11, Keras 2.2 and Sklearn 0.19.

Table 2 shows the performance evaluation of the machine learning mechanism for the Breast Cancer Wisconsin data set. The ROC curves are given in Fig. 5 accordingly.

Table 2. Performance evaluation of machine learning mechanisms

Different models	Sensitivity	Specificity
SVM	94.44%	92.68%
Logistic Regression	94.37%	90.48%
Decision Tree	91.89%	92.31%
Random Forest	90.79%	94.59%
Deep Neural Network	**98.53%**	**91.11%**

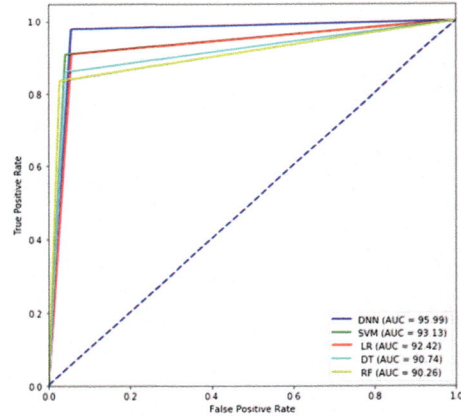

Fig. 5. ROC curves for the machine learning mechanisms

4   Conclusion

In this article, we investigated five machine learning mechanisms for the classification of breast cancer malignancy. While the data set is limited in size, this study yields competitive results with other state-of-art techniques and may provide useful *second opinion* to radiologists for breast cancer diagnosis.

Conflict of Interest. The authors declare that they have no conflict of interest.

References

1. Bray, F., Ferlay, J., Soerjomataram, I., et al.: Global cancer statistics 2018: GLOBOCAN estimates of incidence and mortality worldwide for 36 cancers in 185 countries. CA Cancer J. Clin. **68**(6), 394–424 (2018)
2. Cortes, C., Vapnik, V.: Support-vector networks. Mach. Learn. **20**(3), 273–297 (1995)
3. Boser, B.E., Guyon, I.M., Vapnik, V.N.: A training algorithm for optimal margin classifiers. In: COLT 1992 Proceedings of the Fifth Annual Workshop on Computational Learning Theory, Pittsburgh, Pennsylvania, United States, pp. 144–152 (1992)
4. Breiman, L.: Classification and Regression Trees. Routledge, New York (2017)
5. Breiman, L.: Random forests. Mach. Learn. **45**(1), 5–32 (2001)
6. McCulloch, W.S., Pitts, W.: A logical calculus of the ideas immanent in nervous activity. Bull. Math. Biophys. **5**(4), 115–133 (1943)
7. Krizhevsky, A., Sutskever, I., Hinton, G.E.: ImageNet classification with deep convolutional neural networks, neural information processing systems. In: NIPS 2012 Proceeding of the 25th International Conference, Lake Tahoe, Nevada, United States, vol. 1, pp. 1097–1105 (2012)
8. Breast Cancer Wisconsin (Diagnostic) Data Set. https://archive.ics.uci.edu/ml/datasets/Breast+Cancer+Wisconsin+(Diagnostic)
9. Vert, J.P., Tsuda, K., Schölkopf, B.: Kernel Methods in Computational Biology. MIT Press, Cambridge (2004)
10. de Boer, P.T., Kroese, D.P., Mannor, S., et al.: A tutorial on the cross-entropy method. Ann. Oper. Res. **134**(1), 19–67 (2005)
11. Breiman, L.: Bagging Predictors. Mach. Learn. **24**(2), 123–140 (1996)
12. Fawcett, T.: An introduction to ROC analysis. Pattern Recogn. Lett. **27**(8), 861–874 (2006)

A New Numerical Simulation Process for Footwear Slip Resistance Analysis

Shu-Yu Jhou[1], Wei-Chun Hsu[2], and Ching-Chi Hsu[1(✉)]

[1] Graduate Institute of Applied Science and Technology,
National Taiwan University of Science and Technology,
No. 43, Keelung Rd., Sec. 4, Taipei 10607, Taiwan
hsucc@mail.ntust.edu.tw
[2] Graduate Institute of Biomedical Engineering, National Taiwan University
of Science and Technology, Taipei 10607, Taiwan

Abstract. A high number of slip-and-fall incidents result in common injuries of daily life. The design of outsole tread pattern is one of the key factors which had a direct impact on slip resistance performance. The application of numerical simulation is an opportunity for footwear industry to evaluate the multiple outsole tread pattern design and ground condition in a more controlled and efficient manner than mechanical testing in the developing process.

A complex three-dimensional (3D) FE model of the shoe was developed to evaluate the effect of outsole tread pattern design on slip resistance performance during the gait motion. The dynamic plantar pressure distributions were automatically applied as the loading condition in FE model which allowed to interpret the individualized subject condition.

The herringbone tread design and higher real contact area between shoe and ground could achieve better slip resistance performance. The process of this study demonstrates the potential of numerical simulation for evaluating slip resistance performance.

Keywords: Outsole tread pattern · Slip resistance · Finite element analysis · Gait · Plantar pressure

1 Introduction

The most common injuries in daily life result from slip-and-fall accident. In the United States 2016, over 9 million emergency room visits are due to slips and falls according to National Safety Council (NSC). In Taiwan, at 32%, slip and fall injuries are the most frequently reported accidents at work. Footwear factor, the material and tread pattern design of the outsole included, is one of the factors which had direct impact on the slip resistance performance [1]. Setting up the mechanical stander testing or human motion experiment for evaluation of slip resistance performance is time and cost consuming. Developing a numerical simulation is an opportunity to offer the more controlled and efficient manner for footwear industry.

The previous studies have developed the finite element model to predict the coefficient of friction [2, 3]. However, the models have been simplified as a heel pad

© Springer Nature Switzerland AG 2020
K.-P. Lin et al. (Eds.): ICBHI 2019, IFMBE Proceedings 74, pp. 50–56, 2020.
https://doi.org/10.1007/978-3-030-30636-6_7

and a specimen. A case study investigated how the traction-force of entire out sole with five different tread patterns of the boot effected to resist slip in the gaiting direction [4]. However, the loading condition was simplified by using the same uniform pressure. The oversimplified or unaesthetic model and lack of individualized subject condition are common in previous numerical studies. After a high level of technical skills is achieved in certain fields from 3D modeling to computational simulation and motion analysis, we aim to coalesce esthetics and coherence in this footwear traction analysis. We tend to coalesce esthetics and coherence in this study. More specifically, the goal of the current study is to develop the numerical method for evaluating the slip resistance performance during the gait. To do this, we developed a three-dimensional (3D) FE model of the shoe to be applied for various of outsole tread design and density. Numerical analysis considered loading-response, mid stance and push off phase of the gait. The plantar pressure distributions were applied and allowed to interpret the individualized subject condition.

2   Materials and Methods

2.1   Development of Geometry

In this research, instead of the traditional computer aided design programs, we used a state-of-the-art software, Geomagic Freeform (3D Systems, Rock Hill, SC, USA), which is a fast and cost-effective way to create a complex three-dimensional (3D) shoe model (Fig. 1). The shoe model could be imported into ANSYS Workbench 18.2 (ANSYS, Inc., Canonsburg, PA, USA) for tread pattern design and slip resistance analysis. The structure of this 3D shoe-ground model consisted of upper, insole, midsole, outsole and ground (Fig. 1). Figure 2A represents two commonly used outsole tread designs were developed in present study: straight stripe (Design A) and herringbone (Design B). Three tread densities were given to each tread design (Fig. 2B).

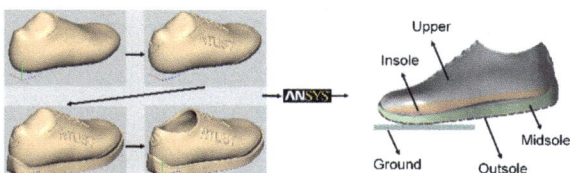

Fig. 1. Development of the shoe model in Geomagic Freeform and the structural composition of 3D shoe-ground model.

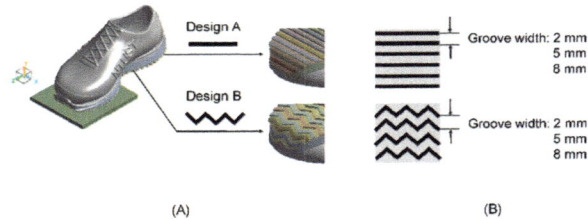

Fig. 2. The outsole tread pattern designs: (A) Two tread designs; (B) Three tread densities to each tread.

2.2 Slip Resistance Analysis

In current study, Ogden Foam 2nd Order material model was used for the footwear and the concrete ground was idealized as homogeneous, isotropic and linearly elastic. The values of the footwear elastomeric foam parameters and material properties of the ground were selected based on previous study [5]. Three phases of human gait cycle were considered: push off, mid-stance, and loading response. The ground was fully constrained throughout simulation while the horizontal displacement was applied to the shoe (Fig. 3A). The dynamic plantar pressures during the gait were recorded by F-SCAN system (Tekscan, Inc., USA). We uased ACT (Application Customization Toolkit), which is time-effective manner to create the automatic pressure application on the FE model as loading condition (Fig. 3B). The The simulation process was divided into two steps: pressure application and shoe movement.

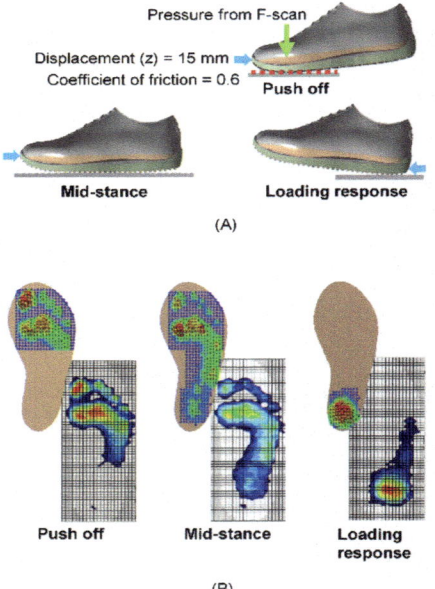

Fig. 3. (A) Boundary and loading condition of three major phases; (B) Plantar pressure application

2.3   Mechanical Testing

In order to validate the results of numerical simulation, the former slip-resistance standard testing ASTM F 1677 for the Brungraber Mark II was performed [6]. The outsole specimen with straight stripe tread design and herringbone tread design were developed to measure the coefficient of friction between the outsole specimen and walkway surface in dry conditions. The configuration of the mechanical testing and the outsole specimen are reported in Fig. 4.

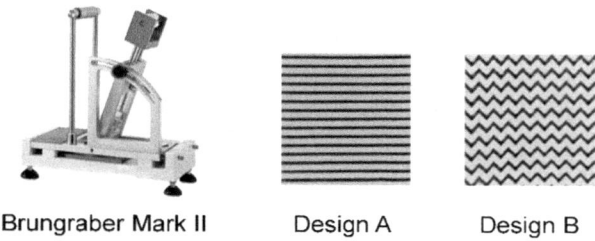

Brungraber Mark II   Design A   Design B

Fig. 4. Mechanical testing and the outsole specimen.

3   Result and Discussion

3.1   Finite Element Model Validation

Eighteen finite element models including two tread designs with three tread densities in three positions were developed in present study. Each finite element model contained approximately from 899,000 to 972,000 nodes and from 436,000 to 465,000 elements. The nonlinearities from material properties, large deformations and friction conditions were considered. The reaction force of the moving surface of the shoe converged properly. According to the results of the mechanical testing from Footwear & Recreation Technology Research Institute, herringbone tread pattern (Design B) had the higher value of coefficient of friction compared with that of straight stripe tread pattern (Design A). The FE results of reaction force were found to be reasonably complied with the mechanical testing observations.

3.2   Effects of Tread Density

The effects of tread density on reaction force were compared based on the same outsole tread design. As shown in Fig. 4, the maximum reaction force in the moving direction decreased when tread density decreased among both Design A and Design B. The dense density of outsole tread pattern (groove 2) showed the highest reaction force in the moving direction for both two designs. Therefore, the outsole tread pattern with dense density led to a better slip resistance performance. The results of maximum reaction force during three phases of human gait cycle revealed the same trend.

3.3   Effects of Tread Design

The effects of tread pattern design on reaction force were compared based on the same width of the tread and the groove. As shown in Fig. 5, the maximum reaction force in the moving direction showed that the herringbone tread pattern (Design B) had the higher value of reaction force compared with straight stripe tread pattern (Design A). The results of maximum reaction force during three phases of human gait cycle revealed the same trend.

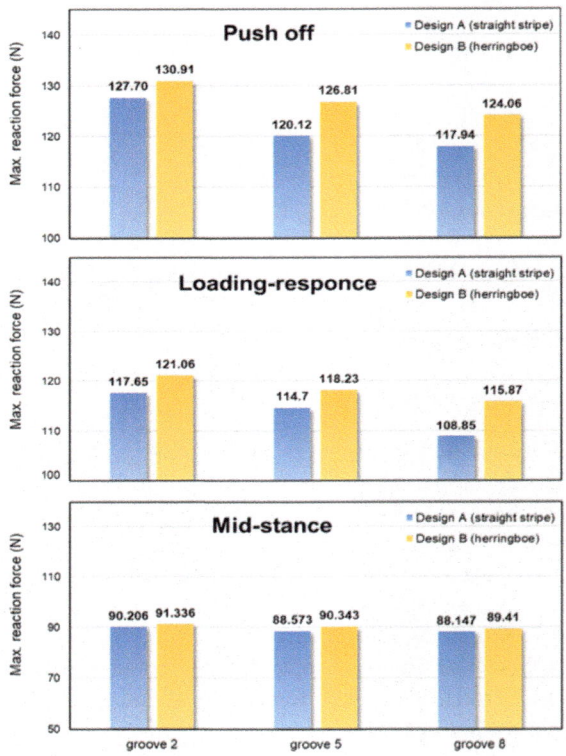

Fig. 5.   The results of maximum reaction force during push off, loading-response and mid-stance

3.4   Real Contact Area

For the plastic material, the real contact area (green line) is the main contributor to the friction force (Fig. 6). The greater real contact area between the shoe and ground has greater reaction force.

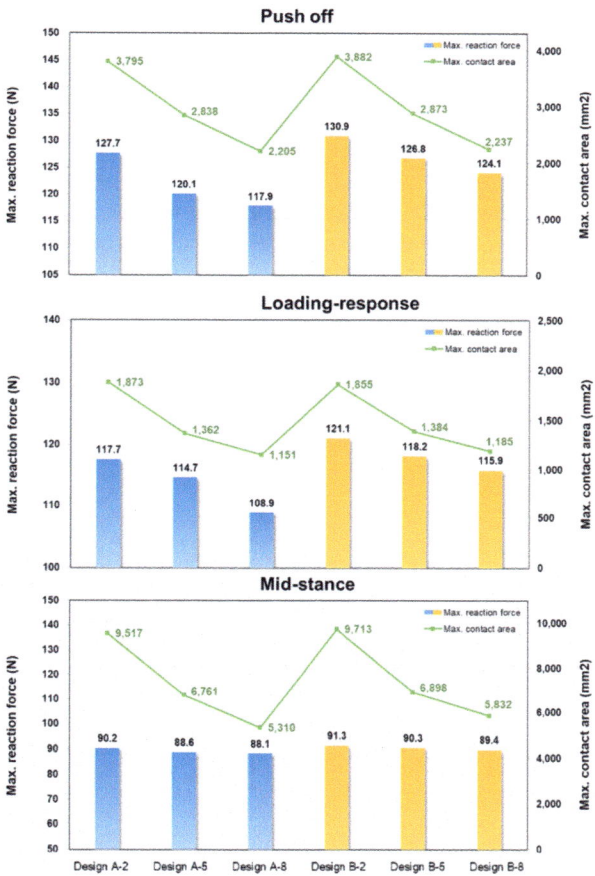

Fig. 6. The results of maximum reaction force and contact area during push off, loading-response and mid-stance

4 Conclusions

The herringbone tread design and higher real contact area between shoe and ground could achieve better slip resistance performance. This study demonstrates the potential of computational technology for evaluating slip resistance performance. The simulation process could be applied further on the product development in the early design phase in footwear industry.

Acknowledgment. This study was supported by Footwear & Recreation Technology Research Institute, Taiwan.

Conflict of Interest. The authors declare that they have no conflict of interest.

References

1. Courtney, T.K., et al.: Occupational slip, trip, and fall-related injuries–can the contribution of slip-periness be isolated? Ergonomics **44**(13), 1118–1137 (2001)
2. Moghaddam, S.R.M., et al.: Predictive multiscale computational model of shoe-floor coefficient of friction. J. Biomech. **66**, 145–152 (2018)
3. Li, K.W., Chen, C.J.: The effect of shoe soling tread groove width on the coefficient of friction with different sole materials, floors, and contaminants. Appl. Ergon. **35**(6), 499–507 (2004)
4. Sun, Z., Howard, D., Moatamedi, M.: Finite element analysis of footwear and ground interaction. Strain **41**, 113–117 (2005)
5. Cheung, J.T., Zhang, M.: Finite element modeling of the human foot and footwear. In: ABAQUS Users' Conference 2006 (2006)
6. ASTM F1677-05.: Standard test method for using a portable inclineable articulated strut slip tester (PIAST) (Withdrawn 2006). ASTM International (2005)

A Numerical Study of Different Hallux Valgus Treatments Using Three-Dimensional Human Musculoskeletal Lower Extremity Models

Kuan-Ting Huang[1], Kao-Shang Shih[2], and Ching-Chi Hsu[3(✉)]

[1] Department of Mechanical Engineering,
National Taiwan University of Science and Technology,
Taipei 10607, Taiwan, R.O.C.
[2] Department of Orthopedic Surgery, Shin Kong Wu Ho-Su Memorial Hospital,
Taipei 111, Taiwan, R.O.C.
[3] Graduate Institute of Applied Science and Technology,
National Taiwan University of Science and Technology,
No. 43, Keelung Rd., Sec. 4, Taipei 10607, Taiwan, R.O.C.
hsucc@mail.ntust.edu.tw

Abstract. Hallux valgus (HV) was one of the most frequent human foot deformities. The aim of this study was to evaluate mechanical responses and stabilities of the plate implants and Kirschner wire (KW) after the distal metatarsal osteotomy in HV treatment by using finite element (FE) analysis. A three-dimensional FE model of lower extremity was developed to evaluate the four plate fixation methods and three KW fixation methods in weight bearing. The results showed that all the plate fixations revealed better first metatarsal stability than KW. For the result of the contact pressure, the 6-holes-6-screws dynamic compression plate implant had highest result than others plate implant. Adding the bandage to the KW fixation had a highest result in all implant.

Keywords: Hallux valgus · Finite elements analysis · Kirschner wire · Plate fixation

1 Introduction

Hallux valgus is the commonest forefoot deformity [1]. Different treatment methods have been applied to fix this problem including osteotomy fixation plates, Kirschner wires, and bunion splints [2, 3]. Past studies have investigated the biomechanics of hallux valgus with different treatments using numerical and/or experimental approaches [1, 4]. However, there are rare studies that evaluated each treatment method using a realistic musculoskeletal lower extremity model. Thus, the purposes of this study were to develop a more complete three-dimensional human musculoskeletal lower extremity model and to evaluate the strengths and limitations of different hallux valgus treatment techniques.

© Springer Nature Switzerland AG 2020
K.-P. Lin et al. (Eds.): ICBHI 2019, IFMBE Proceedings 74, pp. 57–62, 2020.
https://doi.org/10.1007/978-3-030-30636-6_8

2   Method

Proximal metatarsal osteotomy is the most effective technique for correcting hallux valgus deformities. However, these surgeries are technically demanding and prone to complications, such as nonunion, implant failure, and unexpected extension of the osteotomy to the tarsometatarsal joint [5]. Mild deformities are best treated by distal first metatarsal osteotomies [6].

The distal osteotomy fixation plate designs included 4-hole plate with 4 screws (Fig. 1B), 6-hole plate with 4 screws (Fig. 1C), 6-hole plate with 6 screws and dynamic compression holes (Fig. 1D), and 6-hole plate with 6 screws and locking compression holes (Fig. 1E). All the fixation devices were assembled into the musculoskeletal lower extremity model (Fig. 1A). The dynamic compression screw telescopes and provides fixation while allowing impaction to occur at the fracture during healing and weight bearing.

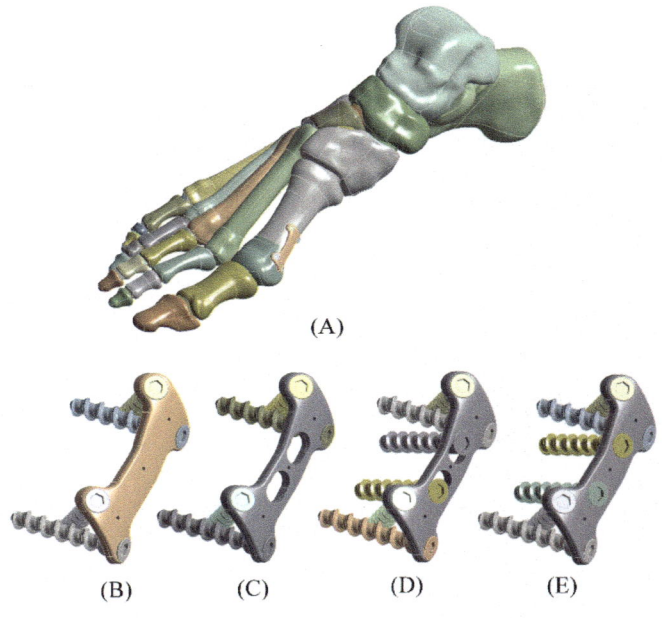

(A)

(B)   (C)   (D)   (E)

Fig. 1. Plate implants: (A) Plate implant treatment; (B) 4H4S; (C) 6H4S; (D) 6H6S-D; (E) 6H6S-L.

Three types of osteotomy fixation with Kirschner wire, a Kirschner wire only (Fig. 2B), a Kirschner wire with a bandage (Fig. 2C) and a Kirschner wire with a fiberglass (Fig. 2D) were developed using SolidWorks. Kirschner wire were assembled into the musculoskeletal lower extremity model in above models (Fig. 2A).

Sixteen types of the foot ligaments were considered and simulated using tension-only spring elements [7]. The finite element models of the lower extremity with

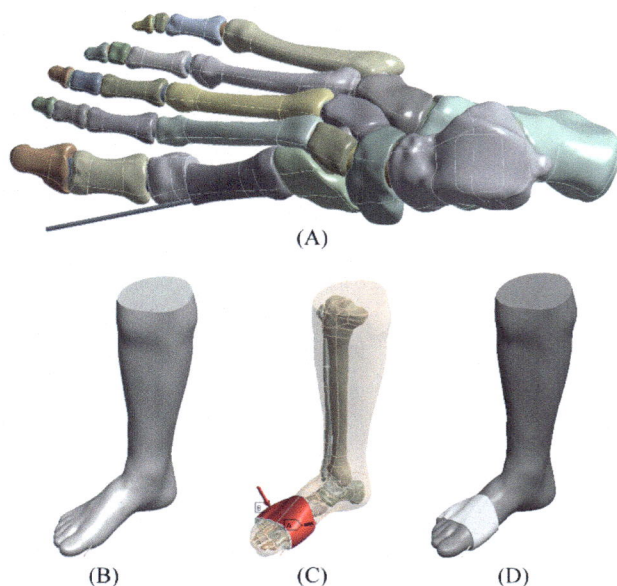

(A)

(B)   (C)   (D)

Fig. 2. Kirschner wire fixations: (A) KW treatment; (B) KW only model; (C) KW with the bandage model; (D) KW with the fiberglass model.

different hallux valgus treatments were developed using ANSYS Workbench 19.2. The proximal tibia was fully constrained, the osteotomy plane was frictionless, all implants were contact, and an Achilles tendon was simulated by applying a tendon force [4]. A ground reaction force was applied to a moveable ground [4]. Boundary conditions of bandage were referenced Mao et al. [1].

In the post-processing, the stress and fixation stability between the first metatarsal and implant, and the contact pressure between osteotomy plane were calculated and discussed.

3   Result and Discussion

All the plate fixations revealed better first metatarsal fixation stability (lower bone deformation) than the KW. It was surprising that both KW-B and KW-F significantly improved the fixation stability compared to the KW (Fig. 3). For the results of the bone stress, the 6H6S-D and 6H6S-L had lower first metatarsal stress compared to the other treatments, due to KW-B and KW-F have more restrict that increase the bone stress (Fig. 4). For the results of the implant stress, 4H4S has lowest stress, all of the stress of plate implants were lower than Kirschner wire treatment, using outer fixations improve reducing implants stress (Fig. 5). The 6H6S-D showed highest contact pressure compared to the other plate fixations, contact pressure of Kirschner wire treatment were obviously greater than plate treatment (Fig. 6).

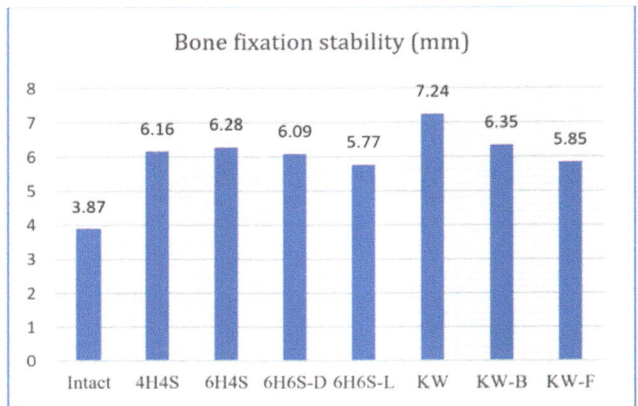

Fig. 3. First metatarsal fixation stability.

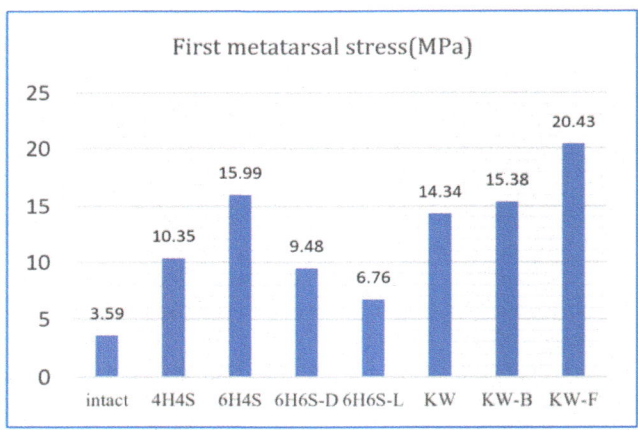

Fig. 4. First metatarsal maximum principle stress.

Adding the bandage to the KW treatment could reduce the implant stress and increase first metatarsal fixation stability, and had highest contact pressure in all treatment.

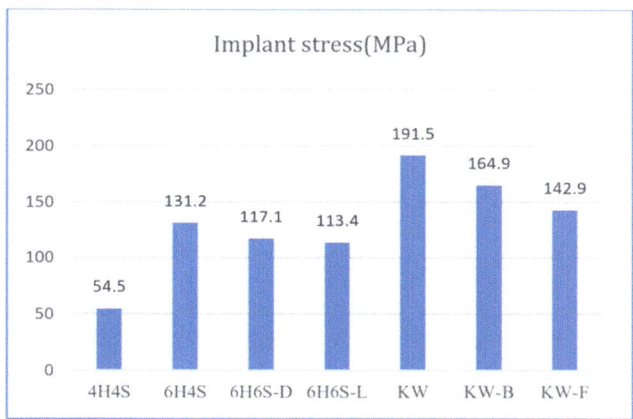

Fig. 5. Implant maximum principle stress.

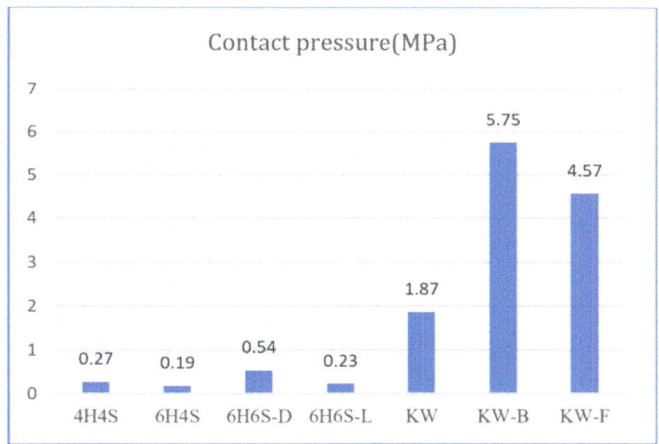

Fig. 6. Contact pressure on the fracture surface.

4   Conclusion

The strengths and limitations of different hallux valgus treatments could be evaluated using a realistic human musculoskeletal lower extremity model. The conclusions of this study are summarized as follows:

1. The 6H6S-D had better fixation stability, lower implant stress, and highest contact pressure compared to the other plate treatments.
2. Adding the bandage to the KW treatment could improve the fixation stability and reduce the implant stress, and had highest contact pressure in all treatment.

This study could provide surgeons some useful information and theoretical basis in the biomechanics for the treatment of hallux valgus.

Conflict of Interest. The authors declare that they have no conflict of interest.

References

1. Mao, R., Guo, J., et al.: Med. Eng. Phys. **46**, 21–26 (2017)
2. Giannini, S., Ceccarelli, F., et al.: Tech. Foot Ankle Surg. **2**(1), 11–20 (2003)
3. Saragas, N.P., et al.: Foot Ankle Int. **30**(10), 976–980 (2009)
4. Wong, D.W.C., Wang, Y., et al.: J. Biomech. **48**(12), 3142–3148 (2015)
5. Erdil, M., Ceylan, H.H., et al.: J. Foot Ankle Surg. **55**(1), 35–38 (2016)
6. Wülker, N., Mittag, F., et al.: Deutsches Ärzteblatt Int. **109**(49), 857 (2012)
7. Ligaments of the Foot and Ankle Overview. https://www.footeducation.com/page/ligaments-of-foot-and-ankle-overview

Point-of-Care Testing System of Uric Acid for the Prevention from Urolithiasis Recurrence

Lin-Chen Yen[1(✉)], Cheanyeh Cheng[2], Wen-Yaw Chung[1], and Vincent Tsai[3]

[1] Department of Electronic Engineering, Chung-Yuan Christian University, Taoyuan, Taiwan, R.O.C.
linda50929@gmail.com
[2] Department of Chemistry, Chung-Yuan Christian University, Taoyuan, Taiwan, R.O.C.
[3] Ten-Chan General Hospital, Taoyuan, Taiwan, R.O.C.

Abstract. In this study, a simple, novel and inexpensive third generation electrochemical uric acid (UA) biosensor based on three-electrode point-of-care test strip was proposed. On the low-cost screen-printed three silver-based electrodes test strip, the Ag/AgCl reference electrode was first formed by simple electrodeposition with one silver electrode, then the working electrode was prepared by the successive coating of redox mediator, polymer hydrogel, and uricase onto the surface of another silver electrode, the third bare silver electrode was served as the counter electrode to complete the uric acid test strip, which has the advantages of lower oxidation potential, faster response time, higher sensitivity, and wider detecting range.

The three-electrode uric acid test strip specifically and directly senses uric acid in the test sample, and the signal is promptly transferred to the amperometric readout circuit that a stable bias voltage is applied by a bandgap circuit. After initial processing, the analog signal is converted to a digital signal which is calculated with the algorithm of microcontroller to produce a value of user-readable mode. Finally, the digital result is displayed on the liquid-crystal-display (LCD) panel. The complete set of uric acid point-of-care testing system will be used to assess the uric acid condition in the urine of a urolithiasis patient and will be helpful in the diagnosis of urolithiasis.

This uric acid biosensor can be used for testing uric acid either in urine or blood specimen. As combined with other biosensors such as calcium ions, pH, and conductivity, etc., it can be extended to develop a multi-parameter detection system and apply for the prevention of urolithiasis recurrence.

Keywords: Uric acid · Point-of-care testing · Urolithiasis · Screen-printing test strip · Ag/AgCl reference electrode · Redox mediator · Uricase · Polymer hydrogel · Three-electrode biosensor · Amperometric readout circuit · Urine

K.-P. Lin et al. (Eds.): ICBHI 2019, IFMBE Proceedings 74, pp. 63–71, 2020.
https://doi.org/10.1007/978-3-030-30636-6_9

1 Introduction

The uric acid level in serum and in urine are in the respectively ranges of 24–76 ppm and 36–740 ppm for healthy person. If uric acid concentration exceeds the normal level, it will lead to hyperuricosuria and hyperuricemia. Over the last few decades, the prevalence and the recurrence of urolithiasis has been increasing. Uric acid calculi account for a significant percentage of urinary stones. Thus, the concept of in-home care for monitoring at any time become more important. There will be a new trend in the development of cheaper, faster, and smarter point-of-care testing (POCT) devices for resolving the established clinical practice and the rapid detection of analytes near to the patient.

At present, several commercial products sensed by the invasive detection of blood, such as uric acid monitoring system. It's painful for patients to collect sample in every detection, so that the development of non-invasive uric acid monitoring device becomes more important. There are three kinds of non-invasive methods for monitoring uric acid level shown as Table 1.

Table 1. Non-invasive methods for monitoring uric acid level

Item	Test paper	SERS	Electrochemical biosensor
Detection mechanism	Compare the dipstick color to the corresponding color on the chart	The structural detection of substance analyzed by vibrational spectroscopy technique	Convert the biological information to electronic signal
Advantage	1. Convenient detection method 2. Wide sensing range	1. Microanalysis 2. High specificity, high sensitivity and short response time in detection	1. High specificity, high sensitivity and Short response time in detection 2. Simple operation 3. Low-cost method for producing
Disadvantage	1. Easier to make artificial error in determination 2. Unable to get accurate values	1. Need to dilute sample 2. Technology integration is difficult	1. High redox potential 2. Poor stability and activity of biomolecules
Technical improvement	Use computer vision algorithms to solve artificial error in determination	Use paper as substrate to make technology integration easier	1. Use immobilization techniques to make biomolecules stable and active 2. Use redox mediator to get lower redox potential
Example	Healthy.io: At-Home Urinalysis Testing [3]	Progresses of Preparation and Applications of Paper-Based Surface-Enhanced Raman Scattering Substrate [4]	Our research

We considered that quantized data of measurement is necessary for accurate determination, and it will be more convenience for user if the sample pre-processing isn't needed. Those are the reasons why electrochemical biosensor is chosen. In this study, biosensor was connected to the system [1], which consist of, front-end readout circuit, analog-to-digital converter (ADC), back-end digital controller with algorithm calibration, peripheral data recording unit, and liquid-crystal-display panel, for completing a POCT system of uric acid shown as Fig. 1.

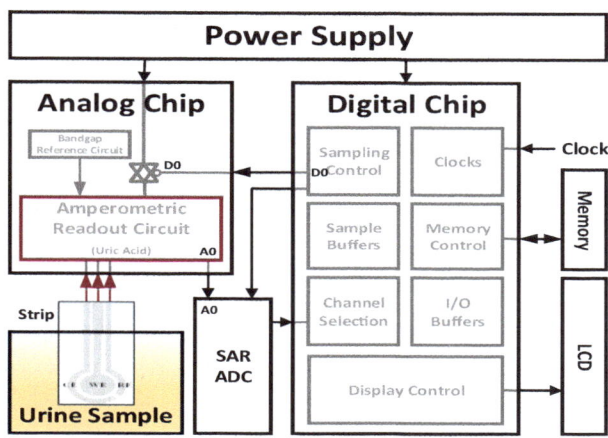

Fig. 1. System structure

2 Methodology

2.1 Sensing Mechanism

The third generation for uric acid biosensor produced by using macromolecules to fix redox mediator and enzyme on the electrode has advantages of lower oxidation potential, faster response time, and higher sensitivity than the first [5] and second [2] generation biosensors. The reactions taking place at working electrode are suggested as followings:

$$\text{Uric Acid} + 2\text{H}_2O + \text{Uricase}_{(ox)}$$
$$\rightarrow \text{Allantoin} + CO_2 + 2\text{H}^+ + \text{Uricase}_{(red)} \tag{1}$$

$$\text{Uricase}_{(red)} + 2\text{FcAld}^+ \leftrightarrows \text{Uricase}_{(ox)} + 2\text{FcAld} \tag{2}$$

$$2\text{FcAld} \leftrightarrows 2\text{FcAld}^+ + 2e^- \tag{3}$$

2.2 Screen-Printed Electrode

AutoCAD, developed and marketed by Autodesk, is a commercial computer-aided design (CAD) and drafting software application. As an alternative to the traditional electrodes, the recent developments in the electrochemical application of screen-printed technology are used to modify the disposable sensors. In this research, the sensor for uric acid amperometric detection based on silver screen-printed electrode (SPE) was designed by using AutoCAD. There are three electrodes on one test strip: working electrode (WE), reference electrode (RE), and counter electrode (CE) (Fig. 2).

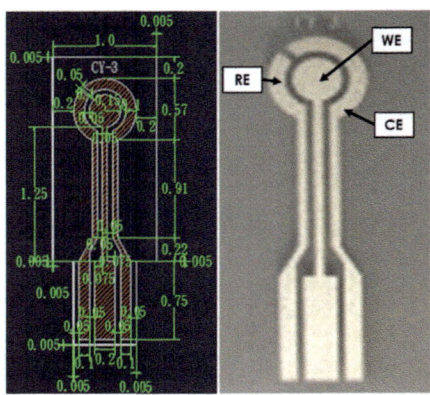

Fig. 2. The 2-D model of SPE and the finished product

2.3 Preparation of Uric Acid Test Strip

The three-step process procedures of the uric acid test strip was shown as Fig. 3. In step I, based on [6], one silver electrode was formed the Ag/AgCl reference electrode by simple electrodeposition in 3.5 M potassium chloride solution with an applied voltage of 2.0 V for 10 min, and then the test strip was immersed in saturated potassium chloride solution for 5 min. After that, the test strip was thoroughly rinsed with deionized distilled water at 100 °C. In step II, the WE was prepared by the coating of 0.0075 mM ferrocene carboxaldehyde (FcAld) dissolved in EtOH/HCl (19.9/0.1, v/v) at 30 °C for 20 min. In step III, The FcAld adsorbed electrode was coated with the mixture with the ratio of 200 μM uricase dissolved in 0.1 M pH 8.5 NaPB to polymer hydrogel/NaPB (1/1.5, v/v) is 1:1 at 30 °C for 30 min. The test strip was stored at 4 °C environment for later experiments.

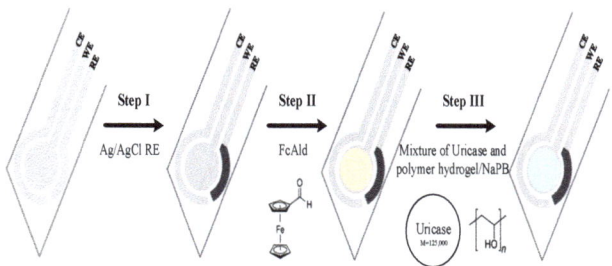

Fig. 3. The three-step preparation for the UA test strip

2.4   Amperometric Readout Circuit

The 3-electrode amperometric sensor readout circuit [10] is shown as Fig. 4. PMOS pass transistor (M0), which can couple the power supply (VDD) rail to the WE without any voltage drop, act as a switch. For reducing the input impedance effectively and getting wider sensing range, the source of PMOS transistor (M3) was connected to CE. The use of high gain folded cascode operational transconductance amplifier (FC-OTA) drove the source of M3, thus the current maintained direction from WE to CE. One self-biased OTA (SB-OTA1) and NMOS transistors (M2, M4 and M5); and the other self-biased OTA (SB-OTA2) and PMOS transistors (M3, M7 and M8) formed the high gain current mirrors copying the current from senor side to the input of integrator (CCII-based current integrated).

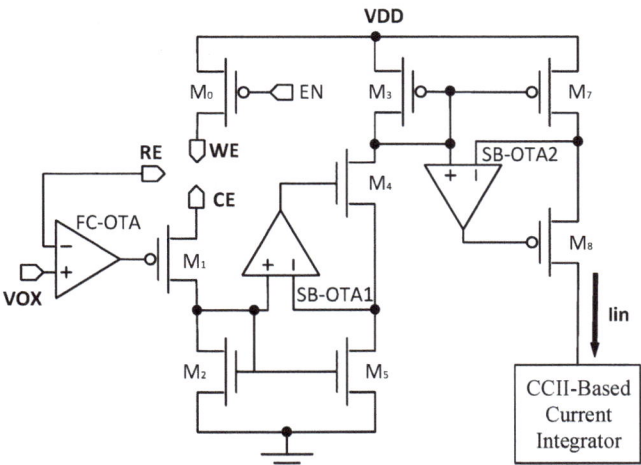

Fig. 4. The 3-electrode amperometric sensor readout circuit

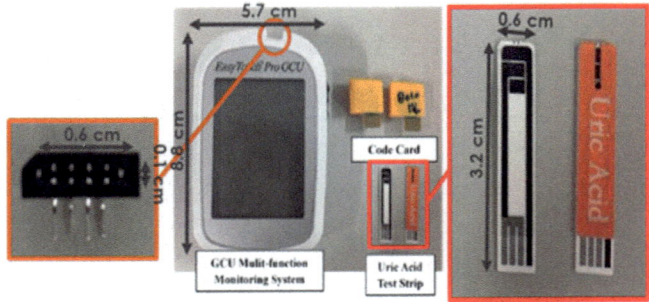

Fig. 5. UA strip and monitoring system

2.5 Commercial Module

Figure 5 shows the uric acid strip and monitoring system provided by Bioptik Technology, Inc. Its sensing range is 20–500 ppm and response time is 6 s. The strip is 2-electrode, disposable and siphon type. The self-made uric acid solutions were tested by commercial module and showed the result in Fig. 6. According to the curve, we can know that the solutions are reliable.

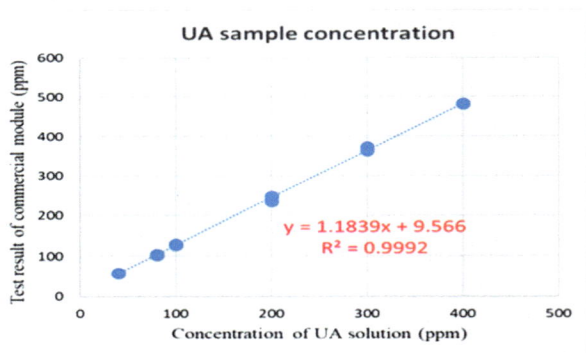

Fig. 6. UA sample tested by commercial module

3 Results

3.1 Cyclic Voltammetry

In Fig. 7, it illustrates the cyclic voltammograms of the UA test strip at six different concentration levels (0, 0.4, 10, 100, 500, 800 ppm) of UA standard solutions in 0.1 M pH 8.5 NaPB were measured by using CV at 35 °C. The oxidation potential of the redox mediator FcAld adsorbed electrode was 0.2533 V. The oxidation potential shifts should be due to the increasing UA concentration. Nevertheless, the results show that both FcAld and Uricase were successfully coated on the silver SPE.

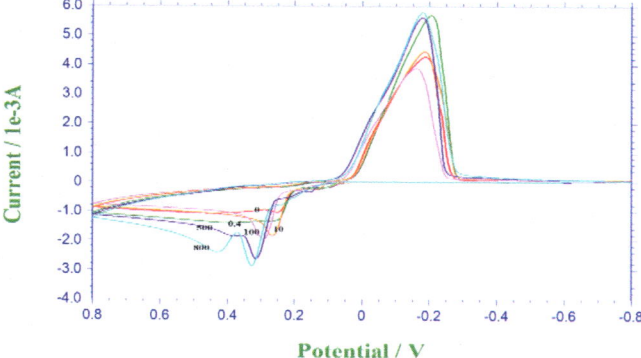

Fig. 7. Cyclic voltammograms of UA test strip for different concentrations of UA standard solutions

3.2   Amperometric Charge-Concentration Curve

The charge-concentration curves are showed in Fig. 8, which are converted by taking current into charge with integral operation. There are two linear regression line of the charge in different concentration ranges of 0–200 ppm and 200–800 ppm. According to different integration time, the test results are provided with different coefficient of determination (R^2) and slope of function. In addition, a value of R^2 is to 1.0 indicates it is a very reliable model for future forecasts and larger value of slope means higher sensitivity. Based on that, we chose 3 s as integration time and whose R^2 are respectively 0.9456 and 0.9921; and whose slope are respectively −0.0025 and −0.0008.

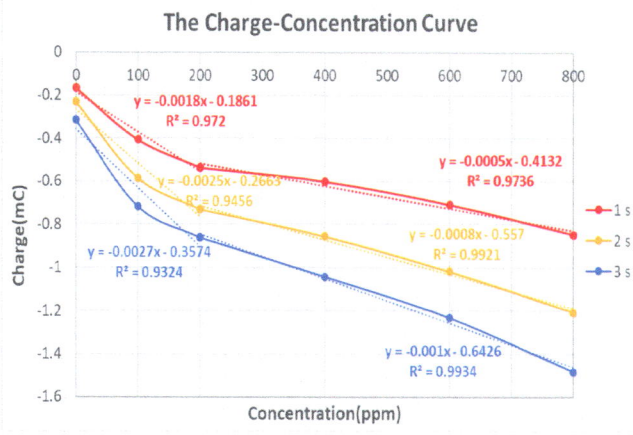

Fig. 8. The charge-concentration curve of UA solutions

4   Conclusions

The research report the third-generation uric acid test strip, which features wide sensing range, short response time, high accuracy, low sample volume, low cost, and disposable. According to preliminary measure results, it is reliable for the detection of UA. By Integrating with self-developed portable device and sensor, it is valuable for POCT application in the prevention from urolithiasis recurrence of patients.

Acknowledgment. The authors would like to acknowledge Bioptik Technology Inc. Taiwan for the technical support.

Conflict of Interest. The authors declare that they have no conflict of interest.

References

1. Silverio, A.A.: A multi-sensor readout interface circuit with system-on-chip implementation applied to urine quality analysis (Doctoral dissertation). Chung Yuan Christian University, Taoyuan, Taiwan (2016)
2. Kao, C.-Y.: Amperometric uric acid biosensor and two-dimensional liquid chromatography-mass spectrometer for urinary uric acid assay (Master's thesis). Chung Yuan Christian University, Taoyuan, Taiwan (2016)
3. Healthy.io at. https://healthy.io/
4. Yue, Y., Guojun, W., Jing, Z., Jianjun, L., Jian, Z., Junwu, Z.: Progresses of preparation and applications of paper-based surface-enhanced raman scattering substrate. Acta Agronomica Sinica **55**(3), 0307011 (2018). https://doi.org/10.3788/cjl201845.0307011
5. Chauhan, N., Pundir, C.S.: An amperometric uric acid biosensor based on multiwalled carbon nanotube–gold nanoparticle composite. Anal. Biochem. **2011**(413), 97–103 (2011)
6. Tsai, C.-M.: The improved study of miniature IrO2/Ta2O5-base potentiometric sensor to carbon dioxide (Master's thesis). National Chiao Tung University, Hsinchu, Taiwan (2009)
7. Chauhan, N., Preeti, P., Pundir, C.S.: covalent immobilization of uricase inside a plastic vial for uric acid determination in serum and urine. Anal. Sci. **30**, 501–506 (2014)
8. Bhawna, Pundir, C.S.: Fabrication of dissolved O_2 metric uric acid biosensor based on uricase bound to PVC membrane. J. Sci. Ind. Res. **69**, 695–699 (2010)
9. Li, C.X., Zeng, Y.L., Tang, C.R.: Glucose biosensor based on Carbon/PVC-COOH/Ferrocene composite with covalently immobilized enzyme. Chin. Chem. Lett. **16**(10), 1357–1360 (2005)
10. Chang, S.-Y.: Multi-parameter system-on-a-chip (SoC) design for the prevention of urolithiasis recurrence (Master's thesis). Chung Yuan Christian University, Taoyuan, Taiwan (2016)
11. Chang, S-Y.: Multi-parameter system-on-a-chip (SoC) design for the prevention of urolithiasis recurrence (Master's thesis). Chung Yuan Christian University, Taoyuan, Taiwan (2016)
12. Cheng, S.-C.: A novel mixed-mode signal processor design by current-mode circuits for biomedical sensing system (Master's thesis). Chung Yuan Christian University, Taoyuan, Taiwan (2009)
13. Chang, S.-K.: Compound circuit for the prevention of urolithiasis recurrence (Master's thesis). Chung Yuan Christian University, Taoyuan, Taiwan (2017)

14. Kuo, C.-N.: Microelectrode arrays for biosensor application (Master's thesis). National Chung Hsing University, Taichung, Taiwan (2014)
15. Chao, C.-T.: Fabrication and test of an amperometric uric acid biosensor (Master's thesis). National Taiwan University of Science and Technology, Taipei, Taiwan (2009)
16. Martin, S.M., Gebara, F.H., Strong, T.D., Brown, R.B.: A low-voltage, chemical sensor interface for systems-on-chip: the fully-differential potentiostat. IEEE Cat. No. 04CH37512 (2004). https://doi.org/10.1109/iscas.2004.1329148
17. Chu, C.-H.: System design and implementation for amperometric electrochemical sensor (Master's thesis). Chung Yuan Christian University, Taoyuan, Taiwan (2011)
18. Lin, L-S.: Selective determination of uric acid in the presence of ascorbic acid at screen-printed carbon electrode modified with electrochemically pretreated carbon nanotube. National Sun Yat-sen University, Kaohsiung, Taiwan (2010)

A Transcutaneous High-Efficiency Battery Charging System with a Small Temperature Increase for Implantable Medical Devices Based on the Taguchi Method

De-Fu Jhang[(✉)], Szu-Ying Kao, Kuan-Ting Lee,
and Chiung-Cheng Chuang

Department of Biomedical Engineering, Chung Yuan Christian University,
Chung Pei Road, Chung Li District, Taoyuan City, Taiwan
y217834@hotmail.com.tw, h76121@gmail.com,
mimi20124@hotmail.com, cheng965@cycu.edu.tw

Abstract. With the rapid development of science and technology in recent years, medical equipment is gradually being implanted in human bodies to allow patients to lead normal lives. Implantable medical devices must function in the body for long periods of time; hence, efficient rechargeable power sources must be developed to non-intrusively recharge these devices. In the charging process, implantable medical devices will damage the surrounding tissue due to the resulting heat generation. In order to enhance the charging efficiency and decrease the temperature variation, a 200-mAh Li-polymer battery was charged by a multistage sinusoidal current with the minimum-ac impedance, and an optimal rapid-charging pattern was identified by the Taguchi method. Experiment results showed that in terms of charging efficiency and battery and tissue temperature control, a multistage sinusoidal current with the minimum-ac-impedance frequency performed best compared with constant current (CC), pulse current, and constant current constant-voltage (CC-CV) charging strategies. In terms of battery temperature variation, compared to the above-mentioned three charging methods, the multistage sinusoidal current method are improved charging temperatures about 1.34 °C, 1.53 °C, and 1.71 °C, respectively; in respect to charging efficiency, efficiency improved about 5.52%, 17.4%, and 5.37%, respectively.

Keywords: Multistage current charging · Minimum-ac-impedance ·
Optimal rapid-charging pattern · Taguchi method · Implanted battery recharging

1 Introduction

With the development of rechargeable power supply and radio frequency (RF) power transmission technology, many implantable medical devices combine wireless power transmission with secondary lithium batteries [1, 2]. Implantable devices generate heat during charging, damaging surrounding body tissues and making patients feel uncomfortable. The effect of device charging on human body temperature control is a very important issue [3]. Therefore, experts and scholars share the common goal of

© Springer Nature Switzerland AG 2020
K.-P. Lin et al. (Eds.): ICBHI 2019, IFMBE Proceedings 74, pp. 72–79, 2020.
https://doi.org/10.1007/978-3-030-30636-6_10

determining how to fully charge implantable devices in the shortest time, decrease the battery temperature variation, and improve charging efficiency.

Nowadays, several charging techniques include constant-trickle-current charging (CTC), constant-current (CC) charging, and constant-current constant-voltage (CC-CV) charging; but these charging strategies' efficiency and battery lifetime are unable to meet the needs of users [4–8]. Chen et al. used a Bode plot to obtain the minimum-ac-impedance frequency (fZmin) and combined fZmin with a sinusoidal current to charge Lithium battery. The experimental results showed that, compared to the CC-CV and pulse current charging strategies, the minimum-ac-impedance frequency had the best charging efficiency and minimal temperature rise during charging [9, 10]. Although experiments show that sinusoidal current with fZmin have better performance, the increase in temperature is greater than 2 °C; if this charging strategy was used with an implantable medical device, it might damage the surrounding body tissue [11]. In this study, in order to decrease the temperature rise and search for rapid-charging pattern, an optimization technique based on the Taguchi method is introduced for rapid-charging with a sinusoidal current charging strategy [12, 13]. A lithium-polymer battery was charged by a multi-stage sinusoidal current with the fZmin and integrated by the Taguchi method. We used a state of charge (SOC) switching multi-stage current to control and terminate the charging process.

2 Experimental Procedure and Materials

Figure 1 shows the flowchart of the battery-charging process in this paper. First, an ac-impedance analyzer measured the ac-impedance spectrum of the Li-polymer battery, and the minimum-ac-impedance frequency was obtained. Then, the estimated SOC, which controls the multi-stage current switching time until the battery is fully charged, was measured from the terminal voltage. Thus, it is important to establish a relationship between the terminal voltage and the SOC. Initially, the Li-polymer was fully discharged and placed in an incubator for an hour at 37 °C. The battery was charged by 1.0C pulse current consisting of a six-minute charge equivalent to SOC 10% increment and one-hour rest until the battery was fully charged (e.g., 4.2 V). In addition, the battery voltage was recorded for every 10% SOC [12]. The experimental results of the Li-polymer battery voltage is illustrated in Fig. 2, which shows the relationship between the battery voltage and SOC.

We proposed a four-stage sinusoidal current charging method where each stage had an SOC range of 25% [12].

At each stage, the battery was charged by a pre-set current.

When the voltage was detected at the next stage of the SOC voltage, the charging current was also transferred. The charging process continued until the battery was fully charged, and then the charging process terminated. Table 1 lists the charging current candidates selected for this study where the charging current at each stage had a different level with a current difference of 0.2C. The charging current at each stage had a current difference of 0.5C. In addition, the charging current at each stage was lower than that of its previous stage.

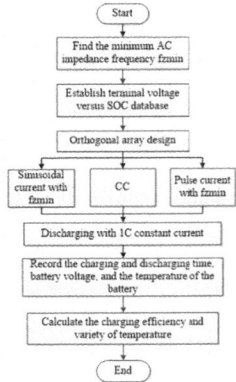

Fig. 1. Flowchart of the experiment

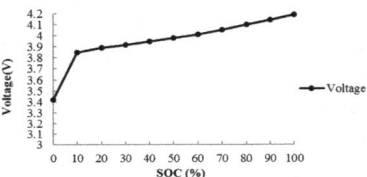

Fig. 2. The relationship of terminal voltage versus SOC

Table 1. Charging current candidates for four charging stages

Stage	I_1	I_2	I_3	I_4
$I^+(1)$	2C	1.5C	1C	0.5C
$I^0(2)$	1.8C	1.3C	0.8C	0.3C
$I^-(3)$	1.6C	1.1C	0.6C	0.1C

By using orthogonal arrays (OAs), the Taguchi method searches the parameters of a small number of experiments. According to the most commonly used standard OAs for experimental design, the search for an optimal charging pattern for this study can be represented by $L_9(3^4)$, where 9, 3, and 4 represent the number of experimental runs, the number of factor levels, and the maximum number of factors that the table can handle, respectively [14]. The charging pattern is shown in Table 2; it is the simplest and most efficient because interactions between the control factors are quasi-uniform in each column. The structure of the charging platform is shown in Fig. 3.

Table 2. $L_9(3^4)$ orthogonal array

	I_1	I_2	I_3	I_4
1	1	1	1	1
2	1	2	2	2
3	1	3	3	3
4	2	1	2	3
5	2	2	3	1
6	2	3	1	2
7	3	1	3	2
8	3	2	1	3
9	3	3	2	1

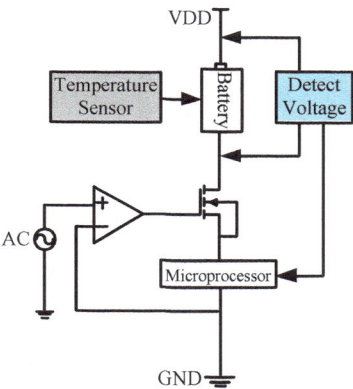

Fig. 3. Battery-charging platform

The minimum-ac-impedance frequency with sinusoidal current was applied at the input. Then a voltage/current converter that contains a FDG311 N and an operational amplifier. The battery voltage was read by a microprocessor and used to control the charging current. Figure 4 shows the flow chart of the experimental procedures for the charging pattern. In the four-stage charging pattern, if the battery voltage reaches SOC 25% (see Fig. 2), the microcontroller will switch to the next stage and the battery will charged by I_2, otherwise, the battery will be charged by I_1. When the battery voltage reaches 4.2 V, the battery is considered to be fully charged. During the entire charging process, the charging time, battery temperature, battery voltage, and charging current were recorded. When the battery voltage achieved the full charge of 4.2 V, it was discharged with 1C constant current until the battery voltage dropped to 3.0 V, and the discharging time was recorded. The total charging capacity Qin can be calculated as

$$Qin = Iin \times Tin \qquad (1)$$

where Iin is the average charging current and Tin is the charging time. Finally, the battery-charging efficiency was calculated according to [10]

$$\text{"}\eta\text{="} \ \text{"Qout"} / \text{"Qin"} \ \times 100\% \tag{2}$$

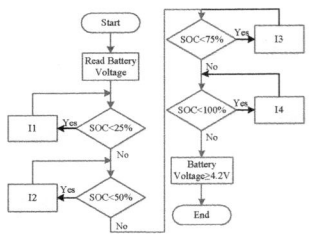

Fig. 4. Flowchart of the microcontroller

3   Experimental Results

The battery selected for this experiment was a new SLT402030 (200-mAh) Lithium-ion polymer battery. Figure 5 shows the ac-impedance spectrum of the Li-polymer battery measured by the CH Instruments CHI6273E (CHI 600E Series) ac-impedance analyzer. The ac-impedance spectrum showed that the minimum-ac-impedance frequency was 10.01 kHz.

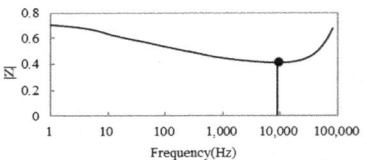

Fig. 5. AC impedance spectrum of the Li-polymer battery

We used the Taguchi method to search for and realize the optimal rapid charging pattern, and used the minimum-ac-impedance frequency to charge the battery. Experimental results are shown in Tables 3, 4, and 5. The optimal charging patterns are noted in Table 3, Table 4, and Table 5 as experiments no. 5, no. 9, and no. 9, respectively.

Table 3. Experimental results for sinusoidal current

	Charging time(s)	Discharging time(s)	Charging efficiency (%)	Temperature variation (°C)
1	3890	2895	85.4	2.74
2	5727	2992	93.7	2.3
3	9791	2833	97.9	1.8
4	13671	3064	99.7	2.75
5	4340	2849	99.7	1.83
6	5631	2920	91	2.76
7	5501	3040	93.3	2.22
8	13222	3148	98.5	3.11
9	4044	2669	99	3.58

Table 4. Experimental results for constant current

	Charging time(s)	Discharging time(s)	Charging efficiency (%)	Temperature variation (°C)
1	3332	2651	98.94	2.22
2	5753	2942	95.97	1.84
3	13169	3090	98.2	3.58
4	13423	3083	98.66	3.18
5	4096	2322	97.26	3.18
6	6875	2870	97.65	4.91
7	6469	3387	97.53	3.17
8	18817	2979	92.4	2.75
9	2977	2225	99.49	2.27

Table 5. Experimental results for pulse current

	Charging time(s)	Discharging time(s)	Charging efficiency (%)	Temperature variation (°C)
1	4172	2953	95.92	2.05
2	5631	3087	98.08	1.69
3	14828	3308	99.09	2.13
4	16906	3499	99.10	2.63
5	4313	2866	99.76	3.25
6	5872	3223	99.34	3.70
7	5369	2950	97.64	1.28
8	14531	3469	98.11	1.28
9	4177	3169	98.54	1.66

4 Invitro Experiments

In this study, we used a transcutaneous power supply (bq500210EVM-689 (Tx) and bq51013EVM-725 (Rx), Texas Instruments) with an operational frequency between 110 and 200 kHz, an output voltage of 5 V, and currents up to 1 A. We used 5% solid Agarose to simulate biological tissues to mimic skin heat response during transcutaneous power transmission, and a thermistor (PR222J2) was placed in a battery box and between the receiver and biological tissues, respectively. A booster circuit was connected to the receiver of an output to increase the Vcc of the charging circuit to 6 V. Figure 6 provides a block diagram of the experimental setup. Additionally, the experimental system was placed in an incubator, and the tissue temperature was maintained at 35.5 °C [11]. As the battery was charging, the charging current, battery voltage, battery temperature, and tissue temperature were all being record simultaneously.

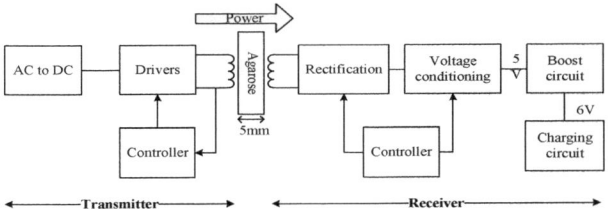

Fig. 6. Block diagram of in vitro experiment

5 Results

In this paper, the optimal experimental results were used in the in vitro experiments. The sinusoidal, CC, and pulse current charging patterns used the optimal results obtained in Sect. 3 (experiments no. 5, no. 9, and no. 9 of Table 3, Table 4, and Table 5 respectively). Table 6 compares the experimental charging time, discharging time, charging efficiency, battery temperature, and tissue temperature performance of the four charging methods. The results confirm that the optimal sinusoidal charging pattern performed best. Although the multistage CC method had better charging and discharging times, the battery and tissue temperatures were higher. In addition, four different charging strategies were used for the in vitro experiments.

Table 6. Different charging strategies in vitro experiments in this study

	Multistage sinusoidal current	Multistage CC	Multistage Pulse current	CC-CV
Charging time(s)	3818	3647	4809	6447
Discharging time(s)	2809	2666	2654	2558
Battery Rising Temp(°C)	1.29	2.63	2.82	3.00
Tissue Rising Temp(°C)	3.50	3.63	3.56	5.47

6 Conclusion

Experiments indicate that the sinusoidal current charging method determined by the Taguchi method provided a higher charging efficiency compared with that of the constant current and pulse current charging strategies. The in vitro experiments showed that a battery charged by a multi-stage sine current performed better than other charging strategies, and the battery temperature increased only 1.29 °C during charging. As a result, the temperature variation of a Li-polymer battery charged by multi-stage sinusoidal current pattern is less than 2 °C. Compared to the multi-stage CC, multi-stage pulse current, and CC-CV charging strategies, the charging efficiency, battery rising temperature, and tissue rising temperature of our proposed charging strategy were all improved. In terms of battery temperature variation, the charging strategy proposed in this paper are improved about 1.34 °C, 1.53 °C, and 1.71 °C, respectively, and charging efficiency are improved about 5.52%, 17.4%, and 5.37%, respectively.

Conflict of Interest. The authors declare that they have no conflict of interest.

References

1. Smith, D.K., Lovik, R.D., Sparrow, E.M., Abraham, J.P.: Human tissue temperatures achieved during recharging of new-generation neuromodulation devices. Int. J. Heat Mass Transf. **53**(15–16), 3292–3299 (2010)
2. Cheng, H.-W., Yu, T.-C., Luo, C.-H.: Direct current driving impedance matching method for rectenna using medical implant communication service band for wireless battery charging. IET Microwaves Antennas Propag. **7**(4), 277–282 (2013)
3. Lovik, R.D., Abraham, J.P., Sparrow, E.M.: Potential tissue damage from transcutaneous recharge of neuromodulation implants. Int. J. Heat Mass Transf. **52**(15–16), 3518–3524 (2009)
4. Cope, R.C., Podrazhansky, Y.: The art of battery charging. In: The Fourteenth Annual Battery Conference on Applications and Advances, pp. 233–235. IEEE (1999)
5. Chi, H.T.Q., Park, D.-H., Lee, D.-C.: An advanced fast charging strategy for lithium polymer batteries. In: IEEE 2nd International Future Energy Electronics Conference (IFEEC), pp. 1–6. IEEE (2015)
6. Lin, C.-H., Hsieh, C.-Y., Chen, K.-H.: A Li-ion battery charger with smooth control circuit and built-in resistance compensator for achieving stable and fast charging. IEEE Trans. Circuits Syst. I-Regul. Pap. **57**(2), 506–517 (2010)
7. Chen, L.-R.: PLL-based battery charge circuit topology. IEEE Trans. Ind. Electron. **51**(6), 1344–1346 (2004)
8. Gao, Y., Zhang, C., Liu, Q., Jiang, Y., Ma, W., Mu, Y.: An optimal charging strategy of lithium-ion batteries based on polarization and temperature rise. In: IEEE Conference and Expo Transportation Electrification Asia-Pacific (ITEC Asia-Pacific), pp. 1–6. IEEE (2014)
9. Chen, L.-R., Wu, S.-L., Chen, T.-R.: Improving battery charging performance by using sinusoidal current charging with the minimum AC impedance frequency. In: IEEE International Conference on Sustainable Energy Technologies (ICSET), pp. 1–4. IEEE (2010)
10. Chen, L.-R., Wu, S.-L., Shieh, D.-T., Chen, T.-R.: Sinusoidal-ripple-current charging strategy and optimal charging frequency study for Li-ion batteries. IEEE Trans. Ind. Electron. **60**(1), 88–97 (2013)
11. Goto, K., Nakagawa, T., Nakamura, O., Kawata, S.: An implantable power supply with an optically rechargeable lithium battery. IEEE Trans. Biomed. Eng. **48**(7), 830–833 (2001)
12. Vo, T.T., Chen, X., Shen, W., Kapoor, A.: New charging strategy for lithium-ion batteries based on the integration of Taguchi method and state of charge estimation. J. Power Sources **273**, 413–422 (2015)
13. Liu, Y.-H., Luo, Y.-F.: Search for an optimal rapid-charging pattern for Li-ion batteries using the Taguchi approach. IEEE Trans. Ind. Electron. **57**(12), 3963–3971 (2010)
14. Liu, Y.-H., Hsieh, C.-H., Luo, Y.-F.: Search for an optimal five-step charging pattern for Li-ion batteries using consecutive orthogonal arrays. IEEE Trans. Energy Convers. **26**(2), 654–661 (2011)

Using Bi-planar X-Ray Images to Reconstruct the Spine Structure by the Convolution Neural Network

Chih-Chia Chen[✉] and Yu-Hua Fang

Department of Biomedical Engineering,
National Cheng Kung University, Tainan, Taiwan
lonal5926@fanglab.bme.ncku.edu.tw

Abstract. The spine-related disease is one of the most common musculoskeletal-related disorder in the world. Although computed tomography (CT) is an outstanding tool for investigating spinal pathology in clinical protocol, the overexposure to radiation dose issue cannot be underestimated. Therefore, the bi-planar EOS X-ray imaging was adopted as the scanning technology, which can capture the anteroposterior (AP) and lateral (LAT) view X-ray images simultaneously with ultra-low radiation doses. High quality and high contrast bi-planar X-ray images would be acquired from the EOS system and these two radiographs enable a precise three-dimensional reconstruction of vertebrae, pelvis and other parts of the skeletal system. To overcome the time-consuming issue of spine reconstruction using the EOS system, a convolution neural network (CNN) was applied to reconstruct the entire spine model. Nowadays, the CNN model has already been adopted in the transformation from 2D image to 3D scenes. Our approach represents a potential alternative for EOS reconstruction while still maintaining a clinically acceptable diagnostic accuracy.

Keywords: EOS system · AP & lateral view · CNN · Reconstruct 3D model

1 Introduction

Traditionally, we usually use the X-ray or CT angiography to get the bone information. X-ray is a low-dose radiation imaging method, but it has two problems. The first problem is that you can't get enough information about the spine because the doctor can only diagnose from the patient's 2D image, but lacks the information in the 3D space. The second problem appears in the process of imaging. During scanning, the patient must maintain the same posture to avoid motion-induced image artifacts. In addition, depending on the X-ray machine, the radiologist may need to take some times to obtain a systemic bi-planar X-ray image. This is undoubtedly a big challenge for patients and radiologists [1]. On the other hand, although CT can obtain complete and detailed bone information, the radiation dose received by patients will be quite high [2]. It will increase the risk of cancer in patients who need regular tracking, and the overexposure to radiation dose issue cannot be underestimated [3, 4]. Therefore, we proposed to the EOS system to reconstruct the spine model. The EOS system was

© Springer Nature Switzerland AG 2020
K.-P. Lin et al. (Eds.): ICBHI 2019, IFMBE Proceedings 74, pp. 80–85, 2020.
https://doi.org/10.1007/978-3-030-30636-6_11

developed by a French company named "EOS imaging" to provide 3D X-ray images and 3D bone structure for preoperative evaluation [5, 6]. The EOS system is currently used in 51 countries around the world, and its technology is quite mature. Through the EOS system, the X-ray images of the anteroposterior view and the lateral direction are simultaneously photographed. Then, the anatomical position of the patient's spine can be reconstructed via the software [7, 8]. EOS X-ray imaging provides a faster, more precise and less radiation dose exposure alternative than traditional X-ray.

Even the EOS system has advantages aforementioned, limitations still existed. In the processing of using the EOS system to reconstruct the whole spine, it is necessary to manually mark the position of each vertebral body, and this process usually takes more than one hour. The main reason is that the bones of the arms and shoulders make it difficult for the vertebral body between T2 and T5 to distinguish its position. It takes more time to adjust the contrast of the X-ray image and estimate the actual position of the vertebral body. In the case of the scoliosis, it is more necessary to align and correct the position of each vertebral body, so the vertebral parameters calculated by the software algorithm can be correct. Such a process, even if a licensed and skilled radiologist may take about two hours to complete the EOS images of a patient, and a few numbers of the patient can be completed in a day. In Taiwan, presently only the National Cheng Kung University Hospital is equipped with the EOS system. Therefore, in order to popularize the EOS system, it is necessary to significantly reduce the time taken for the EOS system to perform the alignment. In our study, we attempt to use the convolution neural network (CNN) to accelerate the reconstruction speed of spine and have a promising result [9–11].

2 Materials and Methods

2.1 Dataset

This study acquires data from "The Cancer Imaging Archive (TCIA)" which is an open-access database of medical images for cancer research. Data within the archive is organized into collections which typically share a common cancer type and/or anatomical site. The majority of the data consists of CT, MRI, and nuclear medicine (e.g. PET) images stored in DICOM format. All data are anonymized in order to comply with the Health Insurance Portability and Accountability Act and National Institutes of Health data sharing policies. We take 90 spine models for training and 10 for testing.

2.2 Tomographic Iterative GPU-Based Reconstruction Toolbox

To get bi-planar images, Tomographic Iterative GPU-based Reconstruction Toolbox (TIGRE) will be used to generate the projection images, which is a MATLAB toolbox for fast and accurate 3D tomographic reconstruction. The aim of TIGRE is to provide a wide range of easy-to-use iterative algorithms to the tomographic research community. TIGRE is an open source toolbox which allows everyone for any purpose to use it.

2.3 Preprocessing

In order to train the CNN model, we need the 3D spine model and the corresponding bi-planar images. However, in the current progress, we don't have such many EOS images. Hence in the first preprocessing step, we pick the 3D spine models which are segmented manually from CT data. Second, we will do the forward projection from those 3D spine models to acquire the simulated bi-planar images. Third, we rotate the training data in every 90° for the data augmentation to create more data

2.4 Convolution Neural Network

Our convolution neural network can be divided into two different parts, the encoder part and the generator part. In the current results, the loss of this network will be defined as the mean-square error between the fake models and the spine models which are segmented from the CT data. Finally, we evaluate the performance of CNN by dice score coefficient, structural similarity index (SSIM) and cross-validation.

2.5 Training Detail

We propose our encoder in Fig. 1, The image encoder takes a 64 × 64 image as input and outputs a 128-dimensional vector. It includes 32 × 32, 16 × 16, 8 × 8, 4 × 4 convolution layers, and a fully connected layer. The numbers of channels are [64, 128, 256, 512], kernel sizes [32, 16, 8, 4], and strides [1, 1, 2, 2]. There are ReLU and batch normalization layers between convolutional layers, and we add a sigmoid layer at the end. The anteroposterior view and lateral view images are both 64 × 64 pixels. Using these two images as input, we can get two vectors respectively. Then, these two vectors are combined into a new longer vector which is going to be used later by the generator.

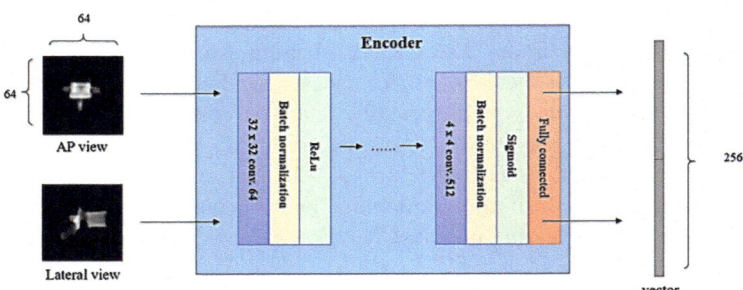

Fig. 1. The architecture of the encoder

Next, the previously combined vector is the input vector of the generator. As shown in Fig. 2, the generator consists of five convolution layers with numbers of channels [512, 256, 128, 64, 1], kernel sizes [4, 8, 16, 32, 64], and strides [1, 1, 2, 2, 2]. There are ReLU and batch normalization layers between convolutional layers, and we add a tanh layer at the end. The input is a 256-dimensional vector, and the output is a $64 \times 64 \times 64$ matrix with values between zero to one, which means the possibility the voxel exists.

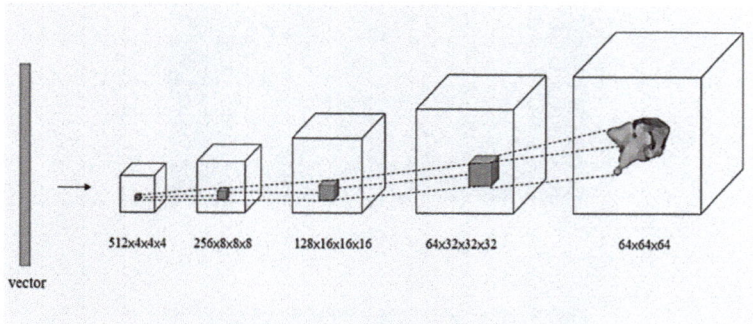

Fig. 2. The architecture of the generator.

3   Results

Figure 3 is the learning curve. In this study, 5-fold validation is used to calculate the indexes of results and average it. The dice score coefficient of testing data is 0.74, and the SSIM is 0.93. The following Figs. 4 and 5 would show one section of the spine for example. We can see that the main place of vertebral body can been simulated well, but the performance of the boundary of the transverse and spinous process is not. The project still has the room for improvement.

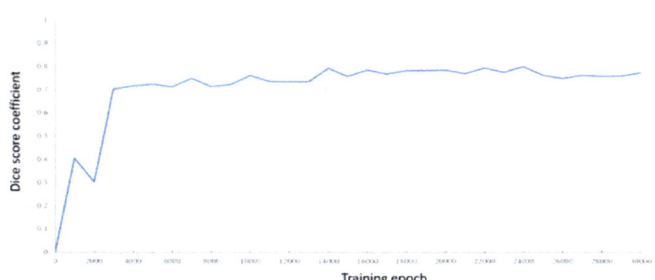

Fig. 3. Learning curve.

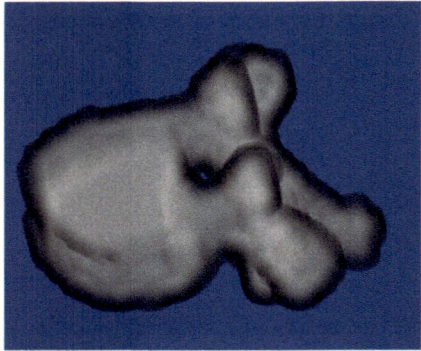

Fig. 4. Original 3D model.

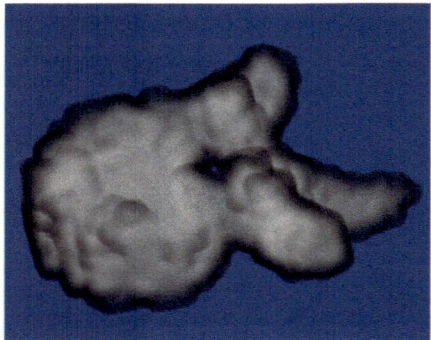

Fig. 5. Reconstructed model.

4   Discussion

In the following step of this project, we have to add more training data. In particular, we have only used one section of the spine as the target of training now, so we should gradually amplify our target to the whole thoracic image. Then, we should use the bi-planar X-ray images and 3D reconstructed model data from the EOS system to make sure that our algorithm can really work. At last, we still have to keep adjusting the loss function, optimizer, and other parameters, and the precision of the reconstructed model is expected to be more improved.

5 Conclusions

From the preliminary result, CNN provides an exceptional diagnosis algorithm for the reconstruction of the spine and vertebral body, which could have profound clinical implications for orthopedists. Our approach still represents a clinically acceptable diagnostic accuracy and potential clinical applicability.

Acknowledgment. This work financially supported by the Ministry of Science and Technology in Taiwan under grant number MOST 107-2221-E-006-167-MY2.

Conflict of Interest. The authors declare that they have no conflict of interest.

References

1. Pearcy, M.J., Portek, I., Shepherd, J.: Three-dimensional X-ray analysis of normal movement in the lumbar spine. Spine (Phila. Pa. 1976) (1984)
2. Brenner, D.J., Hall, E.J.: Computed tomography — an increasing source of radiation exposure. N. Engl. J. Med. (2007)
3. Johnson, J.N., et al.: Cumulative radiation exposure and cancer risk estimation in children with heart disease. Circulation (2014)
4. Berrington De González, A., et al.: Projected cancer risks from computed tomographic scans performed in the United States in 2007. Arch. Intern. Med. (2009)
5. McKenna, C., et al.: EOS 2D/3D X-ray imaging system: a systematic review and economic evaluation. Health Technol. Assess. (2012
6. Melhem, E., Assi, A., ElRachkidi, R., Ghanem, I.: EOS® biplanar X-ray imaging: concept, developments, benefits, and limitations. J. Child. Orthop. (2016)
7. Humbert, L., DeGuise, J.A., Aubert, B., Godbout, B., Skalli, W.: 3D reconstruction of the spine from biplanar X-rays using parametric models based on transversal and longitudinal inferences. Med. Eng. Phys. (2009)
8. Chaibi, Y., et al.: Fast 3D reconstruction of the lower limb using a parametric model and statistical inferences and clinical measurements calculation from biplanar X-rays. Comput. Methods Biomech. Biomed. Eng. (2012)
9. Lin, C.-H., Kong, C., Lucey, S.: Learning efficient point cloud generation for dense 3D object reconstruction (2017)
10. Yang, G., Cui, Y., Belongie, S., Hariharan, B.: Learning single-view 3D reconstruction with limited pose supervision. In: Lecture Notes in Computer Science (including subseries Lecture Notes in Artificial Intelligence and Lecture Notes in Bioinformatics) (2018)
11. Jiang, L., Shi, S., Qi, X., Jia, J.: GAL: geometric adversarial loss for single-view 3D-object reconstruction. In: Lecture Notes in Computer Science (including subseries Lecture Notes in Artificial Intelligence and Lecture Notes in Bioinformatics) (2018)

Biomechanical Analysis of Pullout Strength of Spinal Pedicle Screws with Full Insertion and Back-Out Using Finite Element Method

Yu-You Chen[1], Chian-Yun Hsu[2], Kao-Shang Shih[3], and Ching-Chi Hsu[1(✉)]

[1] Graduate Institute of Applied Science and Technology,
National Taiwan University of Science and Technology,
No. 43, Keelung Road, Sec. 4, Taipei 10607, Taiwan, R.O.C.
hsucc@mail.ntust.edu.tw
[2] Department of Mechanical Engineering,
National Taiwan University of Science and Technology,
Taipei 106, Taiwan, R.O.C.
[3] Department of Orthopedic Surgery, Shin Kong Wu Ho-Su Memorial Hospital,
Taipei 111, Taiwan, R.O.C.

Abstract. Pedicle screws might be backed out after screw insertion. Past studies had evaluated the pedicle screws with full insertion and back-out using experimental approaches. Unfortunately, there is rare study to investigate this problem using numerical approaches. Thus, the purpose of this study was to analyze the pullout performance of spinal pedicle screws with fully inserted setting or backed out using finite element method.

Twelve types of spinal pedicle screws were developed using SolidWorks. Each screw with the full insertion, backed-out 90°, and backed-out 180° were considered to evaluate their pullout performance using ANSYS Workbench. Additionally, a bone compaction technique was developed and applied in the present study.

The results showed that the pullout performance of the conical pedicle screws was significantly reduced compared to that of the cylindrical pedicle screws in situation of screw back-out. Both the screw geometry and bone compaction effect were the key parameters for the evaluation of pullout performance.

Keywords: Pedicle screw · Back-out · Pullout performance · Finite element method

1 Introduction

Pedicle screw and rod fixation system has been widely used for the treatment of spinal disorders [1, 2]. However, the incidence of screw loosening ranges from 0.6% to 11% and might be even higher in osteoporotic spines [3]. Insertional technique of pedicle screws is important in their placement. Conical pedicle screws would be expected to lose pullout strength if they were backed out from full screw insertion. In the past, researchers had evaluated the problem of screw backed-out using experimental approaches. However, the pullout performance of pedicle screws is mainly determined

© Springer Nature Switzerland AG 2020
K.-P. Lin et al. (Eds.): ICBHI 2019, IFMBE Proceedings 74, pp. 86–90, 2020.
https://doi.org/10.1007/978-3-030-30636-6_12

by screw designs, and only limited screw designs were tested and discussed [4]. Computer simulations have become a useful tool in the field of biomechanical engineering and can be used to analyze all possible screw designs [4, 5]. Unfortunately, there is rare study to investigate the pullout strength of pedicle screws with full insertion and back-out using numerical approaches. Thus, the purpose of the present study was to evaluate the pullout performance of spinal pedicle screws with full insertion and back-out using finite element method.

2 Materials and Methods

2.1 Designs of Spinal Pedicle Screws

Twelve types of spinal pedicle screws with an outer diameter of 6.5 mm were divided into three groups with an inner diameter of 3.9, 4.4, and 4.9 mm at the screw tip, respectively (Fig. 1). Each group comprised four types with different core tapering that began at the screw tip in Design A, E, and I; at 1/3 length from screw tip in Design B, F, and J; and at 2/3 length in Design C, G, and K. Design D, H, and L have no core tapering design, and they are a cylindrical pedicle screw. The other design variables of spinal pedicle screws were kept constant. All the screw models were created using SolidWorks.

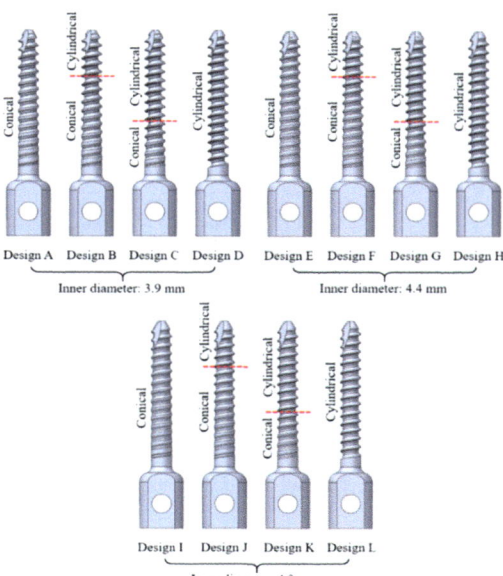

Fig. 1. Twelve designs of spinal pedicle screws

2.2   Finite Element Analysis

The finite element analyses of the spinal pedicle screws were conducted using commercial software ANSYS Workbench 19.2. The finite element model consisted of a
spinal pedicle screw and a cylinder of cancellous bone. The screws were assumed
inserted in the center of the cylinder with a diameter of 30 mm. The material properties
of the screws and bone were assumed to be linear isotropic. The elastic modulus was
114 GPa for pedicle screws and 137.5 MPa for bone. Poisson's ratio was 0.3 for both
screws and bone. To model the foam compaction effects, the elastic modulus of the
bone surrounding the conical core were adjusted according to the density change of the
bone around that core (Fig. 2). The boundary condition was full constraint at the
surface of the bone. The loading condition was an axial displacement applied to the end
surface of the pedicle screw (Fig. 2). The interface between the pedicle screw and bone
was assumed to be frictionless contact. In post-processing, the total reaction force on
screws was calculated to assess the pullout performance.

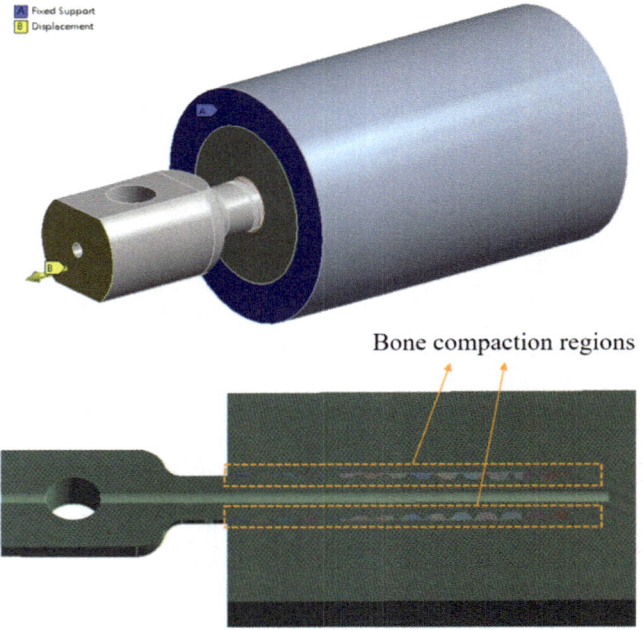

Fig. 2. The loading and boundary conditions of the finite element models.

3   Results and Discussions

All the finite element models were successfully meshed and solved. Each finite element
model contains more than 600,000 nodes and 300,000 elements. Convergence analysis
was conducted by adjusting the element size. The total reaction force and displacement
converged properly. The variations due to different element sizes were less than 1%.

The displacement distribution of the pedicle screw with full insertion, backed-out 90°, and backed-out 180° was obtained. The deformation of the screws was negligible (Fig. 3A).

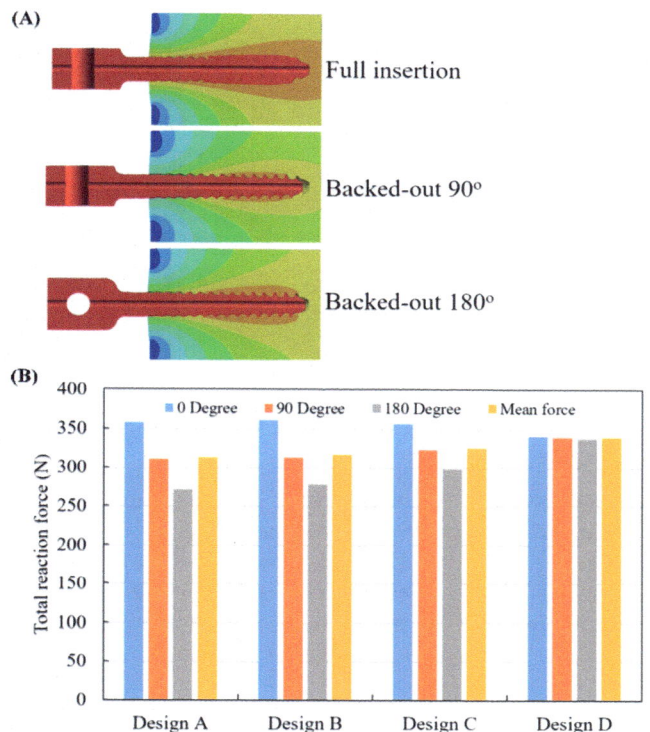

Fig. 3. (A) The displacement distribution; (B) The total reaction force.

Design D, which is a cylindrical pedicle screw, has a minor effect on the total reaction force if the screw back-out was considered. However, the total reaction force of Design A, B, and C was significantly reduced after screw back-out. It was noted that the pullout performance of Design A was significantly reduced after the screw back-out compared to the other screw designs (Fig. 3B).

The mean total reaction force of all the spinal pedicle screws was also calculated (Fig. 4). All the cylindrical pedicle screws (Design D, H, and L) revealed higher mean total reaction force compared to the full conical pedicle screw (Design A, E, and I) and partial conical pedicle screws (Design B, C, F, G, J, and K).

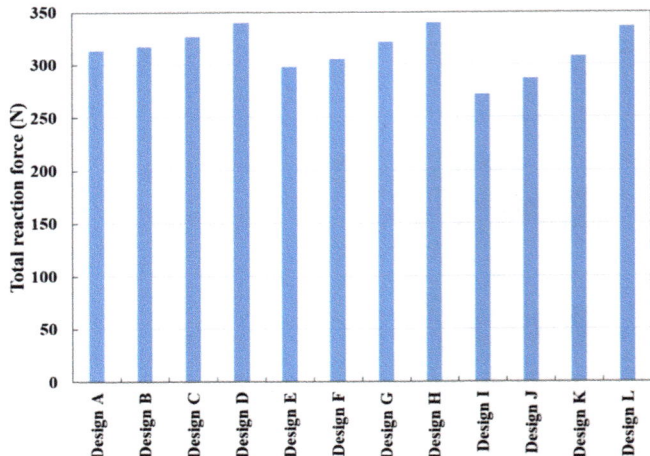

Fig. 4. The total reaction force of twelve spinal pedicle screw designs.

4   Conclusions

The spinal pedicle screws with full insertion and back-out can be successfully analyzed and evaluated using finite element method. The pullout performance of the conical pedicle screws was significantly reduced compared to that of the cylindrical pedicle screws in situation of screw back-out. Both the screw geometry and bone compaction effect were the key parameters for the evaluation of pullout performance.

Acknowledgment. This study was supported by Industrial Technology Research Institute, Taiwan.

Conflict of Interest. The authors declare that they have no conflict of interest.

References

1. Verlaan, J.J., Dhert, W.J.A., Oner, F.C.: Intervertebral disc viability after burst fractures of the thoracic and lumbar spine treated with pedicle screw fixation and direct end-plate restoration. Spine J. **132**, 217–221 (2013)
2. Silbermann, J., Riese, F., Allam, Y., et al.: Computer tomography assessment of pedicle screw placement inlumbar and sacral spine: comparison between free-hand and O-arm based navigation techniques. Eur. Spine J. **20**, 875–881 (2011)
3. Paré, P.E., Chappuis, J.L., Rampersaud, R., et al.: Biomechanical evaluation of a novel fenestrated pedicle screw augmented with bone cement in osteoporotic spines. Spine **36**, E1210–E1214 (2011)
4. Chao, C.K., Lin, J., Putra, S.T., et al.: A neuro-genetic approach to a multiobjective design optimization of spinal pedicle screws. J. Biomech. Eng-TASME **132**, 091006 (2010)
5. Chen, C.S., Chen, W.J., Cheng, C.K., et al.: Failure analysis of broken pedicle screws on spinal instrumentation. Med. Eng. Phy. **27**, 487–496 (2005)

A Free-Hand System of the High-Frequency Single Element Ultrasound Transducer for Skin Imaging

Wei-Ting Zhang[1]($\boxtimes$), Yin-Chih Lin[2], Wei-Hao Chen[1],
Chia-Wei Yang[1], and Hui-Hua Kenny Chiang[1,2]($\boxtimes$)

[1] Department of Biomedical Engineering, National Yang-Ming University,
No. 155, Sec. 2, Linong Street, Taipei, Taiwan (ROC)
{visionary840911,hkennychiang3}@gmail.com
[2] Biomedical Engineering Research and Development Center,
National Yang-Ming University, No. 155, Sec. 2, Linong Street,
Taipei, Taiwan (ROC)

Abstract. Ultrasound (US) imaging is a non-invasion and non-radiation medical imaging system. One of them, the single-element transducer has significant potential in the medical device. As compared to an array transducer, it could reduce the size of the imaging system. For example, the ultrasound needle for epidural anesthesia and eyeball.

In this study, we develop a free-hand US system on skin imaging. Using the 20 MHz high-frequency single element ultrasound transducer on the skin scanning. The high-frequency ultrasound could provide an excellent resolution to 0.1 mm. The bandwidth of the transducer is 20%, and the Insertion loss (IL) is $-$31.9 dB, and the Electromechanical coupling factor (K_t) is 0.72. Meanwhile, the free-hand apparatus which based on the optical tracking sensor is designed and applied in this system. It is convenient for scanning the skin surface.

This control and display panel is designed by the LabVIEW software. The inboard filter and Hilbert transformation are used to eliminate the environment noise. To solve the problem of unstable scanning speed, the interpolation method with one order is used to fit and smooth the image. Therefore, the high-quality ultrasound images could be applied in the skin scanning.

Keywords: Ultrasound · Free-hand · High-frequency ·
Single element transducer · Skin imaging · Imaging system · Medical device ·
Dermatology · Interpolation

1 Introduction

This research develops a free-hand scanning ultrasound transducer with a 20 MHz high-frequency image transducer and an optical sensor scanning system. The handheld scanning system uses the optical sensor Capclip from Japan Elecom to detect the walking distance and provide ultrasonic transducer displacement. Different from the traditional use of motor movement, the scanning system can be smaller in size, no longer limited to large areas, but also can scan high curved areas, and the application range is wider.

© Springer Nature Switzerland AG 2020
K.-P. Lin et al. (Eds.): ICBHI 2019, IFMBE Proceedings 74, pp. 91–99, 2020.
https://doi.org/10.1007/978-3-030-30636-6_13

High frequency ultrasound has higher resolution than conventional fundamental image. It can show the image of tissue clearly and it is widely used in the field of ophthalmology, dermatology, microcirculation, etc. However, in the past it was not quite easy to produce a transducer and the signal to noise ratio (SNR) was too low. Therefore, high frequency ultrasound was not generally used in the to clinical diagnosis.

In this research, we propose to use a high frequency ultrasound transducer of 20 MHz.

2 Methods and Materials

2.1 Ultrasound Theory

Ultrasonic waves are sound waves that belong to mechanical waves and transmit energy through the vibration of molecules. More than the frequency that can be heard by the human ear, the frequency above 20 kHz is called ultrasonic. Sound waves are also transmitted at different speeds in different media. The wave speed can be expressed by the frequency and wavelength of the wave:

$$C = f \times \lambda \tag{1}$$

C is the speed of sound, f is the frequency, and λ is the wavelength. In human tissue, the propagation speed is about 1450 m/s. Because the speed of wave transmission is different in different media, the acoustic impedance of each substance is also different. Ultrasonic waves produce reflection phenomenon under the difference of acoustic impedance of different interfaces, which is an important basis for ultrasonic diagnosis. Acoustic impedance is the resistance that ultrasonic waves need to overcome when transporting between substances, usually expressed as Z, and can be obtained from the density of the medium and the speed of transmission:

$$Z = \rho \times C \tag{2}$$

Z represents Acoustic impedance (Rayles), ρ represents Density of medium (Kg/m^3), and C represents Speed of Sound (m/s) in the medium.

Ultrasound transducers operate through a piezoelectric effect, a phenomenon in which mechanical energy is exchanged with electrical energy. The piezoelectric material emits ultrasonic waves through the electrical energy to generate ultrasonic waves. When the sound waves pass through different media, there are different reflection phenomena. After receiving the reflected signals, the transducers are converted into electrical energy and presented in an amplitude manner. Different piezoelectric materials have different conversion capabilities. At the resonant frequency, the ability to convert mechanical energy with electrical energy is called the electromechanical coupling coefficient K_t. The higher the K_t value, the better the piezoelectric conversion effect. In addition, by controlling the thickness of the wafer, we can make single crystal materials of different frequencies. The thinner the wafer, the higher the frequency of the transducer.

2.2   Ultrasound Transducer Manufacture

The Lead Magnesium Neonate-Lead Titanate (PMN-PT) crystal is used as an active layer in this transducer. This transducer has the highly sensitive to pick the reflected US signal. The Parylene layer and the mixed of 301-1 and Au powder spray as a matching layer to reduce the interface reflection. Furthermore, E-solder 3022 is used as a backing layer to increase the damping ratio to reduce the residual oscillation. The impendence match circuit is used for the performance enhancement.

The electric and optical properties of the transducer is listed in Table 1. According to the geometrical size and theoretical calculation, the spatial resolution and Depth of Field (DOF) is 0.35 mm and 5 mm. The bandwidth could be increase from 15% to 25% after the impendence matching circuit, as shown in table. It implied that the dermatologic tissue is located in the reasonable range of the transducer.

Table 1. Material of 20 MHz transducer

		Layer1	Layer2	Crystal	Backing layer
20 MHz	Material	Parylene	301-1 & silver	CTS, PMN-PT	E-solder 3022
	Thickness (µm)	16	24	92.5	980

2.3   Impedance Matching Network

Since the performance of the ultrasound transducer mainly depends on the energy transfer, the internal resistance of the ultrasonic actuator is mostly 50 Ω; while the ultrasonic transducer has different impedances of each transducer due to the different conditions of the process, in order to make the ultrasonic wave To achieve maximum performance, we use an L-type impedance matching circuit. We used the Agilent 4294 A to measure the impedance of the ultrasonic transducer, select the impedance value at the resonant frequency, and then design the impedance matching circuit by SMITH CHART to achieve 50 Ω ∠ 0° at the resonant frequency.

Figure 1 is the miniaturization impedance matching network.

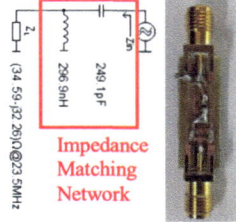

Fig. 1. Matching network design and circuit

2.4   Optical Tracking System

The optical sensor is mainly composed of four core components, which are a light-emitting diode, a lens assembly, an optical engine, and a control wafer (Fig. 2).

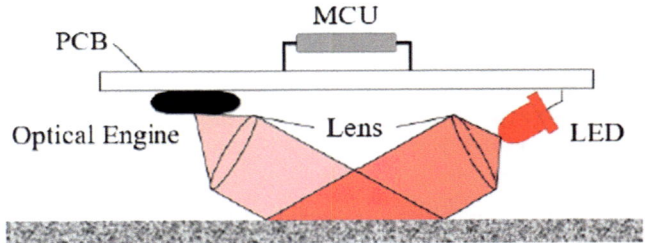

Fig. 2. Structure of optical tracking system

When the sensor moves, the imaging sensor records a continuous pattern, and then analyzes the front and back of each picture through a "digital signal processor" (DSP) to determine the direction and displacement of the sensor. This gives the value of the movement in the x, y direction of the sensor. It is then transmitted to the sensor's Micro Controller Unit via the SPI. The processor of the sensor processes these values and passes them to the host computer. The traditional photodetector sampling frequency is about 2000 Frames/sec, which means that it can only acquire and process 2000 images in one second.

3   Experiment and Discussion

3.1   Transducer Specifications

The skin imaging transducer requires a high frequency to increase the axial resolution. Therefore, the 20 MHz PMN-PT is used, and the Superficial Musculo-Aponeurotic System (SMAS) layer is about 4.5 mm below the skin. To remove the excitation oscillation generated by the ultrasonic excitation and protect the transducer, a layer is placed in front of the transducer. 1 mm Ultrasonic gel pad (Parker Laboratories Inc.), so the design focus distance is 5.5 mm (Table 2).

Table 2. Specifications of transducer

Frequency	20.0 MHz
Diameter	1.3 mm
Focal distance	5.49 mm
Beam width (−6 dB)	0.35 mm
Field depth (−6 dB)	From 3.65 mm
	To 10.96 mm

3.2   Free-Hand Single Element Ultrasound Transducer System

The ultrasound transducer is excited by the pulse wave transmitting receiver (pana-metrix 5800PR, Olympus) to receive the analog signal, and then converted from the analog signal to the digital signal by the oscilloscope (HDO4034-ND, Teledyne LeCroy) to the computer for signal processing, and the optical sensor Transfer mobile information via Bluetooth to the computer for integration.

The free-hand single-element scanning transducer has built-in Bluetooth 3.0 to transmit the optical tracking sensor's mobile information to the computer. No additional wiring is required. Simply attach an optical tracking sensor to the existing transducer to facilitate the experiment (Fig. 3).

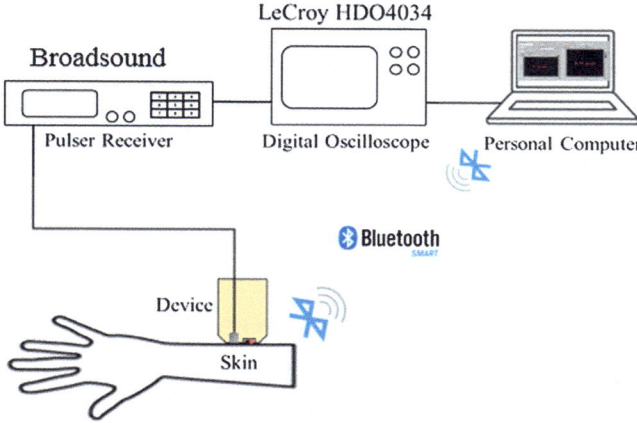

Fig. 3. System architecture

3.3   System Software Architecture

In the software part, use LabVIEW from National Instruments as a program development tool.

The system is executed in a personal computer, and the programmable control hardware is an optical sensor and an oscilloscope, and digitally analyzes the data collected by the hardware listed above, and draws images of different modes and displays them on the program, as shown in the Fig. 4.

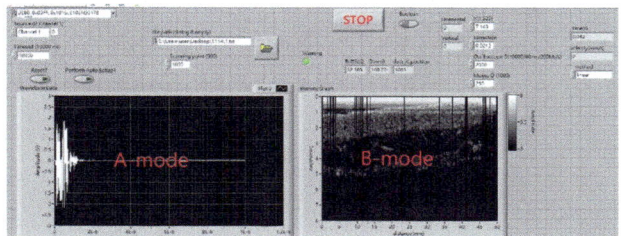

Fig. 4. Interface of LabVIEW program

3.4   Algorithm

The free-hand scanning system, unlike motor scanning, can move at a constant speed, so that each data has the same displacement and easy movement with different speeds and accelerations. In order to solve this problem, we use optical sensors to detect the moving distance. The system uses the displacement value detected by the optical sensor, and then obtains the correct signal position by conversion. According to the different speeds caused by the handheld scanning, each data can be displayed in the correct position.

The system first initializes a fixed matrix, the X axis is the echo signal, the Y axis is the number of sampling points of the oscilloscope, the absolute position of the signal is converted by the displacement value obtained from the optical sensor, and the echo signal is processed into the phase. The corresponding position constitutes a B-mode image.

The displacement value detected by the optical sensor is its resolution, which is not the actual distance. It must be converted to the actual distance value.

4   Result and Conclusion

4.1   Ultrasound Transducer Performance Verification

The Free-hand holder is designed and fabricated, as shown in Fig. 5(a). To avoid the block which caused by conductive jelly, the optical tracking is mounted which adjacent to the imaging transducer but not in the path of motion. The sensor is used to track the position directly and precisely. The Lead Magnesium Neonate-Lead Titanate (PMN-PT) crystal is used as an active layer in this transducer. This transducer has the highly sensitive to pick the reflected US signal. The Parylene layer and the mixed of 301-1 and Au powder spray as a matching layer to reduce the interface reflection. Furthermore, E-solder 3022 is used as a backing layer to increase the damping ratio to reduce the residual oscillation. The echo signal and spectrum is displayed in Fig. 5(b).The impendence match circuit is used for the performance enhancement, as shown in Fig. 5(c).

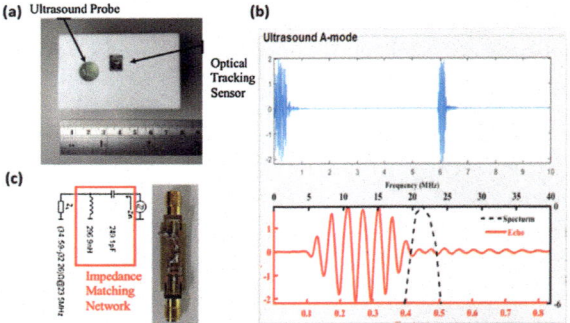

Fig. 5. (a) Appearance of device (b) Fast Fourier Transform of ultrasonic signal (c) Matching network design and circuit

According to the geometrical size and theoretical calculation, the spatial resolution and Depth of Field (DOF) is 0.35 mm and 5 mm. The bandwidth could be increase from 15% to 25% after the impendence matching circuit, as shown in table. It implied that the dermatologic tissue is located in the reasonable range of the transducer.

4.2   Resin-Phantom Testing

The resin-phantom, as shown in Fig. 6(a) which made by 3D Stereolithography (SLA) method is used to verify the feasibility before the scan on human skin. We can use this test to know the resolution of the single element transducer. The Fig. 6(b) shows the regular wave for the phantom. This image shows that this single element transducer has a good resolution.

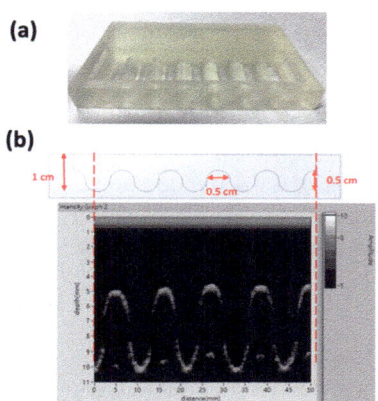

Fig. 6. (a) 3D Stereolithography phantom (b) Scan result of phantom

4.3   Result of Skin Image

There are three layers may be distinguished in human skin: epidermal echo, dermis and subcutaneous issue, which correspond to the anatomical structure. Figure 7 is the scanning image in the arm. It shows the structure of skin from epidermis to subcutaneous tissue. In the surface to below 1 mm. The texture could be clearly observed. In the range of below 1 mm is Epidermis. In the range of below 2 mm to 3 mm is dermis layer, the partial sweat gland, sebaceous gland and hairy are revealed blurrily. In the range of below 4 mm is superficial muscular aponeurotic system (SMAS).

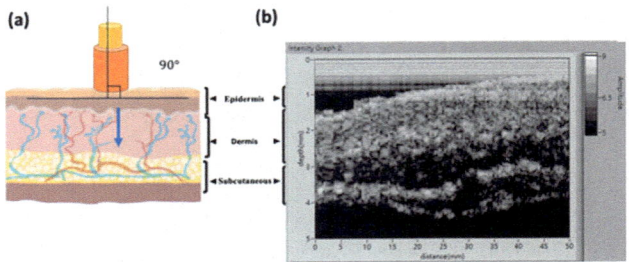

Fig. 7. (a) Structure of skin (b) Scan result of Arm

The face has the characteristic of the high-curved. In order to avoid images distortion, the transducer must be scanned vertical for 90°. Thus, it is difficult to scan using the conventional 1D motor. Figure 8(b) is the US scanning image in the face with the frequency of 20 MHz. Our approach could approach the real curve on the face. The anatomy diagram, as shown in Fig. 8(a), shows the human skin and subcutaneous tissue, but unlike arm scanning, the superficial muscular aponeurotic system (SMAS) layer of the skin scan is exceptionally obvious. SMAS has been mainly located between 4–6 mm under the skin. It is extended by multiple fibers. The dermis layer of epidermis and subcutaneous tissue and muscle of the underlying layer will be responsible for the contraction of facial muscles to the skin-conducting role to maintain facial contours.

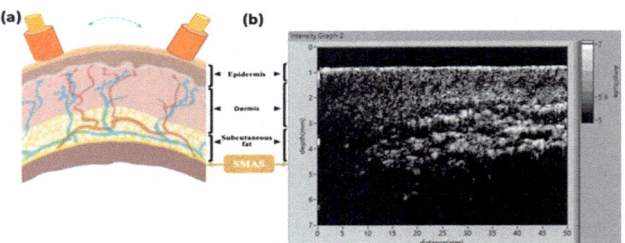

Fig. 8. (a) Structure of skin (b) Scan result of Face

This study develops a free-hand single element ultrasound transducer system using optical tracking method for skin imaging. In the results, the texture of the skin can be clearly seen, and the optical tracking system is used to instantly and correctly form the B-mode image to achieve the goal of precise positioning.

The skin in the human body is uneven, and this system can be used to successfully scan and accurately image, making it easier to observe skin tissue.

In the future, we hope to integrate the system and make the system more complete.

Conflict of Interest. The authors declare that they have no conflict of interest.

Reference

1. Kuhl, C.K., Schrading, S., Leutner, C.C., Morakkabati-Spitz, N., Wardelmann, E., Fimmers, R., Kuhn, W., Schild, H.H.: J. Clin. Oncol. **20**, 8469–8476 (2005)
2. Branney, S.W., Moore, E.E., Cantrill, S.V., Burch, J.M., Terry, S.J.: BSN. J. Trauma Injury Infect. Crit. Care **42**(6), 1086–1090 (1997)
3. Yano, T., Fukukita, H., Ueno, S., Fukumoto, A.: 40 MHz ultrasound diagnostic system for dermatologic examination. In: IEEE Ultrasonics Symposium Proceeding, pp. 875–878 (1987)
4. Garcia-Garcia, H.M., Gogas, B.D., Serruys, P.W., Bruining, N.: IVUS-based imaging modalities for tissue characterization: similarities and differences. Int. J. Cardiovasc. Imaging (2011)
5. Tikjøb, G., Kassis, V., Søndergaard, J.: Ultrasonic B-scanning of the human skin. An introduction of a new ultrasonic skin-scanner. Acta Derm Venereol. **64**(1), 67–70 (1984)
6. Dines, K.A., Sheets, P.W., Brink, J.A., Hanke, C.W., Condra, K.A., Clendenon, J.L., et al.: High frequency ultrasonic imaging of skin: experimental results. Ultrason. Imaging (1984)
7. Yano, T., Fukukita, H., Ueno, S., Fukumoto, A.: 40 MHz ultrasound diagnostic system for dermatologic examination. In: IEEE Ultrasonics Symposium Proceeding (1987)
8. Mozaffari, M.H., Lee, W.-S.: Freehand 3-D ultrasound imaging: a systematic review (2017)
9. Alfageme Roldán, F.: Ultrasound Skin Imaging. Actas Dermo-Sifiliográficas **105**(10), 891–899 (2014)
10. Ng, T.W.: The optical mouse as a two-dimensional displacement sensor. Sens. Actuators A **107**, 21–25 (2003)
11. Zhou, Q., Xu, X.: PMN-PT single crystal, high-frequency ultrasonic needle transducers for pulsed-wave doppler application. IEEE Trans. Ultrason. Ferroelectr. Freq. Control **54**(3) (2007)

Ultrasonography Classification of Obstructive Sleep Apnea (OSA) Through Dynamic Tongue Base Motion Tracking and Tongue Area Measurements

Cyrel Ontimare Manlises[1,2], Jeng-Wen Chen[3,4], and Chih-Chung Huang[1(✉)]

[1] Department of Biomedical Engineering, National Cheng Kung University, Tainan, Taiwan
cchuang@mail.ncku.edu.tw
[2] School of Electrical, Electronics, and Computer Engineering, Mapúa University, Manila, Philippines
[3] Department of Otolaryngology–Head and Neck Surgery, Cardinal Tien Hospital, New Taipei City, Taiwan
[4] School of Medicine, Fu Jen Catholic University, New Taipei City, Taiwan

Abstract. Obstructive sleep apnea (OSA) is a chronic breathing disorder that most of the time people are oblivious of the symptoms which may delay the diagnosis and may lead to long-term health consequences such as cardiovascular and cerebrovascular diseases. Ultrasonography is currently used to discern the real behavior of the upper airway (UA) in patients with OSA. However, previous methods were not enough to reveal the possible pathophysiology and biomechanics of the human UA. The aim of this study is to use the modified optical flow (OF)-based method in tracking the dynamic tongue base motion, utilizing nine tracking points, to effectively classify which group each subject belongs to. The classification groups are normal, mild, moderate, and severe OSA. A total of 82 participants were enrolled in this study. All of them had their B-mode ultrasound image sequences obtained for 10 s. The first 5 s was recorded during eupneic breathing, and the latter part was during the performance of the Müller Maneuver (MM), a simulation of the collapse of the UA while inducing negative pressure. The results demonstrate that the four classifications are significantly different ($p < 0.05$). The normal group has the largest displacement, while the severe OSA group has the smallest. The normal group has the smallest tongue base area (TBA), while the severe OSA group has the largest. Both instances were also observed during the MM. Tongue area measurement during the eupneic breathing for the four groups are 18.63 ± 2.595, 20.25 ± 2.366, 20.34 ± 3.207, and 21.75 ± 2.764, respectively. During the MM, the measurements were 18.54 ± 2.701, 20.16 ± 2.428, 20.32 ± 3.190, and 21.78 ± 2.820, respectively. Noninvasive sonographic evaluation using dynamic tongue motion tracking and tongue area measurements provides quantitative assessments that can be used by the clinician to indicate individualized treatment plan for each OSA patients.

© Springer Nature Switzerland AG 2020
K.-P. Lin et al. (Eds.): ICBHI 2019, IFMBE Proceedings 74, pp. 100–107, 2020.
https://doi.org/10.1007/978-3-030-30636-6_14

Keywords: Obstructive sleep apnea · Modified optical flow-based method · Medical ultrasound · Tongue motion · OSA classification

1 Introduction

Snoring, choking, or gasping for air while sleeping are mostly disregarded because these symptoms are just being attributed to fatigue, and obesity [1–3]. Around 70 to 80% of people are usually oblivious of these symptoms, which may delay the diagnosis and lead to a more serious medical condition [1, 2]. Crucial complications of obstructive sleep apnea (OSA), if not treated immediately in relation to its level of severity, are predominantly cardiovascular diseases [4]. In many different countries and primarily in approximately 3 to 7% of men, this breathing disorder is constantly increasing and pervasive [1, 2, 5]. However, only few can perceive the consequences of having OSA [6]. OSA is a breathing disorder where episodes of apneas and hypopneas occur repeatedly lasting 10 s or more during sleep [7–9]. Sleep study, otherwise known as polysomnography (PSG), plays an important part in diagnosing OSA, as the former is considered the gold standard in the identification of this phenomenon. The patient spends a night at the sleep center of hospitals to establish exactly the level of severity and the physiological state of their body condition. The Apnea-Hypopnea Index (AHI) is one of the PSG metrics that predicts the level of severity of OSA [1]. However, PSG could not provide the biomechanics of the human upper airway (UA), which may be used to discern the possible pathophysiology of OSA. Upon the definition of the dynamic human UA anatomy, biomechanics and pathophysiology will be revealed, and can be further used for the provision of treatment strategies [10, 11].

An imaging modality such as ultrasonography, is currently integrated with PSG to provide a more effective evaluation of the UA in OSA patients. Ultrasonography was able to unveil the anatomic structure and localize the site of occlusion of human UA [9]. Tracking of the dynamic tongue base motion was concluded, and the research was able to indicate biomechanics of the UA and possible pathophysiology of OSA, and provide effect on the diagnosis and management of OSA [8, 9]. The difference in the tongue base motion (TBM) and tongue base area (TBA), during eupneic breathing and after performance of the Müller Maneuver (MM) was ascertained [8]. The MM is a simulation during wakefulness where negative pressure is induced and will cause the collapse and obstruction in the human UA. The MM is also a widely used index in identifying site of obstruction in OSA patients [11, 12]. The distinction between normal and OSA patients when using ultrasonography is perceptible, nevertheless the level of severity is yet to be determined, hence the purpose of this study. Knowing the level of severity of OSA provides more chances in getting specific information and could help the physician to decide which treatment strategy is more appropriate in addressing the level of condition [8].

Using ultrasonography, different optical (OF) methods and approaches were used to track and estimate complex motions in anatomy, such as movement of the heart and blood vessels [13]. Dynamic tongue base motion is variable and more complex, resulting in the development of a modified optical flow (OF)-based method. This modified method has been concluded successfully. It has been used to evaluate the UA and was utilized to distinguish the difference between normal and OSA patients [8]. This study will use the method to distinguish among the four groups of patients, namely normal, mild OSA, moderate OSA, and severe OSA. A 3.5 MHz commercial curve array transducer was used as it is the best tool for deep part measurement, resulting in the measurement of the submental midline sagittal section. A total of eighty-two participants, including 29 normal, 15 mild, 16 moderate, and 22 severe OSA patients, were prospectively enrolled in this study.

2   Materials and Methods

2.1   Study Population

The population for this study was all recruited by the sleep clinic of the Cardinal Tien hospital in Taiwan. A written informed consent from each participants, who should at least be twenty-years old, was obtained. The study was approved by the institutional ethics board committee of the Cardinal Tien hospital. It was also confirmed that each patient received no prior OSA treatment, no history of craniofacial abnormalities, had no craniofacial surgery, no oropharyngeal or laryngeal masses, no burns, trauma or radiotherapy nor active inflammation in the head and neck region, and no other neurologic disorder except OSA. Table 1 shows the summary of the clinical, and demographic data of the study population. The apnea-hypopnea index (AHI) of each patient was measured using standard PSG.

Table 1.   Clinical and demographic data of study population

Parameters	Normal	Mild	Moderate	Severe
Population	29	15	16	22
Gender (M/F)	20/9	10/5	12/4	16/6
Age	55.5 ± 14.2 (29–80)	51.1 ± 13.1 (30–76)	54.6 ± 13.0 (20–69)	49.7 ± 12.4 (26–71)
Weight (kg)	63.1 ± 20.7	75.9 ± 8.3	77.3 ± 17.3	84.7 ± 13.9
NC (cm)	37.7 ± 3.9	38.60 ± 2.3	40.2 ± 3.6	42.2 ± 3.6
AHI	0.8 ± 1.4	9.9 ± 3.3	21.1 ± 4.5	65.5 ± 21.2

M/F = Male/Female; NC = Neck Circumference; AHI = Apnea-Hypopnea Index

2.2   B-Mode Ultrasound Image

While lying in supine position, a 3.5 MHz commercial curve array transducer was placed on the submental midline sagittal section between the hyoid bone and the symphysis of the mandible of each participant. Figure 1a shows how the measurement was performed. The participants were given directions on what to do during the measurement such as to remain still, not swallowing, not talking, and not moving their tongue. An experienced sonographer performed the proper ultrasound procedure from which the transducer was adjusted until a clear curvilinear hyper-echoic stripe of the air–mucosa interface of the tongue base appeared [8, 11]. The recording lasts for ten seconds. The first five seconds was during the eupneic breathing and the subsequent five was during the MM. All participants were given instructions and demonstration on how to perform the MM. Nine tracking points (the blue arrows) were selected from the air–mucosa interface of the tongue base (the red line) to track its motion, as seen on Fig. 1b.

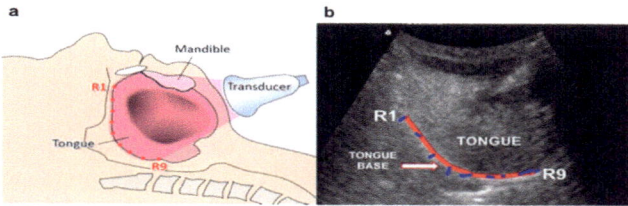

Fig. 1. (a) Submental ultrasound measurement set-up (b) The B-mode ultrasound image of the tongue with 9 tracking points

2.3 Modified Optical Flow (OF)-Based Method

In traditional optical flow (OF) methods such as the Lucas-Kanade method, the motion vector is assumed to be constant within a local window. Tongue base motion is considered hypermobile; and, the locally constant model was not enough to track the tongue base motion, hence the use of a *spatiotemporal-affine model* instead. This method was used to capture local accelerations that are more powerful compared to those captured using the traditional OF method. Additionally, estimation can also be based in multiple frames around a given time point. Large motions such as in the tongue base are difficult to track and are estimated at a fine scale. To address this challenge, the *coarse-to-fine strategy* in space was also applied.

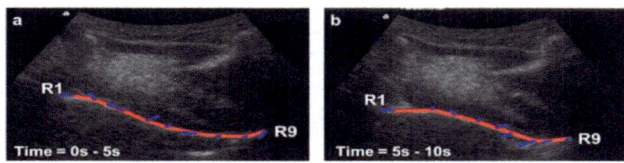

Fig. 2. Tongue base contour during (a) eupneic breathing (b) Müller maneuver

The estimated motion at the coarsest spatial scale will transfer the motion vector to the next finest resolution level, and this will serve as the initial estimate through the use of linear interpolation. Linear interpolation will provide values about the intermediate grid locations. *Geometric moments* and *iterative offset strategy* were added at the latter part of the method to obtain coarser resolution levels, and to estimate large motions more accurately [8, 14].

2.4 Statistical Analysis

One-way ANOVA was used to express all the data in mean ± standard deviation (SD). To determine differences between tracking points, Fisher Pairwise was used. The latter was also used to analyze differences between TBAs of the four groups. The statistical significance was accepted at $p < 0.05$.

3 Results

3.1 Tongue Base Motion Measurements

A modified OF-based method was used to track the nine points which represent the contour of the tongue base. The tongue base contour changed from eupneic breathing (during the first 5 s) to MM (during the last 5 s). As an effect of the performance of MM, Figs. 2a and b demonstrate representative changes in the tongue base contour of a severe OSA patient.

Nine tracking points (R1 to R9), which are presented by different colors, demonstrate the estimated displacement curves that correspond to the tongue base motion. The displacements from each of the groups were estimated in three different terms: lateral (x-direction), axial (z-direction), and total displacement of the nine tracking points.

Total displacement of the nine tracking points was computed using the equation

$$Total\ displacement = \sqrt{D_x^2 + D_z^2} \tag{1}$$

where D_x is the displacement in the x-direction or the lateral displacement, and D_z is the displacement in the z-direction or the axial displacement. Figure 3 shows the estimated displacement motion of the tongue base of a normal patient with respect to time. The negative displacement in lateral movement signifies motion towards the mandible, while in axial movement, it signifies decrease in the size of the tongue base thickness (TBT). Figures 4, 5 and 6 show the estimated displacement motion of the tongue base of mild, moderate, and severe OSA patients with respect to time. The total displacement curves of the four classifications demonstrate that a normal patient has the larger tongue base deformation, while a severe OSA patient has the smallest tongue base deformation. Both of the said instances were observed during the MM, as also claimed by the previous research [8]. A Mild OSA patient has less tongue base deformation compared to a normal patient, while a moderate OSA patient has less deformation compared to a mild OSA patient.

The mean maximum total displacement of the nine tracking points of the four groups were also obtained for comparison and provide more detailed information. Statistically, measurements of the four groups are significantly different at $p < 0.05$. The result demonstrated that tracking points R4 to R6 are significantly different between the normal and severe OSA groups, as also shown by the previous research [8]. Tracking point R8 is also significantly different between the mild and severe OSA groups.

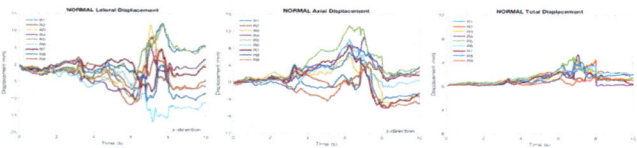

Fig. 3. Normal patient's estimated displacement of nine tracking points (a) Lateral (b) Axial (c) Total displacement

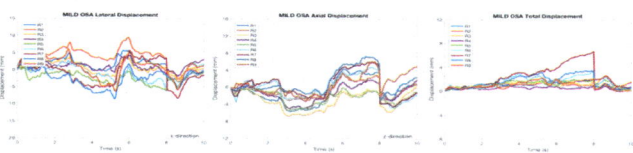

Fig. 4. Mild OSA patient's estimated displacement of nine tracking points (a) Lateral (b) Axial (c) Total displacement

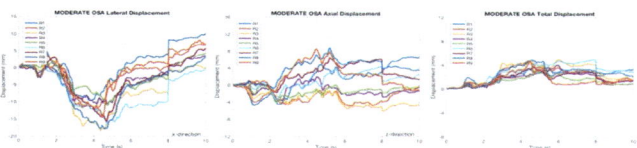

Fig. 5. Moderate OSA group mean estimated displacement of nine tracking points (a) Lateral (b) Axial (c) Total displacement

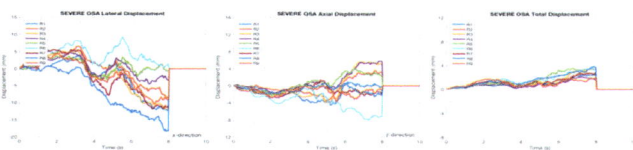

Fig. 6. Severe OSA group mean estimated displacement of nine tracking points (a) Lateral (b) Axial (c) Total displacement

3.2   Tongue Base Area Measurements

The TBA was also measured during the eupneic breathing and after the MM to provide quantitative analysis of the tongue motion. It was measured from the submental section to the tongue base contour as seen on Figs. 7a and b, which also show the changes in the TBA from eupneic breathing to MM.

Sample tongue area variations were illustrated in Fig. 8. Tongue area measurements between the four groups are significantly different at $p < 0.05$. Tongue area measurements during the eupneic breathing for the four groups (normal, mild, moderate, and severe OSA) were 18.63 ± 2.595, 20.25 ± 2.366, 20.34 ± 3.207, and

21.75 ± 2.764, respectively. While during the MM, the measurements were 18.54 ± 2.701, 20.16 ± 2.428, 20.32 ± 3.190, and 21.78 ± 2.820, respectively. It was observed that the normal group has the significantly smallest TBA, while the severe OSA group has the larger TBA among the four groups.

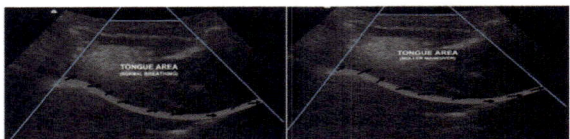

Fig. 7. Tongue area after (a) eupneic breathing (b) Müller maneuver of a severe patient

The sizes of the normal and severe OSA groups are equally the smallest and largest during eupneic breathing and after the MM, as also reinforced by the previous research [8].

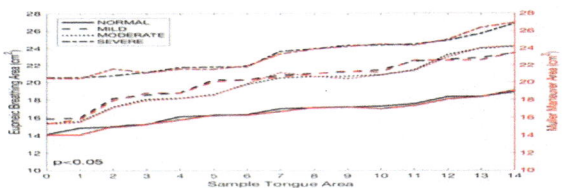

Fig. 8. Tongue area variations between eupneic breathing and MM

4   Conclusions

Tongue base motion is considered hypermobile, thus tracking its motion is extremely challenging. It was also realized that a modified OF-based method is the key to address the challenge in tracking an intense motion. The researchers concluded that a modified OF-based method can effectively demonstrate the differences between the nine tracking points among the four groups of patients with or without OSA, with polysomnography and AHI as the reference standard. It has been proven that the four groups, namely the normal, mild, moderate, and severe OSA were significantly different from each other at $p < 0.05$. Tracking points R4 to R6 are most deformed during the MM in the normal group as compared to the severe OSA group, while tracking point R8 is significantly deformed during the MM in the mild group as compared to the severe OSA group. The racking technique of the modified OF-based method was also used successfully to precisely measure the TBAs during the transition from the eupneic breathing to the MM. The TBAs were smallest in the normal group during the eupneic breathing and the MM, while it is largest in the severe OSA group during the eupneic breathing and during the MM. The results were validated through previous researches.

Acknowledgment. This study was supported by the Ministry of Science and Technology of the Republic of China (Taiwan) under grant MOST 106-2314-B-567-001 and, in part, funded by Cardinal Tien Hospital under grant CTH-107B-2A28 and CTH108B-2A33. No additional external funding was received for this study. The authors are grateful for administrative assistance on this project provided by Chiu-Ping Wang, Shu-Hwei Fan and Po-Cheng Yang. The authors also thank the staff of the Center for Sleep Disorders, Division of Pulmonary Medicine and Department of Medical Imaging of Catholic Cardinal Tien Hospital, for their technical support. They received no additional compensation for their contributions.

Conflict of Interest. The authors declare that they have no conflict of interest.

References

1. Punjabi, N.M.: The epidemiology of adult obstructive sleep apnea. Proc. Am. Thorac. Soc. **5**, 136–143 (2008)
2. Patil, S.P., Schneider, H., Schwartz, A.R., Smith, P.L.: Adult obstructive sleep apnea: pathophysiology and diagnosis. Chest **132**, 325–327 (2007)
3. Gami, A.S., Caples, S.M., Somers, V.K.: Obesity and obstructive sleep apnea. Endocrinol. Metab. Clin. North Am. **32**, 869–894 (2003)
4. Hiestand, D.M., Britz, P., Goldman, M., Phillips, B.: Prevalence of symptoms and risk of sleep apnea in the US population: results from the national sleep foundation sleep in America 2005 poll. Chest **130**, 780–786 (2006)
5. Coughlin, S.R., Mawdsley, L., Mugarza, J.A., Calverley, P.M.A., Wilding, J.P.H.: Obstructive sleep apnoea is independently associated with an increased prevalence of metabolic syndrome. Eur. Heart J. **25**, 735–741 (2004)
6. Stores, G.: Clinical diagnosis and misdiagnosis of sleep disorders. J. Neurol. Neurosurg. Psychiatry **78**, 1293–1297 (2007)
7. Xu, C., Brennick, M.J., Wootton, D.M.: Image-based three-dimensional finite element modeling approach for upper airway mechanics. In: 2005 IEEE Engineering in Medicine and Biology 27th Annual Conference (2006)
8. Chien, C.Y., Chen, J.W., Chang, C.H., Huang, C.C.: Tracking dynamic tongue motion in ultrasound images for obstructive sleep apnea. Ultrasound Med. Biol. **43**, 2791–2805 (2017)
9. Weng, C.K., Chen, J.W., Huang, C.C.: A FPGA-based wearable ultrasound device for monitoring obstructive sleep apnea syndrome. In: 2015 IEEE International Ultrasonics Symposium, IUS 2015 (2015)
10. Faber, C.E., Grymer, L.: Available techniques for objective assessment of upper airway narrowing in snoring and sleep apnea. Sleep and Breath. **7**, 77–86 (2003)
11. Chen, J.W., Chang, C.H., Wang, S.J., Chang, Y.T., Huang, C.C.: Submental ultrasound measurement of dynamic tongue base thickness in patients with obstructive sleep apnea. Ultrasound Med. Biol. **40**, 2590–2598 (2014)
12. Mattos Soares, M.C., Raposo Sallum, A.C., Moraes Gonçalves, M.T., Martinho Haddad, F. L., Gregório, L.C.: Use of muller's maneuver in the evaluation of patients with sleep apnea - literature review. Braz. J. Otorhinolaryngol. **75**, 463–466 (2009)
13. Duan, Q., et al.: Region-based endocardium tracking on real-time three-dimensional ultrasound. Ultrasound Med. Biol. **35**, 256–265 (2009)
14. Sühling, M., Arigovindan, M., Jansen, C., Hunziker, P., Unser, M.: Myocardial motion analysis from B-mode echocardiograms. IEEE Trans. Image Process. **14**, 525–536 (2005)

A Novel Multi-direction Adjustment Strategy for Reducing Ghost Artifact in Body Tomosynthesis

Yu-Ching Ni[1,2(✉)], Chia-Yu Lin[1], Chia-Hao Chang[1], Fan-Pin Tseng[1], Sheng-Pin Tseng[1], and Keh-Shih Chuang[2]

[1] Health Physics, Institute of Nuclear Energy Research, 1000 Wenhua Road Jiaan Village, Longtan District, Taoyuan, Taiwan (ROC)
janet@iner.gov.tw
[2] Department of Biomedical Engineering and Environmental Sciences, National Tsing-Hua University, Hsinchu, Taiwan (ROC)

Abstract. Digital tomosynthesis (DT) reduces tissue overlap and provides tomographic images of high quality with clinically acceptable low radiation dose, it begins to be recognized as an essential diagnostic tool. The scanning direction and model are more flexible in DT. However, scanning parameters of DT are not easy to be determined. In this study, we investigated the effect of dual direction scanning on artifact improvement and the optimization of scanning parameters using the INER Prototype Tomosynthesis scanner. The line-pair shape phantom with 2, 3, 5, 8, 10, 15 mm line widths and 5 mm thickness was used. The projections were acquired with 31 views over a 15° angular range in HF (Head-Foot) direction and RL (Right-left) direction, respectively. 3D images were reconstructed with ML-EM algorithm to evaluate the spread range of ghost artifact with various sweep methods (HF, RL and Dual) and object sizes. Moreover, the projection number ratios (PNR) in dual directions were also evaluated for the influence on artifacts. Under single direction sweep (HF or RL), the spread range was wide when the sweep direction paralleled with the shape direction of object (SDO); the spread range was narrow when the sweep direction is perpendicular to the SDO. The spread range of dual scan was unaffected by the SDO. The PNR in dual directions revealed a similar trend to single direction sweep when the ratio is not equal to one. Based on the above experimental results, we proposed a novel multi-direction adjustment strategy for body tomosynthesis. For the default scanning, the user should choose the isotropic dual direction scan (PNR = 1). After preview, the advanced process can use different PNR depending on the anatomy of interest to improve diagnostic image quality to reduce ghost artifact and distortion.

Keywords: Tomosynthesis · Ghost artifact · Multi-direction scan · TomoDR · Projection number ratio

© Springer Nature Switzerland AG 2020
K.-P. Lin et al. (Eds.): ICBHI 2019, IFMBE Proceedings 74, pp. 108–114, 2020.
https://doi.org/10.1007/978-3-030-30636-6_15

1 Introduction

Since digital tomosynthesis (DT) reduces tissue overlap and provides tomographic images of high quality under clinically acceptable low radiation dose, it is recognized as an essential diagnostic tool. Aside from breast screening, DT is widely used in many regions of the body with arbitrary patient posture [1–3]. During DT imaging, a series of projection images are acquired with a limited angle. These systems can provide CT-like image quality with depth information and less radiation dose. However, the image quality of the traditional DT is limited due to the use of only single-axis scanning geometry. Some structures parallel to the scanning direction are blurring because of ghost artifact [4, 5].

Taiwan TomoDR is an Institute of Nuclear Energy Research (INER) homemade high-quality 3D X-ray imaging modality which can provide high resolution tomosynthesis image with various depth information using limited angle scanning procedure and self-developed image reconstruction algorithm. The scanning direction and model are more flexible in DT. However, scanning parameters of DT are not easy to be determined. In this study, we investigated the effect of dual direction scanning on artifact improvement and the decision of scanning parameters using Taiwan TomoDR.

2 Materials and Methods

2.1 System Description

Taiwan TomoDR as shown in Fig. 1(a), has flexible multi-direction scanning different from commercial scanners (e.g. Shimadzu Safire 17), with more views (61 projections in Head-Foot direction, 31 projections in Right-Left direction) but less radiation dose (0.27 times compared with Safire 17) in chest exam. This imaging system possesses three main features: (1) multiple axes imaging scan, (2) image processing with optimizing scanning conditions to reduce noise, and (3) high performance iterative reconstruction. The leg images acquired by TomoDR (Fig. 1(b)), commercial scanner (Shimadzu Safire 17 Fig. 1(c)), and traditional radiography (Fig. 1(d)), were compared. Locations of special interest in diagnosis such as tibial fracture, distal ankle, and calcaneus-talbicular joint (yellow arrows), were seen more clearly in TomoDR image with dual axes scan. Both traditional radiography and commercial DT scanner that provides only single axis scan had similar performance and were unable to distinguish fractures and joint locations clearly.

3D images were reconstructed using maximum likelihood expectation maximization (ML-EM) algorithm in a $1024 \times 1024 \times 200$ matrix with a $0.5 \times 0.5 \times 0.5$ mm^3 voxel size.

2.2 Phantom Design and Experiment Setup

In order to assess the image quality of the reconstructed images with ghost artifact, we designed a digital phantom with different test objects as shown in Fig. 2. The phantom consists of three major parts, including one circle object, two sets of line pair objects

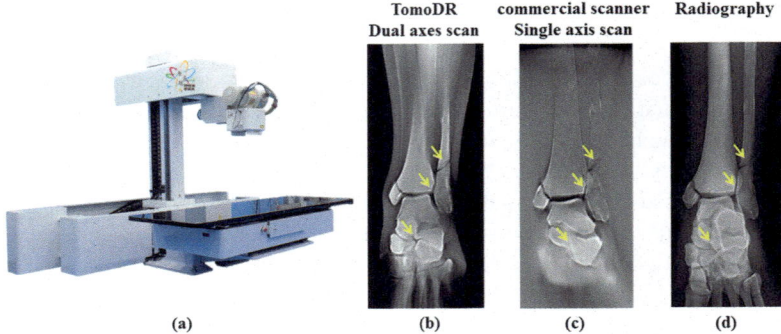

Fig. 1. Appearance of TomoDR and the leg images of different imagers.

(RL-direction and HF-direction), and six groups of pecks objects. The line width of the circle object is 1 mm, and the thickness is 5 mm. The widths of line-pair shape phantom are 2, 3, 5, 8, 10, and 15 mm and the thickness is also 5 mm. The diameter of two sets of peck objects are 2, 3, 5 mm. All objects are made from lead.

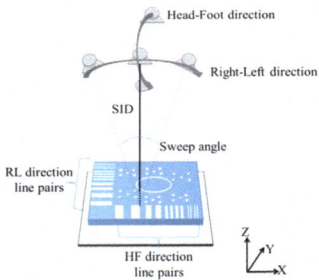

Fig. 2. The geometric setup of imaging the digital phantom.

For the system configurations in the simulated studies, the source to image detector distance (SID) is 1100 mm, the rotation isocenter is on the center of the image detector surface. During the images acquisition process, both the object and the image receptor are stationary, and only the X-ray source moves along head-foot (HF) axis and right-left (RL) axis, respectively. The image detector is a 3072 × 3072 flat panel detector with 0.139 × 0.139 mm^2 pixel size and binning mode of 2 are used. The scanning protocol designs three sweep methods. The HF sweep method is the X-ray source position moving from −7.5° to +7.5° in the HF axis scanning direction. The RL sweep method is similar but in different scanning direction. The dual sweep method combined both HF and RL methods. The projections acquired 31 views over a 15° angular range in all methods. The detail parameters of each sweep methods were listed in Table 1.

Table 1. The imaging parameters of the experiment.

Parameter	Sweep method		
	Head-Foot	Right-Left	Dual
Sweep angle	Head-Foot direction 15°(-7.5°~7.5°)	Right-Left direction 15°(-7.5°~7.5°)	Head-Foot direction 15°(-7.5°~7.5°) Right-Left direction 15°(-7.5°~7.5°)
Projection number	31	31	62
Projection density	2/degree	2/degree	2/degree
Source to image detector distance(SID) (mm)	1110		
Detector matrix size	1536x1536		
Detector pixel size	0.278x0.278 mm²		
Image matrix size	1024x1024x200		
Image pixel size	0.5x0.5x0.5 mm³		
Reconstruction iteration number	40		

2.3   Data Analysis

First, to observe qualitatively the digital phantom with different test objects, including clearly imaged and distortion on focal plane image (X-Y plane) of difference between the single-axis scan (HF and RL) and the dual-axes scan. Then to select the Y-Z plane of the object observed the phenomenon of ghost artifact and quantitatively calculated the line pairs using full width at half maximum (FWHM) to evaluate the range of the artifact spread.

In addition, the dual sweep method can select different number of projections for different sweep directions. The definition of the projection number ratio (PNR) in two axes direction is as follows:

$$\text{Projection number ratio} = \frac{projection\ number\ in\ RL\ direction}{projection\ number\ in\ HF\ direction} \quad (1)$$

3D images of Dual sweep method with various PNR were reconstructed respectively and the ghost artifact and the range of its spread can be compared.

3   Results and Discussions

3.1   Comparison of Single-Axis and Dual-Axes Results

In the focal plane image, all test objects of the digital phantom are clearly seen without distortion. In Y-Z plane image, the extents of ghost artifact in six groups of pecks objects are less obvious. But the circle object and two direction line pairs have similar direction dependence. Therefore, the quantitative analysis is dominated by two sets of line pair objects (RL-direction and HF-direction). Figure 3 shows that even the thicknesses are the same, the bigger objects have more serious spread to out-of-object slices (e.g. Dual scan: 2 mm object becomes 6.81 mm in image; 15 mm object becomes 63.41 mm in image). Besides, the convergent pattern of spread caused by X-ray to image detector beam direction is also shown in Fig. 3.

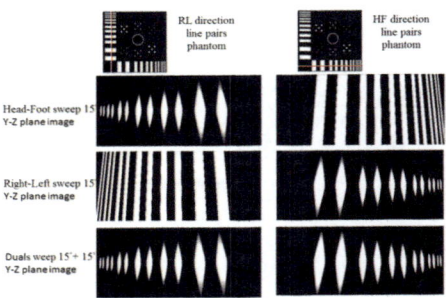

Fig. 3. Y-Z plane images of objects with various shape directions scanned by different sweep methods.

Regardless of HF or RL sweep, the spread range is wide (covering all slices) when the sweep direction is paralleled with the shape direction of object; the spread range is narrow when the sweep direction is perpendicular to the shape direction of object. The spread range of dual scan is unaffected by the shape direction of object (shown in Fig. 4).

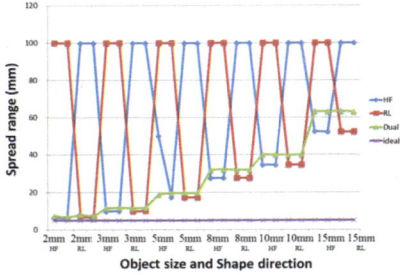

Fig. 4. Spread range of ghost artifact at various object sizes and shape directions.

3.2   Comparison of Dual-Axes with Various PNR

The image of line pair in HF direction is analyzed, and the FWHM of spread range is drawn according to the size of the object for various sweep techniques are shown in

Fig. 5. Compared to PNR = 1, it can be observed that PNR = 2 has a smaller number of total projections, but its image performance in the HF direction is better. This result is in line to the trend of single-axis scan, i.e. the ghost artifact is slighter if the sweep direction is perpendicular to the shape direction of the object. Figure 6 also shows that the image performance is better for PNR = 0.5 when objects are in RL direction.

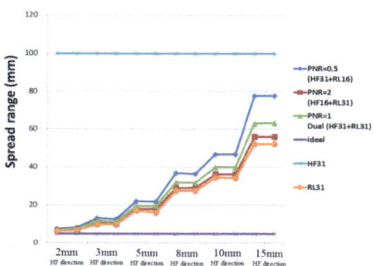

Fig. 5. The relationship of artifact spread range with various size objects in HF direction for various techniques.

It is shown in Figs. 5 and 6 that single-axis scanning (HF or RL) is only advantageous for objects in the vertical direction. For objects in parallel direction the ghost artifact are very serious. However, the dual-axes scanning can be more robust for objects both in vertical and parallel directions. If the PNR were adjusted according to the direction of the object, the artifact can be further reduced to improve the image quality.

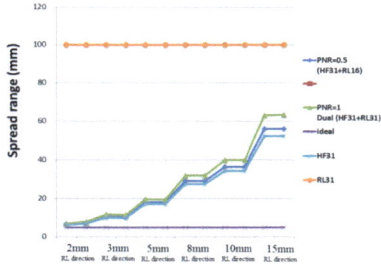

Fig. 6. The relationship of artifact spread range with various size objects in RL direction for various techniques.

4   Conclusions

Based on the above simulated results, we proposed a novel multi-direction adjustment strategy for body tomosynthesis. For the default scanning, the user should choose the isotropic dual direction scan (projection number ratio = 1). After preview, the advanced process can use different projection number ratios depending on the anatomy of interest to improve diagnostic image quality to reduce ghost artifact and distortion.

Conflict of Interest. The authors declare that they have no conflict of interest.

References

1. Dobbins III, J.T., Godfrey, D.J.: Digital x-ray tomosynthesis: current state of the art and clinical potential. Phys. Med. Biol. **48**(19), R65–R106 (2003)
2. Vikgren, J., Zachrisson, S., Svalkvist, A., et al.: Comparison of chest tomosynthesis and chest radiography for detection of pulmonary nodules: human observer study of clinical cases. Radiology **249**(3), 1034–1041 (2008)
3. Gennaro, G., Toledano, A., DiMaggio, C., et al.: Digital breast tomosynthesis versus digital mammography: a clinical performance study. Eur. Radiol. **20**(7), 1545–1553 (2010)
4. Ueno, E., Moribe, Y., Sabol, J.M.: Optimizing parameters for flat-panel detector. Radiographics **30**(2), 549–562 (2010)
5. Zhong, Y., Lai, C.J., Wang, T., et al.: A dual-view digital tomosynthesis imaging technique for improved chest imaging. Med. Phys. **42**(9), 5238–5251 (2015)

Blood Pressure Variation Trend Analysis Based on Model Study

Pei-Ying Chen[1(✉)], Hao-Jen Ting[1], Mei-Fen Chen[1],
Wen-Chen Lin[1,2], and Kang-Ping Lin[1,2]

[1] Department of Electrical Engineering, Chung Yuan Christian University,
Chungli, Taiwan
peggy50231@gmail.com
[2] Technology Translation Center for Medical Device,
Chung-Yuan Christian University, Taoyuan City, Taiwan

Abstract. Hypertension is an important risk factor for stroke and cardiovascular diseases. Ambulatory blood pressure (ABP) measurement is used to estimate the continuous blood pressure. However, the cuff method ABP must have a cuff setting around the upper arm and occluding the arm's blood circulation during the recording period, which makes some of inconveniences, including feel uncomfortable and affects the quality of sleep. The cuff-less method of ABP measurement based on the Pulse Transit Time (PTT) with electrocardiogram (ECG) and photoplethysmogram (PPG) has solved the limitation and presented potential healthcare applications. This study applies five different blood pressure regression models with the major parameter (PTT) and minor parameters (heart rate, pulse wave interval and pulse width) for estimating continuous blood pressure by regression analysis. MIMIC II clinical database is used by the correlation and consistency analysis for different blood pressure models to compare the similarity of the real and estimated blood pressure variation. The best model among the applied blood pressure models is $PTT_{ALL} - BP$ that can perform the average correlation in 0.87 and the average RRratio in 0.68. The blood pressure regression model of $PTT_{ALL} - BP$ provides a successful analysis model for the estimation of long-term monitoring blood pressure trend. monitor for the real and estimated blood pressure have the same trend.

Keywords: Blood pressure variability · Pulse arrival time ·
Cuff-less blood pressure measurement

1 Introduction

Hypertension is a major factor for cardiovascular diseases. Clinical research indicates that the middle-aged person who ages from forty to sixty-nine years. That systolic blood pressure (SBP) rises of 20 mm Hg or diastolic blood pressure (DBP) rises of 10 mm Hg, who will associate with more than a twofold difference in the stroke or cardiovascular disease death rate [1]. According to *American Heart Association (AHA)* guideline was published in 2017 [2], which revised down high blood pressure values. The SBP values were decreased to 130 mmHg and DBP to 80 mmHg, this step hope

© Springer Nature Switzerland AG 2020
K.-P. Lin et al. (Eds.): ICBHI 2019, IFMBE Proceedings 74, pp. 115–121, 2020.
https://doi.org/10.1007/978-3-030-30636-6_17

that the hypertension can manage blood pressure early. The proportion of hypertension who in America is from 32% to 46%.

Circadian rhythm of blood pressure is also a topic that has been widely explored. In different day, blood pressure variation has many characters. Several papers pointed out that normal blood pressure in nighttime will drop by 10–20% of the daytime blood pressure. And, if the nighttime blood pressure drops little or increases, the population of this group has the higher risk of stroke [3, 4]. These evidences have not difficult to find that the stroke risk is more dependent on the blood pressure variation of the day and night [5].

At present, the cuff-less method of blood pressure measurement has features, such as sleeveless, non-invasive, non-inductive and wearable device. The principle of blood pressure is estimated by the negative correlation between blood pressure and Pulse Transit Time (PTT) [6]. PTT decreases while blood pressure rises, and vice versa. And also show about distance that PTT divided by time was called Pulse Wave Velocity (PWV). The value of PTT is measured by Electrocardiogram (ECG) and Photo-plethysmogram (PPG).

In 1878, Moens and Korteweg were established M–K equation models (formula 1) [7]. All of the above show that the relationship between PTT, PWV and BP about the physiology are important factors for arterial wall thickness, blood elastic and blood vessel diameter.

$$PWV = \frac{L}{PTT} = \sqrt{\frac{tE_0 e^{\alpha P}}{\rho d}} \tag{1}$$

Where, L = blood vessel length, t = vascular wall thickness, d = vessel diameter, ρ = blood density, $E0$ = elastic modulus, α = blood vessel modulus, P = blood pressure.

Blood pressure regression models have been continuously proposed, most of that theory extends for time delays or the parameter about correction blood pressure, such as, Xiang's formula in Eq. (2) [8]. Some literatures suggest that high correlation between heart rate variety and blood pressure variety. Therefore, correction of the heart rate was added to the regression model as the formula in Eq. (3) [9].

$$BP = a \cdot Time\,Delay + b \tag{2}$$

$$BP = a \cdot Time\,Delay + b \cdot HR + c \tag{3}$$

2 Methodology

The purpose of this study explores the different PTT measurements to estimate blood pressure. Patient BP data was referred by the online database MIMIC II. Using this database to predict and to compare the blood pressure trends on PTT and some physiological parameters.

This database has more than one ECG signal with different leads, and some data include continuous arterial blood pressure (ABP) signal and PPG signal. Each data has different data length with the sampling rate in 125 Hz. In this study, the ECG, PPG and ABP signals were used to verify the performance for the different cuffless BP regressive models.

There are fourteen subject's BP data shown in Table 1 which presented the average data length in 164 ± 51 min.

Table 1. Subject number and data length

Sample code	Number	Data length (min)	Sample code	Number	Data length (min)
S1	3000063	161	S8	3802888	108
S2	3100033	133	S9	3899400	145
S3	3100140	158	S10	3899730	126
S4	3118326	149	S11	3200516	302
S5	3125881	147	S12	3200829	231
S6	3802508	175	S13	3300565	191
S7	3802623	90	S14	3300592	185

To reduce the general noise in ECG, signals will be processed by a third-order Butterworth low-pass filter with cutoff frequency of 20 Hz. In order to effectively detect the R wave, this study using the algorithm was proposed by Mitra [10]. First, the filtered ECG signal is processed by the first-order differentiator to calculate the slope, then squaring the signal, and then smoothing the signal by a moving average filter, and finally to find the maximum value for locating the R peaks.

To process the PPG and ABP signals is under the same procedure including to select the common feature points, such as the peak value of the signal, the valley value and the maximum slope point. The ABP signal will take the peak as the value of the systolic blood pressure.

Pulse transit time, heart rate, pulse width and pulse wave interval were put into the blood pressure regression model as corrections. And using correction S wave in ECG as the PTT start time which is shown in Fig. 1.

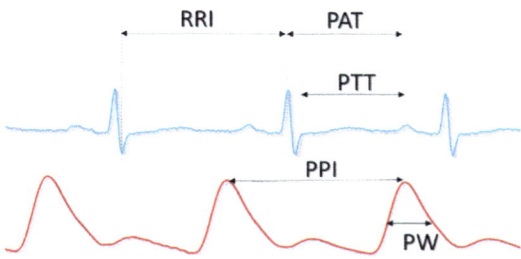

Fig. 1. Characteristic parameters of blood pressure regressive analysis model.

Based on the results proposed by some researches, this study referred five different blood pressure regression models, and one of the most detail blood pressure regression model used in the past shown in Eq. 4. A simplified equation that modifies the Eq. 4 to Eq. 5 shown in below.

$$BP = a \cdot PAT + b \cdot HR + c \cdot PW + d \cdot AMP + e \cdot PPI \cdot \Delta PAT$$
$$+ g \cdot \Delta HR + h \cdot \Delta AMP + i \cdot \Delta PPI + j \tag{4}$$

$$BP = a \cdot PAT[n] + b \cdot HR[n] + c \cdot PW[n] + d \cdot PPI[n] + e \tag{5}$$

Considering blood pressure liner regression items as little as possible, Table 2 shows the summary of each parameter in different ways of Eq. 5. The five different blood pressure regression models is used with the major parameter (PTT) and minor parameters (heart rate, pulse wave interval and pulse width) through blood pressure regression analysis.

Table 2. Blood pressure linear regression models

Model name	Cuff-less blood pressure models
$PTT - BP$	$BP = a \cdot PTT + b$
$PTT_{HR} - BP$	$BP = a \cdot PTT + b \cdot HR + c$
$PTT_{HR,PPI} - BP$	$BP = a \cdot PTT + b \cdot HR + c \cdot PPI + d$
$PTT_{HR,PW} - BP$	$BP = a \cdot PTT + b \cdot HR + c \cdot PW + d$
$PTT_{ALL} - BP$	$BP = a \cdot PTT + b \cdot HR + c \cdot PW + d \cdot PPI + e$

In order to evaluate the similarity between the true BP variation and the estimated BP variation in each subject's BP data, the recurrence quantification analysis (RQA) method is used. This method is a dynamic system analysis method based on the error normalization formula to calculate the trend consistency of two BP data curves. Equation 6 shows the formula of RQA. The analysis result can be plotted in a pattern called recurrence plot (RP). A threshold is empirically considered as 10% in maximum D to present the value in black if less than the threshold and in white if otherwise. Using the Eq. 7 can transform D into the value shown in RP. The parameter RRratio was applied to present the global feature of the consistency rate shown in Eq. 8.

$$D(i,j) = \sqrt{\frac{[x(i) - x(j)]^2}{var(x)} + \frac{[y(i) - y(j)]^2}{var(x)}} \tag{6}$$

$$RRxy = \frac{1}{N^2} \sum_{i,j=1}^{N} D(i,j) \tag{7}$$

$$RRratio = \frac{RRxy}{RRxx} \tag{8}$$

3   Result

This study proposes five different blood pressure regression models with the major parameter PTT and minor parameters (heart rate, pulse wave interval and pulse width), the blood pressure regression analysis in per min. The results of correlation coefficients are shown in Table 3. The best result is $PTT_{ALL} - BP$ in the correlation coefficient 0.87.

Tables 3. Results of correlation coefficients and **RRratio** between the true BP and estimated BP in different cuff-less blood pressure models

Model name	Correlation coefficient	RRratio
$PTT - BP$	0.71 ± 0.12	0.53 ± 0.14
$PTT_{HR} - BP$	0.78 ± 0.08	0.57 ± 0.15
$PTT_{HR,PPI} - BP$	0.80 ± 0.09	0.61 ± 0.16
$PTT_{HR,PW} - BP$	0.86 ± 0.07	0.66 ± 0.11
$PTT_{ALL} - BP$	0.87 ± 0.07	0.68 ± 0.13

In the BP trend consistency analysis, both true and estimated BP value is presented in minute for total length of 160 min shown in Figs. 2 and 3. The results showed the consistency of each BP trend by four cases, that were two cases in good estimated BP in Fig. 2, and two cases in poor estimated BP in Fig. 3. The black line was true BP and red line was estimation BP. In Fig. 2, the RRratio presented to the overall trend consistency in 0.78 and 0.95 in the good estimated cases, respectively. In Fig. 3, the RRration showed the poor follow up between true BP and estimation BP with their RRratio in 0.39 and 0.46, respectively.

Figure 4 was the typical result of the Recurrence Plot. In Fig. 4(a), it can be considered as a standard result, because it was a result of self-consistency comparison. Figure 4(b) to (f) showed the results of estimated BP's performance for different models on the same subject's data. The $PTT_{ALL} - BP$ model presented the estimated BP trend in consistency and closed to the true BP trend.

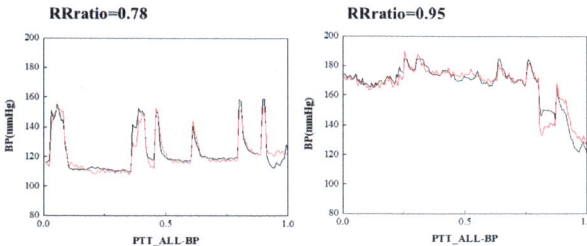

Fig. 2. Two examples of blood pressure trend in good estimation cases and well follow up of long-term BP variation.

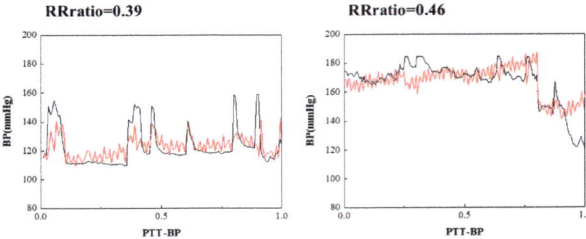

Fig. 3. Two examples of blood pressure trend in poor estimation cases and less follow up of long-term BP variation.

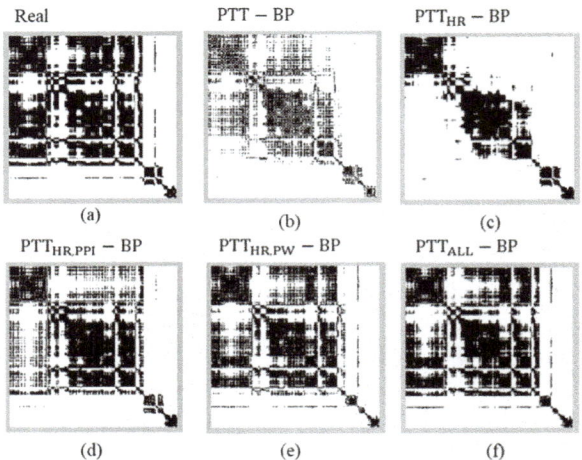

Fig. 4. Examples of the recurrence plot of different blood pressure trend estimations. (a) shows the consistency result of the real BP trend comparing to itself. (b)–(f) show the consistency result of the real BP trend comparing to the estimated BP trends estimated by five different BP models.

4   Conclusions

Five cuff-less estimated BP models based on PTT as the key parameter have been evaluated to analysis the BP trend in long-term BP monitoring. The estimated BP trend will directly present the BP variation of continuous BP. Among five different cuff-less blood pressure models, the model of $PTT_{ALL} - BP$ performed the well BP follow up capability in estimating the continuous BP.

Since the MIMIC II clinical database, all data sampling resolution is acquired in 125 Hz. Higher signal resolution will be much helpful on the regressive analysis to obtain better estimated BP and BP trend. Accurate BP trend will directly be helpful to analysis the BP variation which can be another important BP feature to the stroke prevention.

Conflict of Interest. To the best of our knowledge, the named authors have no conflict of interest, financial or otherwise

References

1. Lewington, S., et al.: Age-specific relevance of usual blood pressure to vascular mortality: a meta-analysis of individual data for one million adults in 61 prospective studies. Lancet **360** (9349), 1903–1913 (2002)
2. Brook, R.D., Rajagopalan, S.: ACC/AHA/AAPA/ABC/ACPM/AGS/APhA/ASH/ASPC/ NMA/PCNA guideline for the prevention, detection, evaluation, and management of high blood pressure in adults. A report of the American college of cardiology/American heart association task force on clinical practice guidelines. J. Am. Soc. Hypertens. **12**(3), 238 (2018)
3. Verdecchia, P., Schillaci, G., Porcellati, C.: Dippers versus non-dippers. J. Hypertens. Suppl. **9**(8), S42–S44 (1991)
4. Verdecchia, P., Porcellati, C.: The day-night changes in ambulatory blood pressure: another risk indicator in hypertension? G. Ital. Cardiol. **22**(7), 879–886 (1992)
5. Marler, J.R., et al.: Morning increase in onset of ischemic stroke. Stroke **20**(4), 473–476 (1989)
6. Mukkamala, R., Hahn, J., Inan, O.T., Mestha, L.K., Kim, C., Hakan, T.: Toward ubiquitous blood pressure monitoring via pulse transit time: theory and practice. IEEE Trans. Biomed. Eng. **62**, 1879–1901 (2015)
7. Westerhof, N., Stergiopulos, N., Noble, M.I.M.: Snapshots of Hemodynamics: An Aid for Clinical Research and Graduate Education. Springer, Boston (2010)
8. Chen, M.W., Kobayashi, T., Ichikawa, S., Takeuchi, Y., Togawa, T.: Continuous estimation of systolic blood pressure using the pulse arrival time and intermittent calibration. Med. Biol. Eng. Comput. **38**, 569–574 (2000)
9. Cattivelli, F.S., Garudadri, H.: Noninvasive cuffless estimation of blood pressure from pulse arrival time and heart rate with adaptive calibration. In: Proceedings of the 6th International Workshop Wearable Implantable Body Sensor Networks, pp. 114–119 (2009)
10. Sadhukhan, D., Mitra, M.: R-Peak detection algorithm for ECG using double difference and RR interval processing. Procedia Technol. **4**, 873–877 (2012)

Raman Spectroscopic Urine Crystal Detection and Clinical Significance Study on Urolithiasis Management

Chih-Hao Wang[1]([⊠]), Jing-Xiang Zeng[2], Pin-Chuan Chen[2], and Hui-Hua Kenny Chiang[1]

[1] Department of Biomedical Engineering, National Yang-Ming University, No. 155, Sec. 2, Linong Street, Taipei, Taiwan
wang228jason@gmail.com
[2] Department of Mechanical Engineering, National Taiwan University of Science and Technology, Taipei, Taiwan

Abstract. Urolithiasis is a common disease with high recurrence rate. According to the record, the prevalence rate of urolithiasis is about 4–15% in Asia, Europe and America while the recurrence rate of urolithiasis is more than 50% after the treatment. The research done by the University of Chicago indicates that the presence of crystals in urine is an important factor of stone formation. Previous studies also conclude that the compound of crystals and stones are highly correlated. Therefore, it is important to analyze urine crystals accurately to prevent potential stone formation.

Our Raman spectroscopic urine crystal detection system features the specially designed microfluidic chip with a chamber, the patented technology of crystal collection using Fe_3O_4 nanoclusters and the 785-nm excitation wavelength automatic Raman microscope we constructed. This system can instantly extract crystals from urine, and the composition of crystals are determined accurately by Raman spectroscopy. It will be a much more powerful and more efficient tool on urine crystal analysis.

The clinical significance study of urine crystals on urolithiasis management mainly focuses on the relationship between morphology including auto-fluorescence of urine crystals and urolithiasis. The urine samples and renal calculi from urolithiasis patients were collected from Taipei Veterans General Hospital and Taipei City Hospital and all the samples were analysized with our Raman spectroscopic urine crystal detection system. Statistically, the pre-surgery urine samples of urolithiasis patients tend to have more atypical crystals in shape, composition and auto-fluorescence incidence than non-patients'. Our data indicates that the pattern of urine crystals plays a significant role in clinical urolithiasis management.

Keywords: Raman spectroscopy · Urolithiasis · Urine crystal · Microfluidic chip · Auto-fluorescence

© Springer Nature Switzerland AG 2020
K.-P. Lin et al. (Eds.): ICBHI 2019, IFMBE Proceedings 74, pp. 122–128, 2020.
https://doi.org/10.1007/978-3-030-30636-6_18

1 Introduction

Urolithiasis has become a common disease in modern world. Patients with urolithiasis may suffer severe pain, nausea, vomiting, infection in urinary system and hematuria. The prevalence rate of urolithiasis in Asia, Europe and America is about 4–15% [1] while a higher prevalence rate of 5–19% with a 60–80% life time recurrence rate appear in the "stone belt" in Asia [2]. According to a national survey done in Taiwan, 9.6% of population suffered urolithiasis throughout their lifetime [3]. The probable factors of urolithiasis include genetics, dietary habits, climate, economy/education level, age and gender. The local prevalence rate is higher in warmer or higher economy/education level place. In recent years, the high prevalence rate area is expanding due to global warming and the prevalence rate is growing in Europe due to growing affluence. The aging of population also plays a role in growing prevalence rate [2].

Urinary stones can be categorized into seven types as listed in Table 1. In most countries of Asia, calcium oxalates (75–90%) such as calcium oxalate monohydrate (COM) and calcium oxalate dihydrate (COD) is the most common type of stones. Uric acid (UA, 5–20%) and calcium phosphates (6–13%) such as hydroxyapatite (HAP) and dicalcium phosphate dihydrate (DCPD) are second most, followed by struvite (2–15%) and cysteine (0.5–1%) [2]. Different clinical treatments are applied on certain type of stones for stone elimination and prevention of recurrence. The research done by the University of Chicago indicates that the presence of crystals in urine is an important factor of stone formation [4]. Previous study done by Lu *et al.* [5] also concludes that type of urine crystals is highly related to urinary stone components (90.4%) for urolithiasis patients. We can evaluate one's stone component by analyzing their urine crystals. Therefore, it's important to analyze urine crystals accurately to prevent potential stone formation.

Table 1. Main urinary stone types and their formulas

Type	Formula
Calcium oxalate monohydrate	$(COO)_2Ca \cdot H_2O$
Calcium oxalate dihydrate	$(COO)_2Ca \cdot 2H_2O$
Hydroxyapatite	$Ca_5(PO_4)_3(OH)$
Dicalcium phosphate dihydrate	$CaHPO_4 \cdot 2H_2O$
Uric acid	$C_5H_4N_4O_3$
Struvite	$MgNH_4(PO_4) \cdot 6H_2O$
Cysteine	$C_6H_{12}N_2O_4S_2$

Current urine crystals identification methods in clinics is morphology under the microscope, however, substance contamination and irregular crystal shapes are huge challenges. It's also difficult to collect irregular crystals from urine for further qualitative analysis. Raman spectroscopy is an advantageous tool on urine crystals identification due to its high specificity, short measurement time and simple sample preparation process. Chiu et al. developed micro-Raman spectroscopy (MRS) system applied on the analysis of micro-stones or stone powders in urine from patients after ureteroscopy lithotripsy. This study concludes that the MRS method is more powerful than FTIR analysis, especially on the identification of the difference between COD and COM, and between HAP and DCPD [6]. In comparison with traditional methods, Raman spectroscopic system could be a proper way for urine crystal detection and analysis.

The process of urinary stone formation can be divided into four steps: supersaturation, nucleation and aggregation, retention and stone formation. Supersaturation occurs when the ratio of urinary calcium oxalate or calcium phosphate concentration to its solubility, tubular fluid in the loop of Henle may provide such condition. With the existence of condensation nucleus, it could lead to nucleation and crystallization in supersaturated tubular fluid, and the urinary crystal promoters and exhibitors are accounted for further crystals aggregation and metabolism. Some of aggregated crystals, or we called micro-stones, may attach to the renal tubule wall and cause retention [7].

Due to several studies on calcium oxalate stones formation, COD crystal is the regular form for human oxalate metabolism while the existence of COM crystal is a dangerous sign of probable urolithiasis. Urine crystal exhibitors tend to make calcium oxalate crystallized in the form of COD but not COM. COD phantom is also found in certain kind of COM stones, which revealed that the transformation from COD to COM happens in vivo with increasing retention time because COM is a relatively more stable form of calcium oxalate compound [8]. All the process of urinary stone formation mentioned above are arranged and presented in Fig. 1.

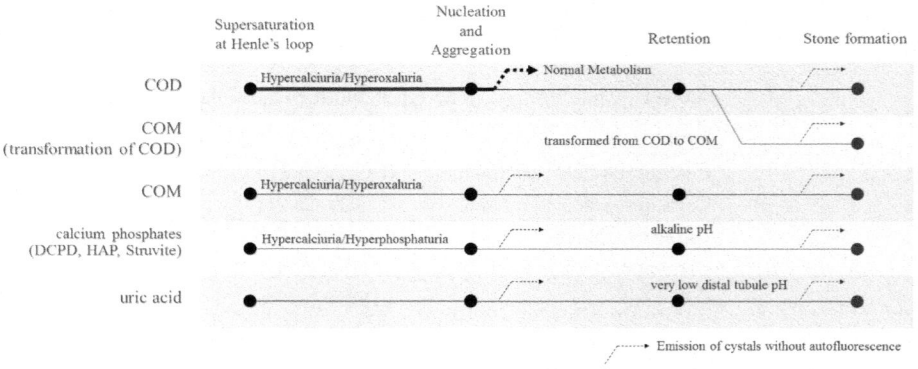

Fig. 1. Process of urinary stone formation.

2   Materials and Methods

2.1   Sample Preparation

The samples are divided into two groups, patient (P, 11 samples) and nonpatient (N, 42 samples). The patients' pre-surgery urine samples and renal calculi were collected from both Taipei Veterans General Hospital and Taipei City Hospital. All of these patients were diagnosed with urolithiasis by urologist. Samples of nonpatients, that didn't have any medical history of urolithiasis, were collected from their first morning urine. All urine samples were sealed in germ-free containers and analyzed in 24 h. Solid renal calculi were stored in germ-free containers for further analysis.

2.2   Urine Crystal Extraction Method (Preprocessing)

The patented technology of urine crystals extraction using Fe_3O_4 nanoclusters was used for urine preprocessing [9]. These urine crystals extractor and 1 ml urine sample are mixed in a 1.5 ml microcentrifuge tube. A magnet was then used to extract the Fe_3O_4 nanoclusters bounded crystals toward tube wall, and all the other substances were removed. The crystals on tube wall were then gathered by adding 10 μl ddH_2O. The final solution with extracted crystals was put on the slide for further analysis.

Another preprocessing method is presented in a specially designed microfluidic chip. This chip features a milling acrylic slide between two quartz slides. The milling acrylic slide contains a microfluidic system with inlet, outlet and a elliptical hole as a gathering site. The 3D image was shown in Fig. 2. We can directly extract urine crystals from the mixture of urine and Fe_3O_4 nanoclusters by passing the microfluidic system with magnet below the gathering site. This preprocessing method is effective but the following result were done by the previous method due to consistency.

2.3   Raman Spectroscopic System

We develop a Raman spectroscopic system for urine crystal detection and analysis that contains a excitation source of a 785-nm laser (LASOS, Germany) with adjustable output power up to 70 mW. A 785-nm high pass filter (Semrock, Rochester, NY, USA) was used to reject the excitation light entering the spectrometer system. A group of filters (D, E and F in Fig. 3) were used for mercury excited red light fluorescence observation and were be switched on when needed. The Raman system was coupled with a microscope (Olympus BX 53) and a camera (Canon EOS 700D) for examining the bright field and fluorescence field images.

The Raman signals from samples were collected by a detection module consisting of a Raman imaging spectrograph (Acton LS785, Princeton Instrument, NJ, USA) mounted on a PIXIS charge-coupled detector with 1340×400 pixels. A 100x microscope objective was used for focusing the laser beam on the sample. We also created a program with a graphical user interface in LabVIEW for camera-management and sample positioning.

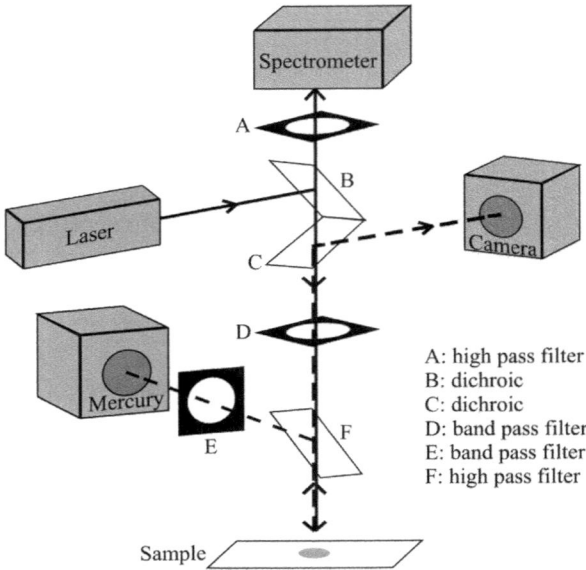

Fig. 2. Raman spectroscopic system for urine crystal detection

3 Results

The Raman spectrum data were analyzed with Originlab 9 and the spectrum fingerprint was compared to reference data for component identification [10–13]. For the patient group (Group P), all 11 urine samples had crystals and 6 of them were fully correlated to stone types, 1 of the other patients was 2/3 correlated, 2 were 1/2 correlated, 1 was 1/3 correlated while one presented zero correlation. Detailed information of Group P's urine crystal and stone type were listed in Table 2 and the presence of typical COD in urine wasn't count in the correlation when there was no COD stones in the calculi sample because it's produced by regular oxalate metabolism.

Table 2. Types and correlation of urinary crystals and stones in Group P.

Sample	Crystal type(s)	Stone type(s)	Correlation
P1	COD, HAP	COM, COD, HAP	66.7%
P2	COM	COM	100%
P3	UA	UA	100%
P4	COM, COD	COM, COD	100%
P5	COD	COM, COD, HAP	33.3%
P6	COM, HAP	COM, HAP	100%
P7	COM	COM, COD	50%
P8	UA	COM, UA	50%
P9	HAP	COM, COD, HAP	33.3%
P10	UA	UA	100%
P11	HAP	HAP	100%

For the nonpatient group (Group N), 9 of 42 had crystals in urine (21.4%) and 8 of them are typical COD crystals. Only one sample had COM crystals with autofluorescence.

We discovered that some urine crystals, including typical COD and other atypical types, had autofluorescence with excitation band around 590 nm and it may be a important factor to indicate a urolithiasis problem. Figure 3 shows the difference of Group P and Group N on the percentage of "rate of crystal incidence" and "rate of autofluorescence or atypical type crystal". With the assistance of fluorescence image, the difference between two groups became larger.

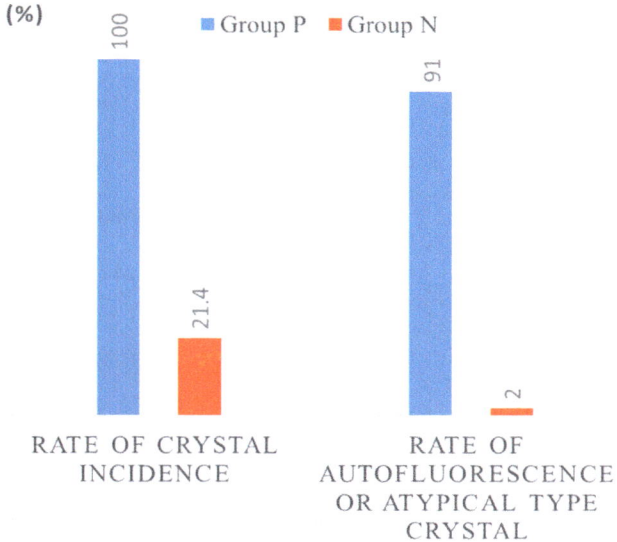

Fig. 3. Group P and Group N on the percentage of "rate of crystal incidence" and "rate of autofluorescence or atypical type crystal"

4 Conclusion and Discussion

By using the Raman spectroscopic urine crystal detection system, seven most common types of urinary stone in urolithiasis patients can be determined accurately. Especially on the identification of COD and COM, which is important for urolithiasis management but cannot be clearly identified by methods in clinics nowadays. It provides a better way for the analysis and study on urine crystals.

The presence of autofluorescence in urine crystals was another important discovery in this study. Typical COD crystals without autofluorescence may refer to a regular metabolism while atypical type crystals, including COD with autofluorescence and other six types of crystals, may indicate a problem of urolithiasis. The resource of autofluorescence in urine crystals has not been well studied yet, it could be proteins or ions that exist in urine and take part in the stone formation process like promoters or inhibitors. As the result, combining the urine crystals' Raman spectrum data and fluorescence image we brought out a more powerful standard that revealed the clinical significance of potential urolithiasis.

Conflict of Interest. The authors declare that they have no conflict of interest.

References

1. Liu, Y., et al.: Epidemiology of urolithiasis in Asia. Asian J. Urol. **5**(4), 205–214 (2018)
2. Fisang, C., Anding, R., Müller, S.C., Latz, S., Laube, N.: Urolithiasis—an interdisciplinary diagnostic, therapeutic and secondary preventive challenge. Dtsch. Arztebl. Int. **112**, 83–91 (2015). https://doi.org/10.3238/arztebl.2015.0083
3. Yu, D.-S., et al.: Epidemiology and treatment of inpatients urolithiasis in Taiwan. Formos. J. Surg. **49**(4), 136–141 (2016)
4. Kidney Stone Guide Book, Kidney Stone Evaluation and Treatment Program. https://kidneystones.uchicago.edu/kidney-stone-book/
5. Lu, S.H., et al.: Urinary crystals in patients with and without urolithiasis. Chin. J. Urol. **5**(3), 163–168 (1994). 中華泌尿科學會雜誌
6. Chiu, Y.-C., Yang, H.-Y., Lua, S.-H., Chiang, H.K.: Micro Raman spectroscopy identification of urinary stone composition from ureteroscopic lithotripsy urine powder. Raman Spectrosc. **41**, 136–141 (2010)
7. Ratkalkar, V.N., Kleinman, J.G.: Mechanisms of stone formation. Clin. Rev. Bone Miner. Metab. **9**(3–4), 187–197 (2011)
8. Costa-Bauza, A., et al.: Type of renal calculi: variation with age and sex. World J. Urol. **25**(4), 415–421 (2007)
9. Chiu, Y.-C., et al.: Enhanced Raman sensitivity and magnetic separation for urolithiasis detection using phosphonic acid-terminated Fe_3O_4 nanoclusters. J. Mater. Chem. B **3**(20), 4282–4290 (2015)
10. Kodati, V.R., Turumin, J.L., Tu, A.T.: Raman spectroscopic identification of phosphate-type kidney stones. Appl. Spectrosc. **45**(4), 581–583 (1991)
11. Kodati, V.R., Tomasi, G.E., Turumin, J.L., Tu, A.T.: Raman spectroscopic identification of cystine-type kidney stone. Appl. Spectrosc. **44**(5), 837–839 (1990)
12. Kodati, V.R., Tu, A.T., Turumin, J.L.: Raman spectroscopic identification of uric-acid-type kidney stone. Appl. Spectrosc. **44**(7), 1134–1136 (1990)
13. Kodati, V.R., Tomasi, G.E., Turumin, J.L., Tu, A.T.: Raman spectroscopic identification of calcium-oxalate-type kidney stone. Appl. Spectrosc. **44**(8), 1408–1411 (1990)

A Real Time Fall Detection System Using Tri-Axial Accelerometer and Clinometer Based on Smart Phones

Yi-Sheng Su[(⊠)] and Shih-Hsiung Twu

Department of Electrical Engineering,
Chung Yuan Christian University, Taoyuan, Taiwan
e271068tw@gmail.com

Abstract. In this paper, we design a method to use smart phone to detect when fall accident happened, it can inform outside people or organization automatically to get help from them.

The smart phone has implemented several sensors, such as the tri-axial accelerometer, electronic compass, global positioning system (GPS) etc. We will use those sensors to do fall detection.

This detection system is used by placing in the waist pocket. Because people activity can be recorded real time by center of gravity in the body. We collect data for normal movements and fall events to setup a database, and then do the data analysis real time to identify if it is normal movement or fall event.

To offload system operation loading and increase the efficiency on the fall detection, this paper will be divided into two parts. In the first part, in order to make the identification more lightweight, the collected data will be used to do the data blurring by weighted moving average. This way can make system easy to comparison and will not lose fall event feature. In the second part, we input the processed data to do fall detection. Three features weightlessness, impact and stillness are used to identify if it is fall event or not. If fall accident is true, system will send warning message and location automatically to the people or organization who we predefined in the system to get help.

The results of our research can be used by everyone and everywhere if wireless network connection is valid. This system can be used in various environments and it is very convenient to hand carry and easy to use. So the acceptance from general people should be very high for them can use this system to get help in time to save their life or mitigate the damage.

Keywords: Real time · Fall detection · Tri-Axial accelerometer · Clinometers · Smart phones

1 Introduction

It is the worldwide trend that more and more people live alone at home, specific for old people. For those people who live alone, sometime they may meet dangerous things happened to them at home, like fall or sick and outside people does not know that to prove help in time. According to World Health Organization (WHO) [1]" data shows

© Springer Nature Switzerland AG 2020
K.-P. Lin et al. (Eds.): ICBHI 2019, IFMBE Proceedings 74, pp. 129–137, 2020.
https://doi.org/10.1007/978-3-030-30636-6_19

that Falls are the second leading cause of accidental or unintentional injury deaths worldwide." When fall accident happened, outside people may not know and cannot provide help in real time. It is high possibility that to cause serious hurt to the people and let them cannot move to use phone to call outside for help. Like broken their bones, brain or spinal trauma, and internal bleeding [2], it is serious to impact old people health and life. According to the accident data from Taiwan related organization report out, fall is the second high accident in Taiwan. From Taiwan Patient safety Reporting system [3], Medication errors are the most frequent event reported to TPR (Taiwan Patient-safety Reporting system) in 2016 (20,245 reported), and second are falls (16,635), as shown in Fig. 1.

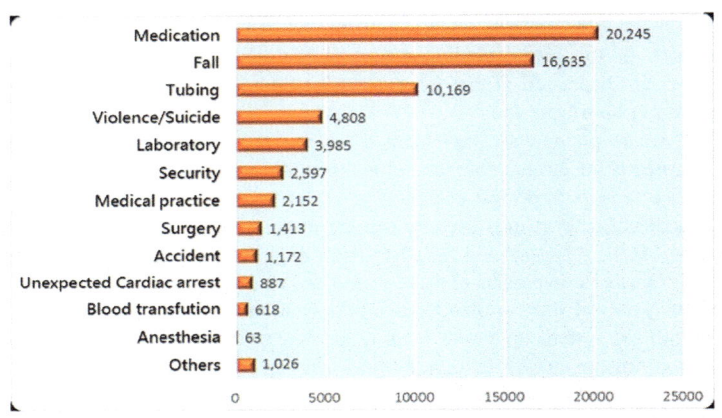

Fig. 1. The types of TPR Reporting Events in 2016 [3]

To protect the people from fall accident and get help in time to save their life or mitigate the damage. Many researches use different methods and technologies for fall detection [4–19]. Fall detection can be grouped into two categories. That is environmental detection system [4–9] and wearable sensor detection system [11–19]:

1. **Environmental detection system**
   This method is placed in the predefined environmental to monitor people activity without wear any type of sensors [4, 5]. Such as image recognition (camera) [6, 7], floor pressure sensor [8, 9], etc. The system can setup in users' home in advance to detect fall accident. The main advantage is that user may not feel uncomfortable since they do not need to wear any sensors with them [10]. But environment detection system needs to design for specific home users with different angels to cover everywhere in the home at different rooms and it has private problem for user [6]. This system only can protect user in predefined space, like home.

2. **Wearable sensor detection system**
   This method just simple to us use sensors like microphone [11], barometric pressure sensor [12], accelerometer sensor [12–17], gyroscope sensor [17], electronic compass etc. Those sensors can be made very small and easy to hand carry by users.

Those wearable devices are low power can continue working for whole day [18]. It is suitable for a mobile detection system. It can be used in various environment. The devices can be placed on leg, hand, chest and waist. But wearing those devices may cause user feel uncomfortable and inconvenience [10].

Smart phone is a mobile device and almost everyone has it now, including old people, it is easy to carry and use [18, 19]. More and more people use smart phone to make phone call or access internet to get the information they need. The mobile phone cost down to everyone can offer to buy it [20]. With the quick development smart phone has several sensors in smart phone, such as the tri-axial accelerometer, electronic compass, global positioning system (GPS), etc. [13–20]. With those sensors, we can analysis the motion signal from human. In this paper, we will use ASUS ZenFone 2 Laser (ZE50kl) mobile phone device, Android 6.0.1 OS. This paper will analysis of five different normal movements [14] and fall event. We purpose a fall detection system based on smart phone angle and acceleration features.

2 Motion Signal Process and Feature Select

In this Chapter, we will introduce the motion signal process and features selection. From Fig. 2, it lists six activities including fall, sit down, jump, lying down, walk and run. When people carry smart phone and enable the detection system, it will record every movement to identify the activity in line with which motion signal in the database. From the Fig. 2, we can see the fall feature is very different from other normal movements. We also can identify that if the same motion signal pattern repeated in short time, then system will identify it is strenuous exercise instead of fall. In order to identify clearly if it is fall event or not, after system recording the motion signals and then it will be compared with database to choose which signal feature is in line with signals system recorded to decide which activity happens.

2.1 Tri-Axial Accelerometer

Accelerometer (G-Sensor), also called gravity sensor, it can do the acceleration detection from any directions. The expression is the axial acceleration magnitude and direction (XYZ). It can detect the forces from both of the gravity and the forces when moving the device. The center of gravity is the balance point for human body. When human body is moving, the center of gravity is near the waist. That's why we will suggest the detection system (smart phone) should be placed in the waist pocket instead of hand or leg. The data signals is a three-dimensional signal X-axis, Y-axis, and Z-axis (as in Fig. 3). The sampled signal is [ax [n], ay [n], az [n]]. To prediget the three-dimensional signal, we will use the one-dimensional signal magnitude vector (SMV) [14] by

$$SMV = \sqrt{a_x^2[n] + a_y^2[n] + a_z^2[n]}, \tag{1}$$

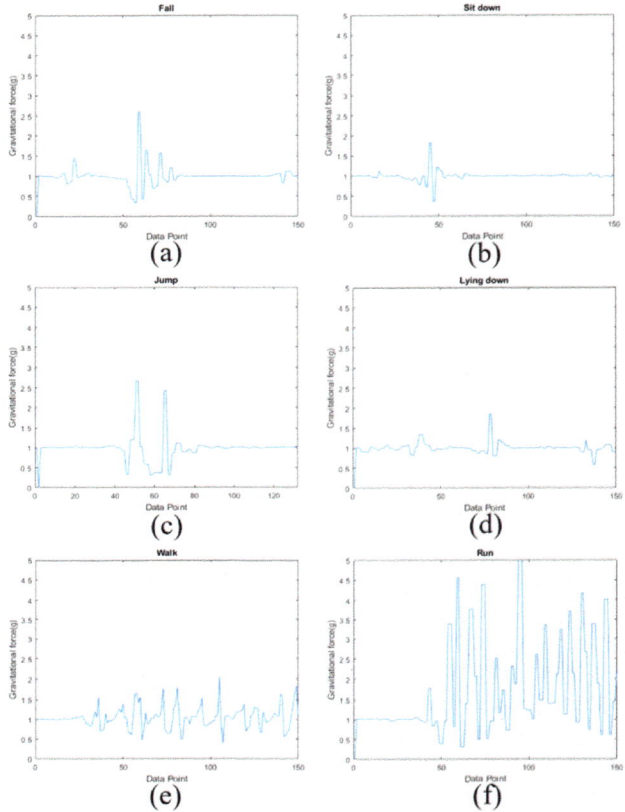

Fig. 2. Six different kinds of activities. (a) Fall. (b) Sit. (c) Jump. (d) Lying down. (e) Walk. (f) Run.

to find out the fall feature. We will observe the fall event motion signal. In the Fig. 2(a), we can see the motion signal at 55th date point, the SMV value is smaller than 1 g. At this time the user body is in a state of weightlessness before landing. In this time period SMV is close to 0.5G. We observe other fall events and find the same characteristic. So we define when SMV smaller than 0.6 g is the weightlessness, and it is the detection system first feature.

2.2   Weighted Moving Average

Now we have the first feature ready to make sure the detection system is more accurate. For next step, we need to find out the second feature. We notice that the fall event happens after weightlessness. The peak values will appear in motion signal after the body is impacted by ground. But it does have problems exist potentially to confuse system to judge if it is fall or not, like the peak values are very often to appear when the body is doing intense exercise to cause the motion signals will be very messy.

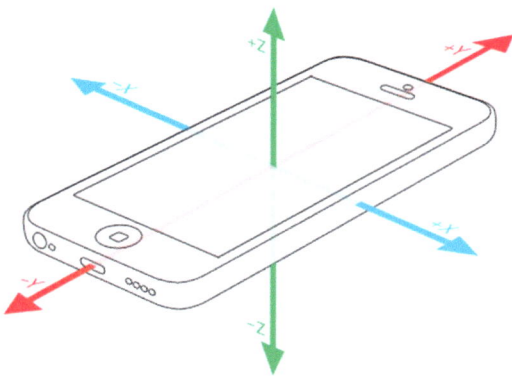

Fig. 3. Tri-axial Accelerometer of Smart phone [21]

It increases the burden of detection system operations and increases the possibility of misjudgment. To offload detection system operation burden and increase the efficiency. We will use weighted moving average (WMA) to process the motion signal,

$$WMA_{t1,n} = WMA_{t0,n} - \frac{Gain*SMV_1}{n} + \frac{Gain*SMV_{n+1}}{n} \tag{2}$$

$$\text{if } SMV > 2.0\,g \text{ } then \text{ } Gain = Impact - weightlessness$$
$$\text{else if } SMV < 2.0\,g \text{ } Gain = 1.$$

Using the moving average process, it can make the motion signal more accurately and can exclude small motion signal noise. But the weakness is that the motion signal peak values can be distortion and lose the fall feature what we are looking for. To retain fall peak values feature, we will give a weighted value, if the SMV value is more than 2.0 g, to give a gain value by impact subtract the weightlessness. The result shows in Fig. 4(b). It just retains fall peak values and make the motion signals cleaner, and then we can compare that with normal movements in Fig. 4(b) and (d). We can define that when the SMV after WMA more than 2.5 g means that it is impacted. And this will be the second feature for the detection system.

2.3 Electronic Compass

After getting above two features, we notice that the fall event after weightlessness and impact. The motion signal will appear horizontal stationary state for a period of time. But this feature has some problems by only using the accelerometer. Detection system can't identify fall or general activity static like jump and run. So we add angle recognition to assist detection system. Smart phone's angle detection uses the electronic compass, we will combine both motion signal and angle information together to detect if is body stillness after the fall event happened. If the motion signal SMV standard deviation equals to 0.1 for 2.5 s after first and second feature and the phone

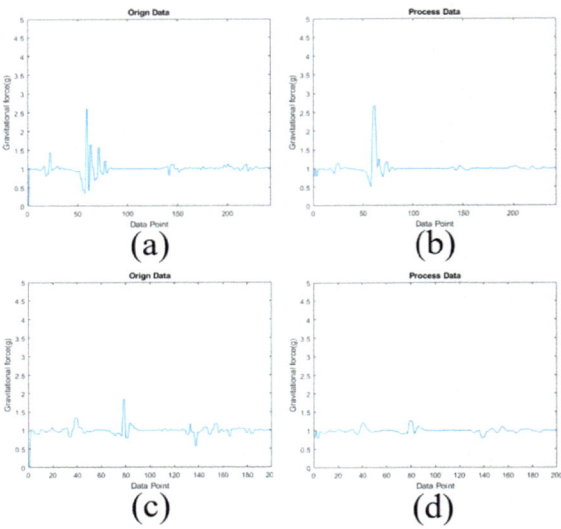

Fig. 4. Comparison motion signal after weighted moving average. (a) Fall original data. (b) Fall process data. (c) Sit original data. (d) Sit process data.

angle smaller than 30°, we can see the SMV and angle comparison in Fig. 5(a) (b). We can use it to identify that the body is at the stillness. And this will be 3rd feature from the detection system.

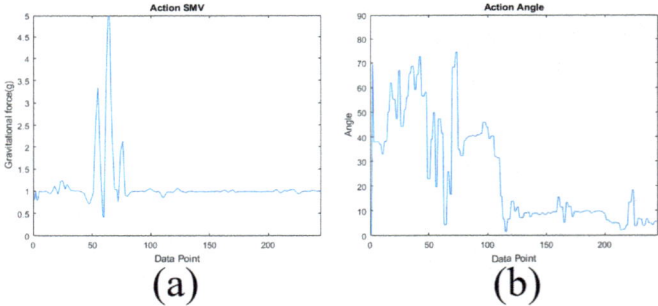

Fig. 5. Comparisons fall event between SMV and angle. (a) Fall event SMV. (b) Fall event angle.

3   Fall Detection Algorithm and Result

We have defined three features to identify fall event versus normal movements. Figure 6 shows the detection flow chart for three features weightlessness, impact and stillness. The first step is to make sure the user body is under weightlessness by detecting SMV value smaller than 0.6 g or not. The second step is to determine the impact on the floor after step 1, it is judged by the peak of the SMV after motion signal data processing the value is over the 2.5 g or not. If the peak over default threshold, the system will identify it is an impact. The third step is to use accelerometer and angle recognition to detect if it is at horizontal stationary state or not after two features were met the conditions. During this step, it also will distinguish the fall event from strenuous exercise. After body impacted within 2.5 s sit will calculate motion signal standard deviation of variation. If standard deviation is smaller than 0.1 and angle recognition is smaller than 30°, the system will define it is stillness. When the three features are all match, the detection system will determine it is a fall event. This algorithm will discriminate fall event from normal movements, including misjudge sitting and lying down. This algorithm can detect fall event effectively. Figure 7 as show the different kinds of test results.

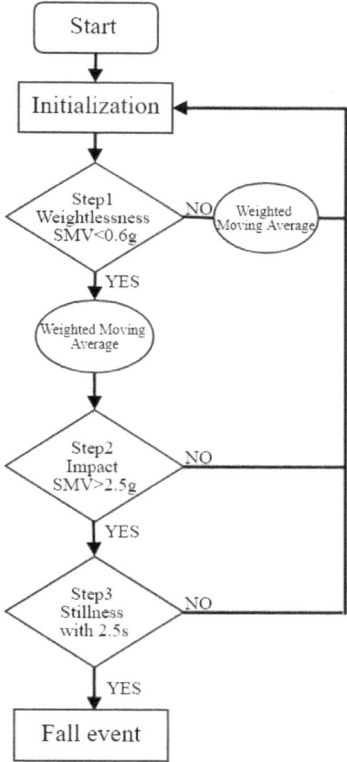

Fig. 6. Fall detection system flowchart.

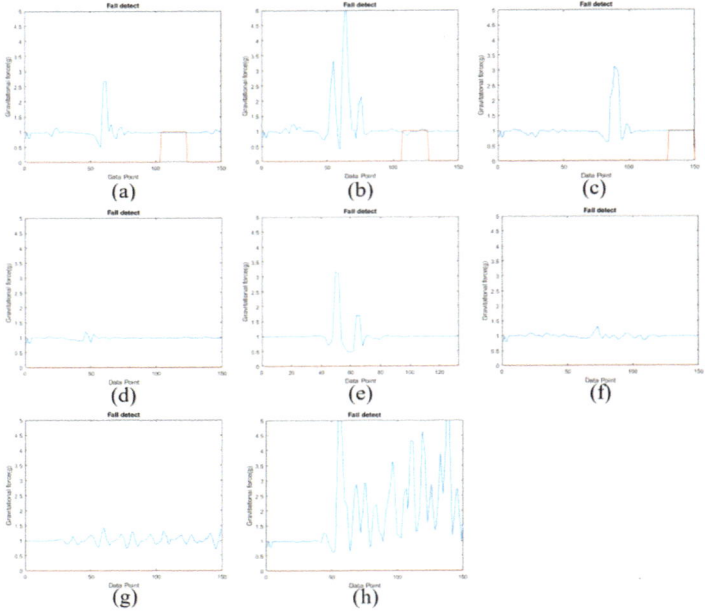

Fig. 7. Fall detect results. (a) Fall. (b) Left fall. (c) Right fall. (d) Sit. (e) Jump. (f) Lying down. (g) Walk. (h) Run.

4   Conclusions

In this paper, we have proposed a fall detection based on smart phone, by installing the system software without adding or modifying hardware. This fall detection algorithm has been implemented to identify three features. Our testing results have shown that this detection system can distinguish people daily living activities and successfully detected three different direction fall events for the forward and lateral (right and left). This design can be used in various environments including indoor and outdoor. The acceptance from general people to use this system should be very high due to no extra cost, easy to handy and easy to use it. For future works, we want to collect more human motion signals from real environment and link the data with machine learning to improve the accuracy of the fall detection system.

Conflict of Interest. The authors declare that they have no conflict of interest.

References

1. Falls WHO, WHO (2018). https://www.who.int/news-room/fact-sheets/detail/falls
2. Health Library. https://www.hopkinsmedicine.org/healthlibrary/conditions/nervous_syste
3. Taiwan Patient-safety Reporting system. http://www.patientsafety.mohw.gov.tw/Content/Messagess/Contents.aspx?SiteID=2&MmmID=621316242156723353

4. Li, K.W., Wen Wang, C., Huang, S.Y.: Subjective rating of floor slipperiness & slip/fall outcomes in a gait experiment
5. Paneerselvam, A., Yaakob, R., Perumal, T., Marlisah, E.: Fall detection framework for smart home. In: 2018 IEEE 7th Global Conference on Consumer Electronics (GCCE), pp. 351–352 (2018)
6. Stone, E.E., Skubic, M.: Fall detection in homes of older adults using the Microsoft Kinect. IEEE J. Biomed. Health Inform. 19(1), 290–301 (2015). Cited by: Papers (165)
7. Agrawal, S.C., Tripathi, R.K., Jalal, A.S.: Human-fall detection from an indoor video surveillance. In: 2017 8th International Conference on Computing, Communication and Networking Technologies (ICCCNT), pp. 1–5 (2017)
8. Rimminen, H., Lindström, J., Linnavuo, M., Sepponen, R.: Detection of falls among the elderly by a floor sensor using the electric near field. IEEE Trans. Inf. Technol. Biomed. 14 (6), 1475–1476 (2010). Cited by: Papers (63)
9. Light, J., Cha, S., Chowdhury, M.: Optimizing pressure sensor array data for a smart-shoe fall monitoring system
10. Demiris, G., Rantz, M.J., Aud, M.A., Marek, K.D., Tyrer, H.W., Skubic, M., Hussam, A.A.: Older adults' attitudes towards and perceptions of smart home technologies: a pilot study. Inf. Health Soc. Care 29(2), 87–94 (2004)
11. Cheffena, M.: Fall detection using smartphone audio features. IEEE J. Biomed. Health Inform. 20(4), 1073–1080 (2016). Cited by: Papers (13)
12. Bianchi, F., Redmond, S.J., Narayanan, M.R., Cerutti, S., Lovell, N.H.: Barometric pressure and triaxial accelerometry-based falls event detection. IEEE Trans. Neural Syst. Rehabil. Eng. 18(6), 619–627 (2010). Cited by: Papers (139), Patents (7)
13. Thammasat, E., Chaicharn, J.: A simply fall-detection algorithm using accelerometers on a smartphone. In: The 5th 2012 Biomedical Engineering International Conference, pp. 1–4 (2012). Cited by: Papers (7)
14. Kau, L.-J., Chen, C.-S.: A smart phone-based pocket fall accident detection, positioning, and rescue system. IEEE J. Biomed. Health Inform. 19(1), 44–56 (2015)
15. Nguyen, T.-T., Cho, M.-C., Lee, T.-S.: Automatic fall detection using wearable biomedical signal measurement terminal. In: 2009 Annual International Conference of the IEEE Engineering in Medicine and Biology Society, pp. 5203–5206 (2009). Cited by: Papers (6)
16. Dumitrache, M., Pasca, S.: Fall detection algorithm based on triaxial accelerometer data. In: 2013 E-Health and Bioengineering Conference (EHB), pp. 1–4 (2013). Cited by: Papers (5)
17. Irwan Nari, M., Suprapto, S.S., Kusumah, I.H., Adiprawita, W.: A simple design of wearable device for fall detection with accelerometer and gyroscope. In: 2016 International Symposium on Electronics and Smart Devices (ISESD), pp. 88–91 (2016)
18. Fang, S.-H., Liang, Y.-C., Chiu, K.-M.: Developing a mobile phone-based fall detection system on Android platform. In: 2012 Computing, Communications and Applications Conference, pp. 143–146 (2012). Cited by: Papers (30)
19. Li, S., Yin, R., Jiang, Y., Qiu, Y., Li, H.: Frequency analysis of fall detection based on Android system. In: 2016 6th International Conference on Electronics Information and Emergency Communication (ICEIEC), pp. 186–189 (2016)
20. Bai, Y.-W., Wu, S.-C., Yu, C.H.: Recognition of direction of fall by smartphone. In: 2013 26th IEEE Canadian Conference on Electrical and Computer Engineering (CCECE), pp. 1–6 (2013). Cited by: Papers (6)
21. Tri-axial Accelerometer picture. https://tw.saowen.com/a/20d36969c163eef7510d7d7af54-6a8ae920479850f576c2d3fe8946fca14fd63

Automatic Classification of Lymph Node Metastasis in Non-Small-Cell Lung Cancer (NSCLC) Patient on F-18-FDG PET/CT

Tsu-Chi Cheng[1]([✉]), Nan-Tsing Chiu[2], and Yu-Hua Fang[1]

[1] Department of Biomedical Engineering, National Cheng Kung University
at Tainan, Tainan, Taiwan
Princesscheng08@gmail.com
[2] Department of Nuclear Medicine, National Cheng Kung University Hospital
at Tainan, Tainan, Taiwan

Abstract. Lung Cancer is a leading cause of death worldwide, and about 85% of lung cancer is non-small cell lung cancer (NSCLC). The staging of lymph nodes in NSCLC patients is extremely important because respective stages require different treatments. FDG-PET/CT is a gold standard for lymph node metastasis staging of NSCLC. However, the results of discriminating lymph node staging on 18F-2-fluoro-2-deoxy-d-glucose (FDG) positron emission tomography (PET)/computed tomography (CT) still needs improvement. In addition to the traditional image parameters of FDG-PET/CT such as standardized uptake value (SUV), there are many other parameters available from FDG-PET/CT images, for example, the lymphatic drainage pathway. For the purpose of a better accuracy on lymph node metastasis diagnosis on NSCLC patient in FDG-PET/CT, this research developed a computer-aided diagnosis (CAD) system to improve the diagnostic efficiency, which achieved an accuracy of 85%, a sensitivity of 82% and a specificity of 85%.

Keywords: Non-small cell lung cancer · F-FDG-PET/CT · Lymph node · Lymphatic drainage pathway · Metastasis

1 Introduction

For the past decades, lung cancer has been the most common cancer and the leading cause of cancer deaths in the world. Non-Small Cell Lung Cancer (NSCLC) accounts for about 85% of all lung cancers. The identification of lymph node in NSCLC is crucial in the staging of a tumor because the state of the lymph nodes is the main determinant of distinguishing and the most important factor in the choice of the therapy [1]. Although CT scans are valuable for the detection of lung cancer, there are still limited in the staging of mediastinal lymph nodes. The sensitivity and specificity of CT scan in identifying metastasis were about 50% and 85%. Recently, 18F-2-fluoro-2-deoxy-d-glucose (FDG) positron emission tomography (PET), has proven to be superior to CT scans in mediastinal lymph node staging in NSCLC patients [2]. The staging of NSCLC lymph node is generally performed through a quantitative assessment using the cutoff value of the maximum standardized uptake value (SUV) [3].

© Springer Nature Switzerland AG 2020
K.-P. Lin et al. (Eds.): ICBHI 2019, IFMBE Proceedings 74, pp. 138–142, 2020.
https://doi.org/10.1007/978-3-030-30636-6_20

However, the diagnostic accuracy of lymph node staging in NSCLC is still not good enough to make decisions for surgery. Many other image parameters from FDG-PET/CT images have been proven that they have the potential to make an improvement of the accuracy of differentiation between metastatic and benign lymph nodes in NSCLC patients. Other than this, texture analysis [4] also can be a way to define lymph node staging [4]. Therefore, this study combined classification tree, a machine learning algorithm with associated learning algorithms that analyze data used for classification and regression analysis, with a variety of image parameters and texture analysis to improve the accuracy in lymph node staging of FDG-PET/CT for NSCLC patients.

Considering that FDG-PET/CT requires better lymph node staging. This study retrospective collected NSCLC patients who had pretreatment FDG-PET/CT and received thoracotomy. To study the appropriate performance of the decision tree with the combination of image parameters. The purpose of the study is to develop the computer-aided diagnosis (CAD) system which obtains a better image discrimination on Non-small cell lung carcinoma lymphatic metastasis in FDG-PET/CT image.

2   Materials and Methods

2.1   Patient Selection

This study retrospectively reviewed the electronic medical records of NSCLC patients in National Cheng Kung University Hospital who underwent F-18-FDG-PET/CT scanning from 2016 to January 2017. The study enrolled 45 patients who had FDG PET/CT imaging before any therapy for NSCLC and underwent thoracotomy and systematic lymph node dissection for NSCLC. For all 45 patients, we recruited 200 benign lymph nodes (LNs) and 22 metastatic LNs.

2.2 ^{18}F-FDG PET/CT

All ^{18}F-FDG PET/CT scans were performed on the PET/CT scanner (Biograph mCT Flow; Siemens Healthcare, Germany). All patients were fasted for about 6 h and a blood glucose level less than 150 mg/dl before injecting with the radiotracer. Each patient was given an intravenous administration of 370 MBq (10 mCi) of ^{18}F-FDG and kept in supine position for 60 min. The CT images were acquired first which patients were breath hold, and CT images were used for attenuation correction and then fusion with PET images. 120 min after ^{18}F-FDG injection the delayed images were obtained.

2.3   Pathologic Results

All patients underwent thoracotomy and lymph node dissection, which recorded the pathologic results and location of the lymph nodes and lung tumors.

2.4   Lesion Manually Segmentation

After the ^{18}F-FDG PET/CT image acquisition from National Cheng Kung University Hospital, all images were reviewed by a nuclear medicine doctor without knowledge of the pathologic results the primary lung tumors and lymph nodes were manually seg-mented by a nuclear medicine doctor who did not know the pathologic results.

2.5   Image Parameters from^{18}F-FDG PET/CT Images

After identifying of lymph nodes and primary tumors, this research analyzed the ^{18}F-FDG PET/CT, images including the following image parameters After identifying of lymph nodes and primary tumors, this research analyzed the ^{18}F-FDG PET/CT, images including the following image parameters: Standardized uptake value (SUV) maximum of both lymph nodes and primary tumor [5], SUV means of both lymph nodes and primary tumor, SUV maximum of lymph nodes on both early and delay images [6], asphericity of lymph node, lymphatic drainage route [7].

2.6   Classifier

For classification, this project used the decision tree as the classifier which incorporated the traditional parameters from FDG-PET/CT images. The data were separated into two sets, a training set, and a testing set. The goal of the decision tree is to generate a model that can distinguish between metastatic or benign lymph nodes. Finally, a decision tree classifier was produced as a binary classifier which can differentiate a metastasis or benign lymph node.

3   Results

To determine the analysis of lymph node staging in patients with NSCLC, a set of 22 malignant lymph nodes and a set of 200 benign lymph nodes of NSCLC patients were used in this experiment. The decision tree classifier allows the detectability of the significant parameters regarding the two-group classification. In order to investigate the suitable performance of the decision tree model, different kinds of image parameters, including the one which only contained single parameters derived from FDG-PET/CT images. All model cohorts were classified into four groups: true positive, true negative, false positive, false negative, based on the results of preoperative PET/CT and the histopathological diagnosis of the resected lymph node. The performance of the single parameters derived from FDG-PET/CT images, including sensitivity, specificity, and diagnostic accuracy, were calculated to evaluate and compare (Table 1).

The decision tree with the implementation of SUV maximum of the primary tumor, asphericity of the lymph node and lymph nodes route had a significantly highest sensitivity value than all the other models. Using the model that comprise SUV maximum of the primary tumor, asphericity of the lymph node and lymph nodes route, the sensitivity, specificity, and diagnostic accuracy were 82%, 85%, and 85% respectively, and the classification tree diagram was shown in Fig. 1.

Table 1. Comparison of each single parameter.

	Accuracy	Sensitivity	Specificity
SUV_{max} of lymph nodes	0.6785	0.7273	0.6300
SUV_{max} of primary tumors	0.6820	0.5909	0.7800
SUV_{mean} of lymph nodes	0.5255	0.9091	0.2700
SUV_{mean} of primary tumors	0.3219	1	0.0200
Lymph nodes volume	0.7685	0.7727	0.6700
Primary tumors volume	0.3859	1	0.0800
Asphericity of lymph nodes	0.7501	0.6818	0.7700
Lymphatic drainage route	0.6575	1	0.3150

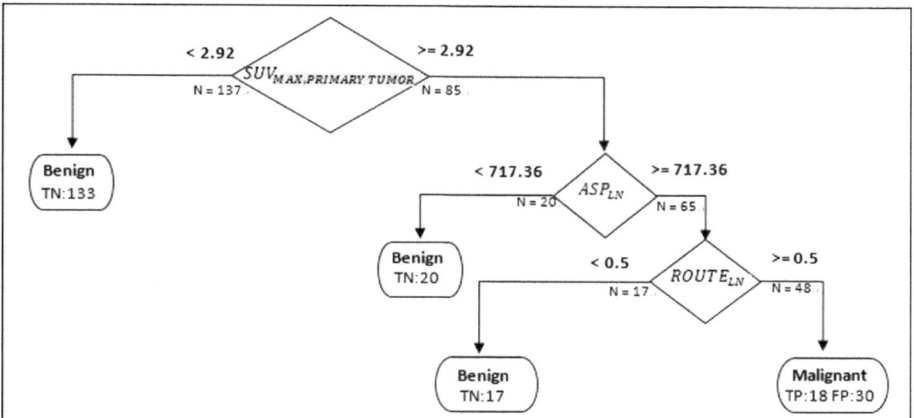

Fig. 1. Classification tree diagram for suitable performance of the decision tree model of distinguishing the LNs.

4   Discussion

FDG-PET/CT is the primary method modality used for NSCLC patients to evaluate lymph nodes and distant metastasis nowadays. However, for the diagnostic of lymph node staging using the cutoff value of SUV in NSCLC is still not enough to make decisions for surgery. For the diagnostic of lymph node metastasis, it is common to have false positive and false negative cases because PET images are based on the fact that FDG is taken up by cells with a higher glycolysis rate and represented as malignant cells. However, active glucose metabolism is not only specific to malignancy, but it can also occur in macrophages and fibroblasts. As for false negative cases may occur from such factors as micrometastasis, likely because of the low volume and low cell concentration. Thus, image parameters are needed. To improve the diagnostic ability of the detecting of lymph node metastasis on FDG-PET/CT image, the image parameters a which have been presented in the foregoing sections were put in the suitable performance of the decision tree model. It was showed that the decision tree model which included the SUV maximum of the primary tumor, asphericity of the lymph node and lymph nodes route which achieved an accuracy of 85%, a sensitivity of 82% and a specificity of 85% had a better diagnostic ability than the other models.

5   Conclusions

In view of that LN metastasis preferentially occurs along the lymph node pathway from the tumor-bearing lobe in NSCLC patients and the present results, the lymph node location is significantly imperative in analyzing the benign and malignant of NSCLC patients' lymph nodes. In conclusion, the present results showed that the computer-aided diagnosis (CAD) system which this research developed provide a way to obtain a better accuracy than by using a quantitative assessment using the cutoff value of the maximum standardized uptake value in lymph node metastasis diagnosis on NSCLC patient in FDG-PET/CT.

Conflict of Interest. The authors declare that they have no conflict of interest.

References

1. Siegel, R.L., Miller, K.D., Jemal, A.: Cancer Statistics, 2017, vol. 67, no. 1, pp. 7–30 (2017)
2. Staging, P., Non, O.F., Cancer, S.L., Tomography, W.P.: Preoperative staging of non–small-cell lung cancer with positron-emission tomography (2000)
3. Schmidt-Hansen, M., Baldwin, D., Zamora, J.: Fdg-pet/ct imaging for mediastinal staging in patients with potentially resectable non–small cell lung cancer. JAMA **313**(14), 1465–1466 (2015)
4. Pham, T.D., Watanabe, Y., Higuchi, M., Suzuki, H.: Texture analysis and synthesis of malignant and benign mediastinal lymph nodes in patients with lung cancer on computed tomography. Sci. Rep. **7**(January), 1–10 (2017)
5. Toba, H., Kondo, K., Otsuka, H., Takizawa, H., Kenzaki, K., Sakiyama, S., Tangoku, A.: Diagnosis of the presence of lymph node metastasis and decision of operative indication using fluorodeoxyglucose - positron emission tomography and computed tomography in patients with primary lung cancer. J. Med. Investig. **573**(3,4), 305–313 (2010)
6. Kasai, T., Motoori, K., Horikosh, T., Uchiyam, K., Yasufuku, K., Takiguchi, F., Kuniyasu, Y., Ito, H.: Dual-time point scanning of integrated FDG PET/CT for the evaluation of mediastinal and hilar lymph nodes in non-small cell lung cancer diagnosed as operable by contrast-enhanced CT. Eur. J. Radiol. **75**(2), 143–146 (2010)
7. Shigemoto, Y., Suga, K., Matsunaga, N.: F-18-FDG-avid lymph node metastasis along preferential lymphatic drainage pathways from the tumor-bearing lung lobe on F-18-FDG PET/CT in patients with non-small-cell lung cancer. Ann. Nucl. Med. **30**(4), 287–297 (2016)

Feasibility Study of Developing a Brain-Dedicated SPECT Scanner

Hsin-Chin Liang$^{(\boxtimes)}$, Yu-Ching Ni, and Hsiang-Ning Wu

Health Physics, Institute of Nuclear Energy Research,
Wenhua Rd, Taoyuan, Taiwan ROC
sjingliang@iner.gov.tw

Abstract. Due to population aging, early diagnosis of neurodegenerative diseases have been noticed. To fulfill such clinical need, developing a hi-performance SPECT scanner for brain function imaging was raised. In this research, a practical scanner geometry was provided and the resolution performance of imaging detectors for composing the scanner was also studied. Consider the resolution and practicality, a cylindrical scanner design, with a detector ring of 48-cm diameter and a rotatable collimator cylinder of 32-cm diameter was chosen for further development. With 1-mm pinholes placing on the collimator cylinder, a FOV (field-of-view) of 21-cm diameter and 15-cm height, also a magnification factor of 0.48 are formed. In such design, the resolution is derived by the intrinsic resolution of imaging detectors. In the aspect of imaging detector unit, three different pixel size were studied. Three GAGG detector units with pixel size of 1.8, 1.5 and 1.2 mm were built and tested. The resultant 2D crystal maps and pixelated energy spectrum were examined to see how crystal pixels being resolved. The outward appearance of the detector unit showed that no peripheral dead space exhibits and thus allows 2D scalable to achieve the scanner building need. The 2D maps of the three detector units all showed successfully distinguished crystal arrays, therefore 1.3 mm resolution for the imaging detector can be achieved at current stage. It means the best scanner resolution at the FOV center of 2.88 mm is expected. In this study, a practical scanner geometry design is made, also its imaging detector unit is developed. Preliminary results show that the best resolution performance is better than 3 mm. Therefore the following task is to design the pinhole collimator pattern, trying to maximize the scanner sensitivity while keeping the resolution around 3 mm.

Keywords: Brain imaging · SPECT scanner · Scanner geometry · Imaging detectors

1 Introduction

Due to population aging, neurodegenerative diseases have become a non-negligible social problem, and thus early diagnosis have been noticed its clinical need [1]. In the current clinical diagnosis means, nuclear medicine based functional imaging has been proved an effective diagnosis tool for such diseases [2]. Therefore, developing a hi-performance SPECT scanner for brain function imaging was raised in our institute. In this research, scanner geometry designs were evaluated, and a practical one was chosen

© Springer Nature Switzerland AG 2020
K.-P. Lin et al. (Eds.): ICBHI 2019, IFMBE Proceedings 74, pp. 143–147, 2020.
https://doi.org/10.1007/978-3-030-30636-6_21

and completed. And also an imaging detector unit which fits the need of scanner composing and the requirement of high resolution performance was developed.

2   Materials and Methods

2.1   Scanner Geometry Description

Several geometrical types including helmet-like and oval cylinder were evaluated. Consider the complexity of reconstruction algorithm, a circular cylinder was chosen for the scanner geometry design. Consider the image resolution of the scanner, a cylinder diameter about half-meter was determined, shown in Fig. 1, with a detector ring of 47.5-cm diameter and a rotatable collimator cylinder of 32-cm diameter. With 45 1-mm aperture, symmetric 60°-cone angle (shown in Fig. 2) pinholes placing on the collimator

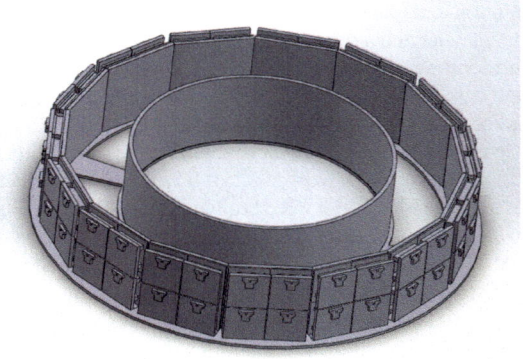

Fig. 1. a Current brain SPECT scanner design.

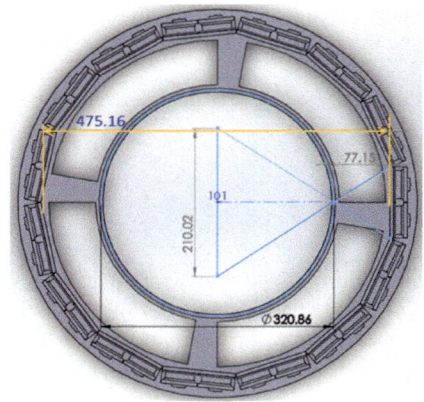

Fig. 2. b Geometric dimension of the scanner design.

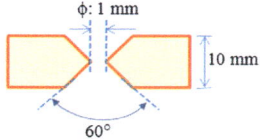

Fig. 3. Cross-section scheme of a pinhole collimator.

cylinder, a FOV (field-of-view) of 21-cm diameter and 15-cm height, also a magnification factor of 0.48 are formed. In such design, the resolution is derived by the intrinsic resolution of imaging detectors. In the scan process, the collimator cylinder stays at 0°, 6°, 12° and 18° to process image acquisition. Therefore, for each set of pinholes, which contains 15 ones, there will be 60 projections in a whole scan process (Fig. 3).

2.2   Development of Imaging Detector Units

The detector ring is composed of 15 imaging detectors, and each detector is composed of 4 imaging units. Each unit is composed of a pixelated GAGG crystal array and an array-type SiPM element (SensL ArrayC 30035-144-PCB). Typical scintillation properties of the material GAGG are listed in Table 1. The choice of above-mentioned materials makes the unit have an imaging area of 50.2×50.2 mm^2. All the gaps between imaging units are equal-spaced, and thus a successive imaging space of the detector ring is expected. Therefore, two requirements for the imaging units are shown, i.e. no peripheral dead spaces to allow 2D scaling and high intrinsic resolution.

Table 1. GAGG:Ce physical properties [3]

Item	Property
Light yield (ph/Mev)	54000
Energy resolution (662 keV)	∼5.6%
Decay time (ns)	90
Density (g/cm^3)	6.6
Effective atomic number	54
Peak emission (nm)	∼540
Self-radiation	No
Hygroscopic	No

For the resolution of the imaging detector unit, three different pixel size detectors were studied. Three GAGG array blocks which have the same size of $50.2 \times 50.2 \times 5$ mm^3 and compose of 1.8, 1.5 and 1.2 mm crystal pixels respectively were tested on the SiPM element. The resultant 2D crystal maps and pixelated energy spectrum were examined to see how crystal pixels being resolved.

3   Results and Discussions

From the outward appearance of the imaging detector unit, shown in Fig. 4, it is exhibited that no peripheral dead spaces and thus allows 2D scaling to achieve the scanner building need. The 2D maps of the three imaging detectors all showed successfully distinguished crystal arrays, which are 26×26 for 1.8 mm pixels, 31×31 for 1.5 mm pixels, and 38×38 for 1.2 mm pixels. One test result is shown in Fig. 5, a high quality 2D crystal map and reasonable gamma energy spectrum can be observed. Due to the pitch size between two crystal pixel centers forward related to the intrinsic resolution of an imaging detector [4, 5], a 1.3-mm resolution (i.e. 50.2 mm/38) for the imaging detector was achieved at current stage. It also indicates that the best scanner resolution at the FOV center of 2.88 mm ($\sqrt{[(1.3/0.48)^2 + 1^2]}$) is expected.

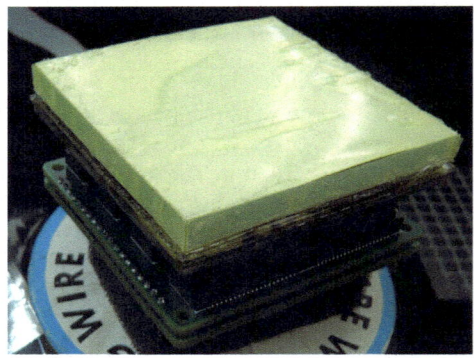

Fig. 4. Outward appearance of the imaging detector unit.

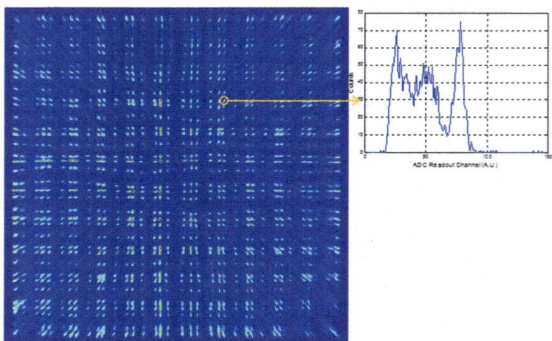

Fig. 5. Imaging detector unit test result. A well-distinguished 2D crystal map (left) and a typical 511-keV gamma spectrum of one selected pixel (right) are shown.

4 Conclusions

In this study, a practical SPECT scanner geometry is evaluated, and also the imaging detector unit which fits the scanner building requirements is developed. Preliminary results show that the best resolution performance is better than 3 mm. Therefore the following task is to put the whole set of design parameters, such as focal length and detector resolution, into a scanner simulation and evaluation process to validate the performances, including image resolution and scanner sensitivity, fitting our original development expectations.

Conflict of Interest. The authors declare that they have no conflict of interest.

References

1. Batsch, N.L., Mittelman, M.S.: World Alzheimer Report 2012. Alzheimer's Disease International (2012)
2. Penny, W.D., Friston, K.J.: Functional imaging. Scholarpedia **2**(5), 1478 (2007)
3. CETC product spec. (2017)
4. Liang, H.-C., Jan, M.-L., Su, J.-L., et al.: Development of an LYSO based gamma camera for positron and scinti-mammography. J. Instrum. JINST **4**, P08009 (2009)
5. Liang, H.-C., Jan, M.-L., Su, J.-L.: Development of a pixelated detector for clinical positron and single-photon molecular imaging. J Med Biol Eng **32**(5), 373–380 (2012)

Development of Urine Conductivity Sensing System for Measurement and Data Collection

Roozbeh Falah Ramezani[1(✉)], Abdul Hadi Nograles[2],
Wen-Yaw Chung[1], Jennifer Dela Cruz[2], Kuan-Hua Li[1],
Chean-Yeh Cheng[3], and Vincent Tsai[4]

[1] Department of Electronic Engineering, Chung Yuan Christian University,
Chung-Li, Taiwan, ROC
s3153079@gmail.com
[2] Department of Electronics Engineering, Mapua University,
Muralla St., Manila, Philippines
[3] Department of Chemistry, Chung Yuan Christian University,
Chung-Li, Taiwan, ROC
[4] Ten-Chen Medical Group, Chung-Li, Taiwan, ROC

Abstract. This paper presents the design of an analog front-end of an electrochemical conductivity sensor. This forms part of a multi-parameter sensing device for use in the detection and diagnosis of urolithiasis in its preliminary stages. The proposed conductivity bio-sensor is used for measuring the concentration of total dissolved salts in urine. It will be combined with FET-based potentiometric sensors for measuring Ca^{2+} and pH, and an amperometric sensor for measuring uric acid into an integrated lab-on-a-chip point-of-care device.

Furthermore, measured data are collected and stored in a database for future use in an AI (Artificial Intelligence) diagnosis system. Such a multi-parameter approach caters for a more effective stone-risk indexing.

The conductivity sensor readout circuit works on the principle of electrochemical impedance spectroscopy. The sample under test (urine) is subjected to a constant sinusoidal current which causes it to develop a potential difference. The sample interface is via four-point gold coated flat electrodes. The true RMS (root mean square) value of current and voltage is measured and impedance magnitude is calculated by dividing voltage to current.

Measurement is iterated for several frequencies in the range between 1.5 kHz and 3.3 kHz. The frequency is selected from prime numbers to avoid harmonics distortion.

The proposed system has been tested in an on-board platform and the results of the measurement are correlated to a commercial conductivity meter device. The developed conductivity sensor and its readout circuitry have potential usage in point-of-care test device for urolithiasis prognosis and screening.

Keywords: Conductometry · Conductivity meter ·
Electrochemical impedance spectrometry · Urine studies · Urolithiasis ·
Point-of-Care · Conductivity sensor

© Springer Nature Switzerland AG 2020
K.-P. Lin et al. (Eds.): ICBHI 2019, IFMBE Proceedings 74, pp. 148–155, 2020.
https://doi.org/10.1007/978-3-030-30636-6_22

1 Introduction

Diagnosis of Urolithiasis (kidney-stone formation) in early stage by testing urine sample using multi-sensor platform is presented in [1]. Improving the accuracy of measured parameters, collection and storing such data contributes to more efficient stone-risk indexing. Multi-frequency bio-impedance measurement is a disruptive technology as it is both non-destructive and relatively simpler to implement especially in portable or point-of-care based systems. This paper presents a novel system for measuring and storing the data of urine sample conductivity. A design of multi-frequency bio-impedance spectroscopy system is presented in [2]. The system is combination of front-end analog signal conditioning circuit and FPGA as digital back-end. The frequency range between 10 kHz and 250 kHz is used in their system. In [3] multi-frequency range between 3 kHz and 1 MHz and mono-frequency of 50 kHz is used for measuring the whole-body and thoracic bio-impedance. A Design of bio-impedance spectrometer for early detection of pressure ulcer with frequency range between 10 Hz and 1 MHz is presented in [4]. Multi-frequency electrical impedance is used for skin cancer identification [5] using 31 logarithmically distributed frequencies between 1 and 1000 kHz. For the circuit interface to the sample under test, a two-point probe setup was used in [5] which makes the implementation simpler whenever the impedance of the sample is larger than that of the electrode's equivalent impedance. However, a four-point probe setup is suggested to have a more accurate reading that is unaffected by electrode impedances as suggested in [1–4].

The block diagram of system presented in this paper is shown in Fig. 1:

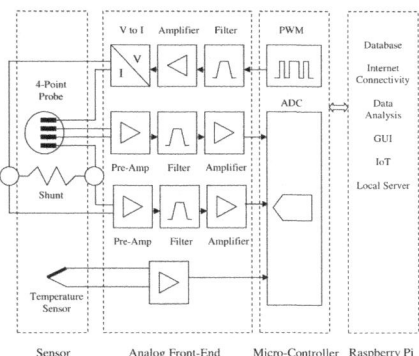

Fig. 1. Conductometric sensor system

Four-point probe forms the urine sample sensor. The desired PWM frequency generated by micro-controller passes through a band-pass filter. The filter outputs a sinusoidal wave that is coupled to an amplifier. Then, the voltage signal is converted to a constant current and fed to the outer probe of the sensor. Such current passes through the urine sample and creates a voltage proportional to its resistance measured between the inner probes. Resistance is function of conductivity and geometry of the sensor.

The voltage signal will pass through pre-amplifier block formed by a high CMRR (Common Mode Rejection Ratio) instrumentation amplifier (IA). The output of the IA passes through a band-pass filter. The succeeding block is a signal conditioning amplifier which brings the signal to the level of ADC (Analog to Digital Converter) input. The microcontroller uses the ADC measured value for calculating the amplitude of impedance of the sample.

In addition, the micro-controller communicates with a Raspberry Pi single-board computer through SPI (Serial Port Interface). Raspberry Pi acts as local server that keeps the database, analysis the data, provides internet connectivity. It also acts as GUI (Graphic User Interface) for overall system.

2 Methodology

Our preliminary tests of several samples include KCl, NaCl solution and urine shows decrease of impedance against increase of frequency that agrees with the results in [1] and [2]. Thus the simplified equivalent circuit shown in Fig. 2 is used for total impedance of sample. Conductivity of sample is measured by the system while eliminating the effect of parasitic capacitance.

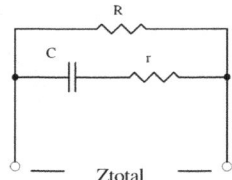

Fig. 2. Electrical equivalent circuit of the sample

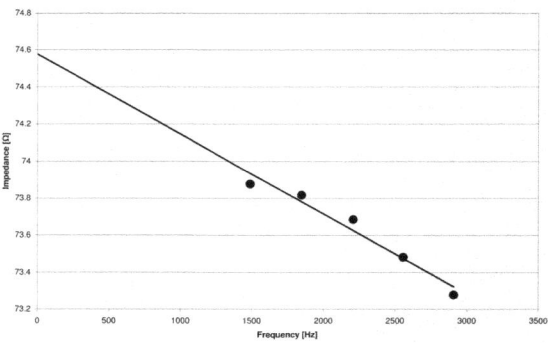

Fig. 3. Impedance of 0.1 M KCL solution at various frequencies

The system measures the impedance in several frequencies and the linear regression line of the impedance in different frequencies is calculated. The Y-intercept of the linear regression (at zero frequency) is the sample resistance as shown in Fig. 3 Conductance is obtained by inversing the resistance, and after multiplying it by the cell constant, the conductivity is calculated.

3 Measurement Range

The conductivity results from 20 urine sample test of three volunteers were taken. In order to find the range the samples are taken randomly during the day. Our test results in Table 1 show the urine conductivity range between 3.13 mS/cm and 19.20 mS/cm. The study of 2000 urine sample presented in [6] shows the urine conductivity range between 1.1 mS/cm and 33.9 mS/cm. Our system is designed to operate in range between 0.1 mS/Cm and 50 mS/cm.

Table 1. Urine sample conductivity

Urine Sample	Conductivity [mS/Cm]	Remark
1	10.18	
2	12.48	
3	10.56	
4	14.10	
5	14.38	
6	13.08	
7	16.74	
8	19.20	Max.
9	15.68	
10	13.31	
11	11.43	
12	8.84	
13	13.78	
14	14.21	
15	7.42	
16	3.13	Min.
17	18.74	
18	8.42	
19	13.14	
20	11.49	

4   Sensor

A gold coated PCB is used as four-point probe that forms sensor for this system. The four-point probe is selected due to its higher accuracy compare to two-point probe. Two-point probes are suitable for measurement of high-impedance and low-conductance samples since the error is negligible. In low-impedance high conductance samples the separation between current feeding and voltage reading circuits of four-point probe reduces error in measurement. Measuring the impedance of the sample between two inner connections is desired. The voltage of inner connectors is measured while current is fed through outer connectors to the all sensing parts. Although sensors could be designed with any arbitrary shape and geometry in this paper only the bar-shape and circular sensors and their cell constant is presented.

4.1   Bar-Shape Sensor

Electrical equivalent circuit of bar-shape conductivity sensor is shown in Fig. 4:

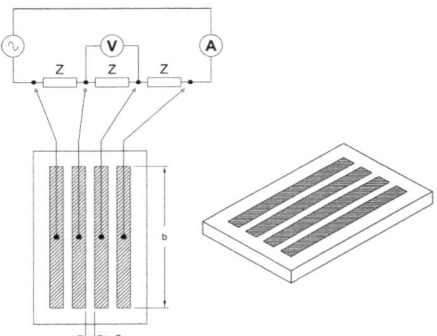

Fig. 4. Bar-shape conductivity sensor

Resistance of sensing section of bar-shape sensor is calculated using (1):

$$R = \rho \frac{a}{bt} \tag{1}$$

R is the resistance in Ω, ρ is the resistivity in Ω-m, a is the sensing part width in m, b is sensing part length in m and t is combined thickness of copper and its gold coating in m.

4.2   Circular Sensor

The electric field in the corner edges of bar-shape sensor is not uniform and caused error in measurement. Circular conductivity sensor shown in Fig. 5 eliminates such error by creating uniform electrical field in whole sensing area.

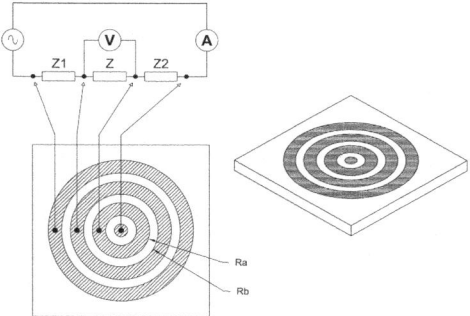

Fig. 5. Circular conductivity sensor

Resistance of sensing part in circular sensor is calculated using (2):

$$R = \frac{\rho}{2\pi t} \ln \frac{R_b}{R_a} \tag{2}$$

R is the resistance in Ω, ρ is the resistivity in $\Omega\text{-}m$, R_a is the sensing part inner circle radius in m, R_b is sensing part outer circle radius in m and t is combined thickness of copper and its gold coating in m.

5 Analog Front End

The analog front end of the system consists of four signal conditioning sections. The first section converts receiving digital PWM signal from microcontroller to sinusoidal constant current. The second section receives the input signal from sensor voltage probes. It will be sent to microcontroller ADC input after amplification and filtering. The third section is similar to second section except receives its input signal from shunt resistor in series with sensor current feed circuit. The fourth section is amplifier and low pass filter for the temperature sensor that will be connected to another microcontroller ADC channel.

6 Digital Back End

Digital back end of the system is a 32-bit Cortex-M0 + ARM microcontroller. It has 8-channel 12-bit SAR ADC with conversion rate up to 1 Msps. The sinusoidal signal from analog front end is fed through ADC after gain and offset adjustment. The ADC input signal voltage level should remain between 0 and 3.3 V that dictates DC offset of 1.75 V with maximum amplitude of 1.75 V for sinusoidal signal. The sampling rate is adjusted to 250Ksps which provide more than 64 samples per cycle for the highest frequency of 3.3 kHz. The samples from ADC then fed through fast digital IIR high-pass filter for removing the DC offset. True RMS values of both sinusoidal signals are calculated by firmware in microcontroller.

In addition, base PWM signal with desired frequency is made using microcontroller timer and connected to analog front end through GPIO.

Furthermore, the temperature sensor DC signal is measured by microcontroller and used for temperature compensation.

Microcontroller performs the calibration process and store the measured value. Communication with single board computer is maintained through SPI.

7   Database and Connectivity

A Raspberry Pi single board computer acts as the gateway of the system. Thanks to its Linux operating system several applications could be run on Raspberry Pi simultaneously.

Serial Port Interface (SPI) is used for low level communication with microcontroller. Calibration commands, adjustments, measurement data and other specific data will be exchanged between microcontroller and Raspberry Pi.

MySql is used as database server. The data are stored in two separate databases for security reason. One secure database with limited access holds patient information. It links to the other database through an ID record. The test results database keeps patient ID, gender and the birthday year info of each patient along with urine test results, test time and date and general condition of patient at the time of test.

Apache 2 html server is used as local server, while combined with PHP it provides GUI for the overall system.

Connection to internet through Wifi or Ethernet converts the whole system to an IoT device that allows storage of data on cloud or access to the system via secure internet connection.

8   Conclusions

Preliminary test results from KCl solution shows improvement in reliability and accuracy of conductivity measurement. Such multi-frequency measurement system combined with data collection and storing system will provide essential point of care solution for diagnosis of kidney-stone in early stages.

Most of existing commercial conductivity meter are using two-point probe as sensor. In addition measurement is performed in single or few frequencies only. Result is considered valid if the difference between such measurements is less than predefined error.

This paper presents utilizing of four-point circular probe which has significant contribution to improve the accuracy of overall system. Furthermore, the system is using innovative approach of multiple impedance measurement in different frequencies and calculates the conductivity at zero frequency. Direct measurement at zero-frequency is not possible due to electrolysis of sample.

The novel concept that presented in this paper will be implemented on a single chip in future.

Acknowledgment. The authors would like to express their deep gratitude to Ten-Chen Hospital Group, Chung-Li for medical issue consulting, Holtek Semiconductor Inc for providing support of digital hardware and Dr. Angelito Silverio for his great help of paper editing.

Conflict of Interest. The authors declare that they have no conflict of interest.

References

1. Silverio, A.A.: A Multi-Sensor Readout Inter-face Circuit with System-On-Chip Implementation Applied to Urine Quality Analysis (Doctoral dissertation). Chung Yuan Christian University, Taoyuan (2016)
2. Chung, W.Y., et.al.: Design of a multi-frequency bio-impedance spectroscopy system analog front-end and digital back-end with on-chip implementation. In: Proceedings of the 2015 International Symposium on Bioelectronics and Bioinformatics, October 2015
3. Nescolarde, L., et.al.: Whole-body and thoracic bio-impedance measurement: hypertension and hyperhydration in hemodialysis patients. In: Proceedings of the 29th Annual International Conference of the IEEE on Engineering in Medicine and Biology Society, pp. 3593–3596 (2009). https://doi.org/10.1109/iembs.2007.4353108
4. Yang, Y., Wang, J.: A design of bio-impedance spectrometer for early detection of pressure ulcer. In: 27th Annual International Conference of the Engineering in Medicine and Biology Society, 2005, IEEE-EMBS 2005, pp. 6602–6604 (2005). https://doi.org/10.1109/iembs.2005.1616014
5. Aberg, P., et al.: Skin cancer identification using multi-frequency electrical impedance – a potential screening tool. IEEE Trans. Biomed. Eng. **51**(12), 2097–2102 (2004). https://doi.org/10.1109/TBME.2004.836523
6. Fazil Marickar, Y.M.: Electrical conductivity and total dissolved solids in urine. Urol. Res. **38** (4), 233–235 (2010). https://doi.org/10.1007/s00240-009-0228-y

Spectrogram and Deep Neural Network Analysis in Detecting Paroxysmal Atrial Fibrillation with Bottleneck Layers and Cross Entropy Approach

Edward B. Panganiban[1,2,3(✉)], Wen-Yaw Chung[1],
and Arnold C. Paglinawan[2]

[1] Department of Electronic Engineering, Chung-Yuan Christian University,
Chung-Li, Taiwan, R.O.C.
[2] School of Electrical Electronics and Computer Engineering, Mapua University,
Intramuros, Manila, Philippines
[3] College of Computing Studies, Information and Communication Technology,
Isabela State University, Echague, Isabela, Philippines
ebpanganiban@isu.edu.ph

Abstract. Paroxysmal AF (PAF) is a form of atrial fibrillation (AF) that is generally clinically silent and undetected. AF is a type of heart disease called cardiac arrhythmia. Automatic detection of AF could make a significant contribution to early diagnosis, control and prevention of chronic AF complications. In this paper, authors presented a novel algorithm through spectrogram and deep learning neural network analysis in detecting paroxysmal AF from image data segments. This method does not require the detection of P and/or R peaks which is a preprocessing step required by many existing algorithms. The PAF Prediction Challenge Database from Physionet.org were used as learning set which composed of 50 record sets. These records were converted into 7,000 PAF and 964 healthy data segments. Each data segment has 5 mins-duration and converted it to graph images. These graph images are then converted into spectrogram to visualize the frequency band present in the spectrum. In this process, ECG numerical values were interpreted into spectrogram form. Spectrogram images are cropped to remove unnecessary markings from the graphing and spectrogram processes. Cropped spectrogram images are then grouped into separate folders according to type. The produced datasets are then fed into training using 500,000 training steps. The algorithm is integrated with TensorFlow CPU version 1.5 and Inception V3 model to take advantage of its astonishing way on how it analyzes images. The deep learning neural network involves a bottleneck layer which uses lesser neurons to reduce the number of feature maps in the network to get the best loss during training. In order to have a faster learning rate, the cross-entropy cost function was used. The final accuracy test from the training reached as high as 96.8%. An actual test for identified PAF and healthy datasets from Physionet.org were performed and all are correctly predicted and thus could be able to classify other different diseases based from converted ECG numerical values. Furthermore, this paper established a low-powered workstation's requirement for implementation because it only requires at least a dual core processor and 2 GB of RAM.

© Springer Nature Switzerland AG 2020
K.-P. Lin et al. (Eds.): ICBHI 2019, IFMBE Proceedings 74, pp. 156–165, 2020.
https://doi.org/10.1007/978-3-030-30636-6_23

Keywords: Spectrogram · Paroxysmal Atrial Fibrillation · Deep learning · Cross entropy · Bottleneck

1   Introduction

According to studies, there are about 0.5% of the world's population has Atrial Fibrillation (AF) and 17% of people aged 85 or above are AF patients [1]. In the United States of America., the number of AF patients will increase by 250% or more than 5.6 million people by 2050 [2]. AF is an irregular heartbeat called arrhythmia which may lead can lead to various heart-related conditions such as blood clots, stroke, and heart failure [3]. Paroxysmal Atrial Fibrillation (PAF) is a type of AF that occurs sometimes then stops by itself then returns to normal heart rhythm. This type of AF is more symptomatic that other types such as persistent AF, long-standing persistent AF and permanent AF. Persistent AF needs medication or a special type of electric shock to help the heart return to normal rhythm, while long-standing and permanent AF cannot be corrected by these treatments [4, 5].

AF can cause death if left untreated because it can damage the heart's structure. Since most AF patients do not feel any symptoms, early detection may help prevent paroxysmal AF which can lead to more serious type of AF. One of the procedures needed for the diagnosis of this type of heart disease is through electrocardiography (ECG) by checking the heart's electrical activity [6]. Medical practitioners need to have in-depth skills and professional knowledge to accurately interpret ECG [7]. In addition, it is time consuming to visually inspect ECG signals [8].

Recent studies showed that there are several methods on how AF episodes were detected based from ECG data. Some of these studies rely on the absence of P-waves [9], R-R irregularities, or a combination of these characteristics, density histogram of R-R intervals, short data segments among others [10]. These were then processed in several algorithms like a machine learning through wavelet transform and support vector machine [8]. Some methods eliminates the need for P-peak or R-Peak detection which is a pre-processing step in detecting AF [8].

Synthesizing these studies, the authors established a novel algorithm in detecting PAF based from ECG data through the application of spectrogram and deep learning analysis with the integration of bottleneck layers and cross entropy approach. In this new approach, it eliminates the need for ECG visual inspection like P-peak or R-peak detection. It can also help an early and accurate detection of AF by identifying the abnormal patterns that can be possible through convolutional deep learning analysis. The proposed AF detection method has high accuracy which makes it a suitable choice for practical use.

2   Materials and Methods

Learning Model
The authors established a model in learning datasets from the PAF database. The model is shown in Fig. 1. This diagram contains seven (7) stages which were used in

developing the neural network model in classifying PAF disease. The stages are regrouped into three functions that include pre-processing, spectrogram analysis and deep learning analysis. Pre-processing involved data collection and conversion, spectrogram analysis performed data spectrum analysis, noise filtering and clustering, while deep learning analysis functioned as learning/training and model validation. Each stage has its own function as explained in the next paragraph.

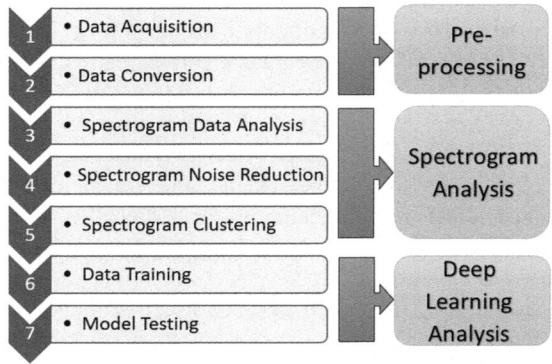

Fig. 1. Learning model

Data Acquisition

Datasets were taken from the physiobank from physionet.org specifically the PAF prediction challenge database. The database downloaded is a two-channel ECG signal in CSV file format and with unaudited beat annotations format. It has learning sets of 50 record sets from 48 different subjects and test set with also 50 record sets from 50 different subjects. Each record is cut up into multiple .TXT file with a 5-mins duration to make it compatible with the next step.

Data Conversion

Data conversion is the process of changing its form into another suitable format. In this step, each .TXT file is then converted into a graphical image based on its numerical values. All .TXT files were processed for data conversion in preparation for its spectrogram analysis.

Spectrogram Data Analysis

Spectrogram is a graphical representation of the range of frequencies of a signal as it varies with time [11]. In this stage, the graphical images are converted into spectrogram to visualize the spectrum frequency band present. These images are analyzed thoroughly to identify the spectrum of frequency band present in the graphical images.

Spectrogram Noise Reduction

Graphical images are susceptible to various types of noise. Image noise is the result of errors in the image acquisition and conversion processes which turn into a change of its real characteristics. Hence, spectrogram noise reduction is important in this stage, specifically to remove the unnecessary markings from the graphing and spectrogram process.

Spectrogram Clustering

The clustering process done in this paper is the grouping of cropped spectrogram images according to its type. There are only two groups classified which are the PAF and healthy records. These records were already filtered in preparation for its training.

Data Training

The datasets which came from the spectrogram clustering underwent into data training for the learning process. In this, it will find patterns, find relationships and evaluate its confidence its identification from the training datasets. Through this, it will help the system develop a model in identifying a PAF disease based from the ECG signal. The test data involved is 10% of the total dataset. The datasets were trained using 500,000 training steps.

Model Testing

This last stage will determine the accuracy of the model. Test images used during the actual test after its training is not part of the training dataset. An actual test for PAF is performed so as to find out the reliability of the model.

Deep Learning Support

The learning environment of the model is combined with the power use of TensorFlow version 1.5. TensorFLow is a machine learning system that usually focuses on the training large data on deep neural networks [12]. This is in particular based on the Inception V3 model of the TensorFLow platform due its learning capability to retrain datasets for the improvement of classification accuracy [13].

Bottleneck neural network is also used in this paper, wherein the authors only used a small number of hidden layers that does not affect its classification accuracy. The advantage of using this is the small number of hidden layers in training the datasets. It is proven that bottleneck features are effective in improving the accuracy of speech recognition, hence, the authors used this additional feature [14].

In order to attain the optimized pattern classification and faster learning rate, cross-entropy loss function is used. This is a refinement of a classification method as also used in a previous study [15].

3   Results and Discussion

Raw Data

Learning datasets will come from the raw data exported from the physiobank atm of PAF prediction challenge database. These records were exported as CSV files which contains two 30-mins and two 5-mins ECG signals. The sample healthy data and PAF data are shown in Figs. 2 and 3 respectively. Those samples represented were cut into 5-min duration only. The height indicates its voltage level and the length is the time.

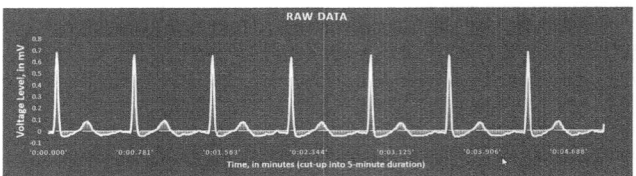

Fig. 2. Healthy raw data

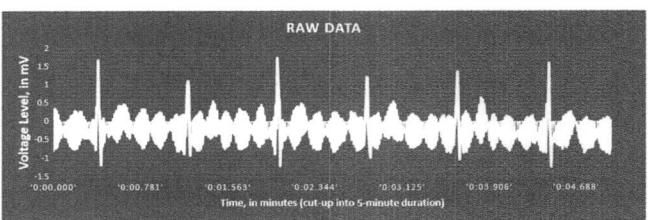

Fig. 3. PAF raw data

Txt Files

The csv files are then converted into txt files which can contain up to 1,000 data values. The number of rows of data differs from each other depending on the exported csv files. These extracted values the variable voltage levels within the duration of 5 min. Figure 4 shows the sample txt files for both healthy and non-healthy (PAF).

File Edit Format View Help	File Edit Format View Help
0.055	-0.795
0.055	0.35
0.055	-0.73
0.055	0.275
0.06	-0.695
0.065	0.19
0.065	-0.54
0.065	0.02
0.07	-0.435
0.075	-0.135
0.075	-0.26
0.075	-0.27
0.075	-0.145
0.075	-0.42
0.075	-0.055
0.075	-0.43
0.075	0.015
0.075	-0.55
0.075	0.035
0.07	-0.67
0.065	0.15
0.055	-0.73
0.05	0.185
0.05	-0.75
0.035	0.275
0.02	-0.745
0.01	0.265
0	-0.725
0	0.215
0	-0.615
-0.01	0.27
-0.025	-0.49
-0.045	

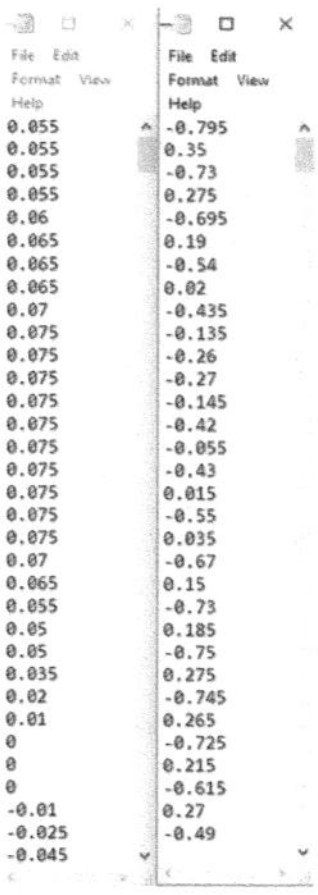

Fig. 4. Sample txt files (a) Healthy (b) PAF

Spectrogram Analysis

The txt files are then fed into spectrogram process and produced an output like what is shown in Figs. 5 and 6. Figure 5 is a sample healthy spectrum of the frequency band represented through a graphical image. The number of rows represents the number of rows of voltage values from a single txt file. The vertical axis represents the normalized frequency output created based from the spectrogram process. Figure 6 is a sample PAF spectrogram image which indicates a lower number of row of data. These spectrogram outputs are the images that are then fed to the deep learning neural network. These images have passed through a noise reduction and clustering. More samples of healthy and PAF spectrogram images are demonstrated in Figures 7 and 8 respectively. Sample test images as shown in Fig. 9 are used to validate the learning model for its accuracy and reliability.

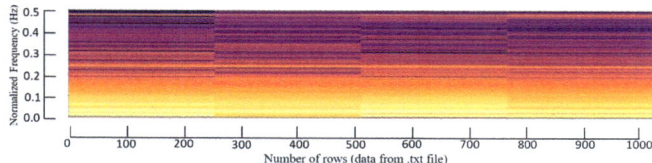

Fig. 5. A 5-min spectrogram input for deep learning analysis (Healthy)

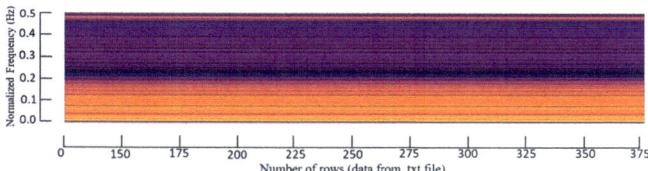

Fig. 6. A 5-min spectrogram input for deep learning analysis (PAF)

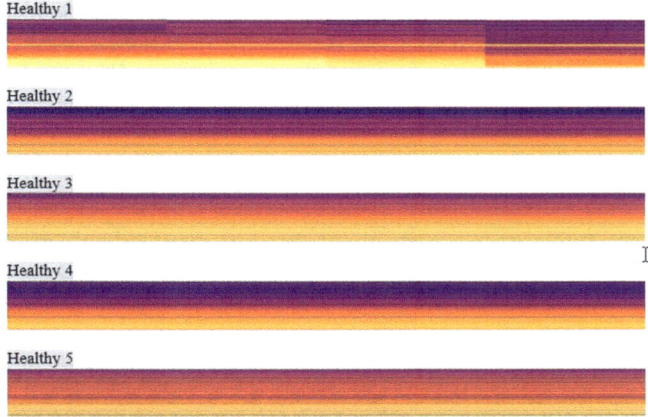

Fig. 7. Sample healthy images from spectrogram process

Fig. 8. Sample PAF images from spectrogram process

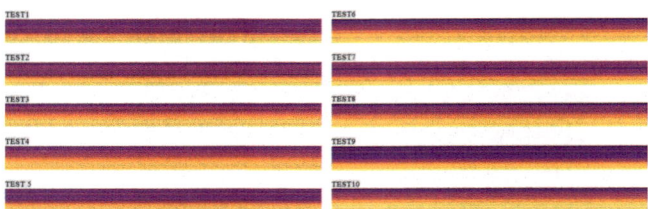

Fig. 9. Test data samples

Data Training Result

After training all the datasets, learning its pattern through deep learning analysis is established. Validation and training accuracy were determined as well as its cross entropy loss. After 500,000 training steps, the model obtained a training accuracy of 96.8%, a validation accuracy of 92.3% and minimal cross entropy loss of 0.197584 only. This means that this algorithm is a reliable approach in identifying PAF and healthy signals. Table 1 illustrates the results of training logs from 25,000 steps up to 500,000 training steps.

Data Testing Result

Test data which comprises 10% from the learned datasets were used to test the algorithm for its reliability in classifying PAF versus healthy signals. It was found out that the learning model is reliable since it can determine correctly what its health status based from the test samples. The result of the test is given in Table 2. This table is only sample taken from 10 test image samples. There is a very small difference only is one sample wherein it is almost in the middle of the classifying score, e.g. test 7. Others, are not confusing because it has large difference of classifying scores. From the ten samples, 6 were identified as having PAF disease while 4 were healthy.

Table 1. Training Result

Training steps	Validation Accuracy	Training Accuracy	Cross Entropy Loss
25,000	70.9%	77.1%	0.389803
50,000	80.8%	85.3%	0.375598
75,000	79.2%	82.1%	0.413507
100,000	74.7%	86.1%	0.385265
125,000	77.9%	85.2%	0.365296
150,000	74.8%	86.3%	0.334466
175,000	77.7%	85.3%	0.357033
200,000	79.4%	86.6%	0.335781
225,000	80.5%	88.7%	0.361666
250,000	80.9%	87.3%	0.355943
275,000	82.4%	89.4%	0.349731
300,000	83.3%	89.4%	0.308340
325,000	85.7%	91.2%	0.274145
350,000	85.8%	91.6%	0.269887
375,000	88.9%	92.7%	0.267745
400,000	90.5%	93.7%	0.252530
425,000	91.8%	94.2%	0.221507
450,000	92.7%	95.4%	0.218415
475,000	92.7%	95.8%	0.204207
500,000	92.3%	96.8%	0.197584

Table 2. Sample test result

Test samples	PAF Score	Healthy Score	Test Remarks
Test 1	0.86	0.13	Correct (PAF)
Test 2	0.93	0.06	Correct (PAF)
Test 3	0.30	0.69	Correct (Healthy)
Test 4	0.60	0.39	Correct (PAF)
Test 5	0.23	0.76	Correct (Healthy)
Test 6	0.70	0.29	Correct (PAF)
Test 7	0.54	0.45	Correct (almost half-way)(PAF)
Test 8	0.72	0.27	Correct (Healthy)
Test 9	0.35	0.64	Correct (PAF)
Test 10	0.14	0.85	Correct (Healthy)

4   Conclusion

A new algorithm in detecting Paroxysmal Atrial Fibrillation (PAF) is established in this paper through the implementation of pre-processing, spectrogram analysis and deep learning analysis. Its final training accuracy obtained is 96.8% with a validation accuracy of 92.3%. The cross-entropy loss reached only 0.197584 and tests were done and accurately classified the health status based on two categories – healthy and PAF. The datasets used came from the PAF prediction Challenge database wherein it includes the healthy, PAF and test datasets. Through the new technologies like TensorFlow platform Inception V3 model, bottleneck features neural network and cross-entropy optimization features, the objectives of this paper were met. Furthermore, this paper established a low-powered workstation's requirement for its development and testing as only requires at least a dual core processor and 2 GB of RAM.

Acknowledgment. The authors would like to thank Chung Yuan Christian University for allowing authors the opportunity to use the Mixed-Mode IC Laboratory in the Department of Electronic Engineering which made this paper possible and attained its objectives. Special thanks also to Mapua University Graduate School Office for the guidance and support given to the researchers.

Conflict of Interest. The authors declare no conflict of interest.

References

1. Heeringa, J., Van Der Kuip, D.A.M., Hofman, A., Kors, J.A., Van Herpen, G., Stricker, B.H. C., Stijnen, T., Lip, G.Y.H., Witteman, J.C.M.: Prevalence, incidence and lifetime risk of atrial fibrillation: The Rotterdam study. Eur. Heart J. **27**, 949–953 (2006)
2. Go, A.S., Hylek, E.M., Phillips, K.A., Chang, Y., Henault, L.E., Selby, J.V., Singer, D.E.: Prevalence of Diagnosed Atrial Fibrillation in Adults. National Implications for Rhythm Management and Stroke Prevention: the AnTicoagulation and Risk Factors in Atrial Fibrillation (ATRIA) Study. JAMA – J. Am. Med. Assoc. **285**, 2370–2375 (2001)
3. Chang, Y., Wu, S., Tseng, L., Chao, H., Ko, C.: AF detection by exploiting the spectral and temporal characteristics of ECG signals with the LSTM model, pp. 1–4. National Chiao Tung University (2018)
4. Shashikumar, S.P., Shah, A.J., Clifford, G.D., Nemati, S.: Detection of Paroxysmal Atrial Fibrillation using Attention-based Bidirectional Recurrent Neural Networks, pp.1–9. arXiv Prepr arXiv180509133 (2018)
5. Chiang, C.E., Naditch-Brûlé, L., Murin, J., et al.: Distribution and risk profile of paroxysmal, persistent, and permanent atrial fibrillation in routine clinical practice: Insight from the real-life global survey evaluating patients with atrial fibrillation international registry. Circ. Arrhythmia Electrophysiol. **5**, 632–639 (2012)
6. Larburu, N., Beregana, T.L.: Comparative Study of Algorithms for Atrial Fibrillation Detection. Publica Univ Navarrensis 142 (2011)
7. Mehall, J.R., Kohut, R.M., Schneeberger, E.W., Merrill, W.H., Wolf, R.K.: Absence of correlation between symptoms and rhythm in "symptomatic" atrial fibrillation. Ann. Thorac. Surg. **83**, 2118–2121 (2007)
8. Asgari, S., Mehrnia, A., Moussavi, M.: Automatic detection of atrial fibrillation using stationary wavelet transform and support vector machine. Comput. Biol. Med. **60**, 132–142 (2015)
9. Aytemir, K., Aksoyek, S., Yildirir, A., Ozer, N., Oto, A.: Prediction of atrial fibrillation recurrence after cardioversion by P wave signal-averaged electrocardiography. Int. J. Cardiol. **70**(70), 15–21 (2007)

10. Dash, S., Chon, K.H., Lu, S., Raeder, E.A.: Automatic Real Time Detection of Atrial Fibrillation. Ann. Biomed. Eng. **37**, 1701–1709 (2009)
11. Xia, Y., Wulan, N., Wang, K., Zhang, H.: Detecting atrial fibrillation by deep convolutional neural networks. Comput. Biol. Med. **93**, 84–92 (2018)
12. Abadi, M., Barham, P., Chen, J., et al.: TensorFlow: A system for large-scale machine learning. Methods Enzymology, pp. 265–283 (2016)
13. Xia, X., Xu, C., Nan, B.: Inception-v3 for flower classification. In: 2017 2nd International Conference Image, of Vision Computing, ICIVC 2017, pp. 783–787 (2017)
14. Yu, D., Seltzer, M.L.: Improved bottleneck features using pretrained deep neural networks. In: Proceedings of Annual Conference of the International Speech Communication Association Interspeech, pp. 237–240 (2011)
15. Shore, J.E., Gray, R.M.: Minimum cross-entropy pattern classification and cluster analysis. IEEE Trans. Pattern Anal. Mach. Intell. **4**, 11–17 (1982)

3D Fluorescence Tomography Combined with Ultrasound Imaging System in Small Animal Study

Shih-Po Su[✉] and Hui-Hua Kenny Chiang

Institute of Biomedical Engineering,
National Yang-Ming University, Taipei, Taiwan
chubby.su2010@gmail.com

Abstract. In recent years, the application of Fluorescence Diffusion Optical Tomography (FDOT) technology in pre-clinical experiments is increasing. It is a non-invasive small animal functional image based on diffusion optical tomography (DOT), which uses photons to absorb and scatter the properties of different materials to reconstruct the structure of the small animal sections. Using this technology can reduce the amount of small animal used and accelerate the research courses from academic researches to clinical applications. However, the potential of this technique is currently limited by its poor spatial resolution. In this work, we develop a dual-modality imaging system combining three-dimensional (3D) fluorescence tomography with ultrasound (US) imaging. This design includes an electron-multiplying charge-coupled device (EMCCD), an ultrasound transducer and a fiber-coupled laser on a planar platform. A customized fluorescence/US system was used to reconstruct the 3D fluorescence tomography from optical surface images in position of the inclusions from US signals by using Near-Infrared Fluorescence and Spectral Tomography (Nirfast). Ultrasound B-mode imaging was used to obtain the structural information to precisely extract the tissue boundary of a sample and improve fluorescence reconstruction. The advantages of using this system are noninvasive, easy-to-use and good contrast to soft tissue. We validated the system with meat and a 4T1 tumor nude mice. From the FDOT image and the line profile, it can be seen that the edge information added to the ultrasound is sharper, and the soft tissue and the tumor can also get good results at the same time. The reconstruction results show the combined fluorescence/US system can effectively localize the tumor and drug metabolism. It is very helpful for the study of tumor location and the development of cancer drugs in the small animal study.

Keywords: Fluorescence Diffusion Optical Tomography · Ultrasound image · Image reconstruction

1 Introduction

1.1 The Fluorescent Diffusion Tomography System

The fluorescence diffusion optical tomography system can be roughly divided into Epi-illumination and Trans-illumination, as shown in Fig. 1. The difference between the

© Springer Nature Switzerland AG 2020
K.-P. Lin et al. (Eds.): ICBHI 2019, IFMBE Proceedings 74, pp. 166–173, 2020.
https://doi.org/10.1007/978-3-030-30636-6_24

two is the light source and image capturing position: the former is the light source and the image capturing system is located at the same side of the object, the latter is the light source and the image capturing system is located on the opposite side of the object. This study used a planar trans illuminated machine architecture [1, 2]. In addition to its advantages of easy operation and lightweight, it can measure deeper tissue through penetrating excitation light.

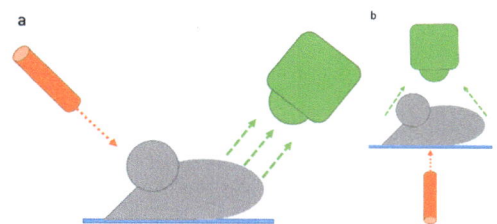

Fig. 1. (a) Epi-illumination and (b) Trans-illumination

1.2   Compound Technology: Fluorescence Diffusion Optical Tomography Combined with an Ultrasound Image

Fluorescence Diffusion Optical Tomography (FDOT) imaging system has been widely used in the clinical development of new drugs, genomics treatment, tumor tracking, infectious disease research, etc. In order to fulfill these medical needs, many researchers have developed different forms of non-invasive imaging systems through anatomical imaging systems combined with FDOT imaging and tumor tracking experiments on the small animal.

Compared with magnetic resonance imaging (MRI) [3–5] and computerized tomography (CT) [6], Ultrasound (US) structural imaging also has considerable advantages: The cost of the Ultrasound system is lower than the cost of CT or MRI.; Ultrasound has good contrast to soft tissue and can provide a real-time image.; Ultrasound has no radiation and easy to use. Because of the above advantages, Ultrasound has become the most important medical image.

Recently, many research teams have used this ultrasound structural image to assist FDOT imaging study. By using 5 MHz, 10 MHz single element ultrasound transducer with the stepper motor to extract the ultrasonic image as the prior image structure to assist fluorescence image reconstruction [7–9]. After processing the Near-Infrared Fluorescence and Spectral Tomography (Nirfast), a functional image of the fluorescence diffusion optical tomography combined with the ultrasonic anatomical image is achieved.

We developed a planar small animal imaging system combining FDOT imaging and ultrasound imaging (US), performing functional and structural image measurement in the air. The stepper motor drives the ultrasound probe and the fiber to perform linear scanning to obtain the fluorescent information and ultrasound images.

2   Materials and Methods

Our study develops a planar system for small fluorescence diffusion optical tomography. It's based on trans-illumination structure, which means the light source and detector are put at opposite sides of objects. During tomographic experiments, the small animal can lie on the holder by the most comfortable way. The excitation light source (660 nm laser) penetrates into the bottom of small animal through an x-y motor platform.

2.1   System Architecture

In this study, the system architecture is shown in Fig. 2. It can capture the functional and structural images of the small animal. The system part of the FDOT image capturing, we use a 660 nm (Cube, Coherent) diode laser and a fiber optic (Silica optical fiber, Polymicro TechnologiesTM) to couple the laser source. The fiber coupling ratio can reach 66%. In optical data acquisition, Using Electron Multiplying Charge Coupled Device (EMCCD) (ProEM: 512B_eXcelon, Princeton Instruments) to detect bands from 300 nm to 1000 nm, the quantum efficiency is 90% or more in the 600 nm to the 700 nm band. The measurement was carried out with a filter (694/44 nm BrightLine® single-band bandpass filter, 664 nm RazorEdge® ultra steep long-pass edge filter, Semrock) to receive the optical parameters at 660 nm and the 705 nm fluorescence signal.

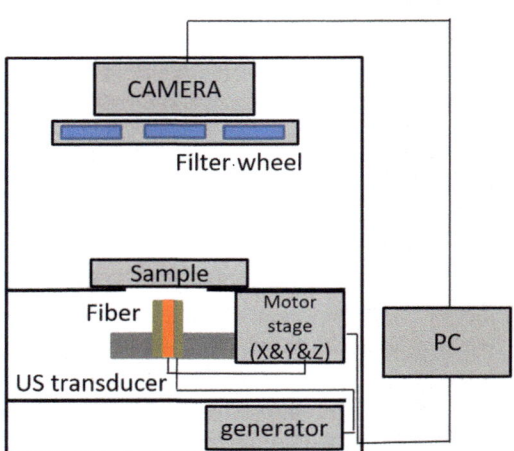

Fig. 2. Dual-mode imaging system diagram

The system part of the ultrasonic signal acquisition, using the ultrasonic transmitter PR5800 (Parametric, Inc) to send signals into a single-element disk ultrasonic transducer (outer diameter ∅ 20 mm/Inside diameter ∅ 5 mm, 10 MHz, f/#: 15 mm). The measured signals are converted to digital signals by an oscilloscope (12-bit ADC resolution, 1.25 GS/s sampling rate, 350 MHz bandwidth) (HDO4034, Lecroy) and transmitted to the PC for processing.

2.2   Experimental Materials

In this study, Alexa Fluor 660 (InvitrogenTM) was used as a cursor. The maximum absorption wavelength was 663 nm, the maximum emission wavelength was 690 nm, the extinction coefficient was 132,000 cm^{-1} M^{-1}, and the original concentration was 0.1 mg/c.c.

2.3   Experimental Methods

2.3.1   Fluorescent Molecular Imaging Procedure

Diffusion optical tomography (DOT) is according to photons different characteristics of absorption coefficient (μ_a), Scattering coefficient (μ_s) and Diffuse coefficient (D). By reconstructing the spatially varying optical coefficients, we can obtain a 2D slice of tomography image.

Fluorescence diffuse optical tomography (FDOT) is based on the DOT algorithm. Furthermore, the absorption of the fluorophore (μ_{af}) and quantum yield (η) is taken into consideration. We use FDOT to calculate the location and the concentration of the fluorophore, which is labeled on the tumor.

The first part, with the excitation light wavelength (660 nm) incident, is matched with the excitation light wavelength bandpass filter to reconstruct the optical parameters (μ_a, μ_s') of the tissue at this wavelength; the second part is incident at the fluorescence wavelength (705 nm). The optical parameters (μ_a, μ_s') at the fluorescence wavelength are reconstructed with a bandpass filter with a fluorescent emission wavelength. Finally, the wavelength of the excitation light (660 nm) is incident, and the band pass filter of the fluorescence wavelength can be used to reconstruct. The position and intensity of the fluorescence ($\eta\mu_{af}$) are the fluorescence diffused optical tomographic image.

2.4   Ultrasound Imaging Capturing

Using the self-written Labview motor control interface, with the Arduino Uno development board and the Easy driver chip are used to drive the single-element ultrasound transducer to scan the target section.

In order to consider the influence of the lateral beam width of the transducer and the walking speed of the motor on the reconstructed ultrasound image quality, this study uses swept-scan for ultrasonic image acquisition. This scanning technique is to transmit ultrasonic pulses while continuously moving the ultrasonic probe to obtain echo information quickly; the distance between adjacent line-of-sight ranges is much smaller than that of the transverse beam so that the sampling volume in the focusing range will overlap. The over-sampling can be obtained in the lateral range. It maintains a high degree of correlation between data and increases the resolution of reconstructed ultrasound images [10–12]. The lateral beam width at the focus point is defined as Eq. (1).

$$R_{lat} = \frac{f \cdot \lambda}{D} \qquad (1)$$

λ is the wavelength of the acoustic wave, f is the focal length, and D is the aperture size of the ultrasound transducer. The center frequency of the probe used in this study was 10 MHz, and the $R_{lateral}$ was about 500 μm. In the actual experiment, every two data were separated by about 100 μm.

3   Results

3.1   Meat Experiment

In order to simulate the scattering of light in real tissue, we embedded an 8 mm diameter centrifuge tube containing uniform fluorescent molecules into pork to verify the feasibility of the system for biological tissue. The trend diagram of the optical contrast signal of pork tissue is shown in Fig. 3.

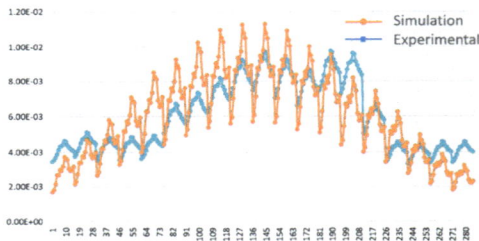

Fig. 3. The optical contrast signal of pork tissue

The motor receives an image every 1 mm, and there are 19 images taken at different light source positions. The orange line segment in the figure is the fluorescent surface signal for setting the known parameters; the blue line segment is the experimental data. Due to the complexity of the composition of living organisms, the actual experimental data and simulated data are not as good as the simulated experiments. It can be observed from the curve of Fig. 3 that the light intensity trend of the data and the actual data is still very similar, and the position of the strongest signal is also the same, but the brightness value is significantly different, and some points are not continuous, which is presumed to be the pork. The degree of light transmission is high, resulting in data interaction.

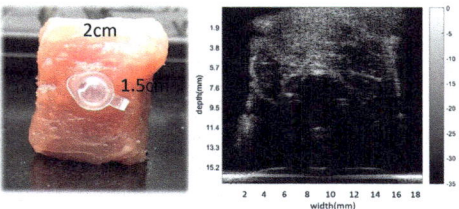

Fig. 4. The image of the pork and its ultrasound image

The structural image of the pork was obtained by scanning a 10 MHz single-element ultrasound transducer. As can be seen from Fig. 4, the contour and internal texture of the meat piece are detailed and visible. Figure 5(a), (b), (c) shows the FDOT reconstruction image of the pork, with the ultrasound image as the prior information. Comparing the results with prior and without prior: the result of no structural information, the light spreads evenly in the pork, because the light transmission of the pork is high, the light source is incident from the bottom, causing some over-exposure at the bottom of the meat. The result of adding structural image reconstruction is similar to the theoretical value, and the position of the cursor and the background can be clearly distinguished.

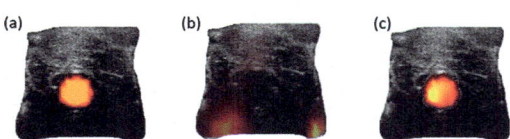

Fig. 5. The FDOT reconstruction image of the pork (a) simulation theoretical value (b) without prior FDOT reconstruction result (c) with prior FDOT reconstruction result

3.2 Mice Experiment

In this nude mouse experiment, BALB/c nude mice were implanted into 4T1 breast cancer cells to the leg for 1-2 weeks, as shown in Fig. 6(a).

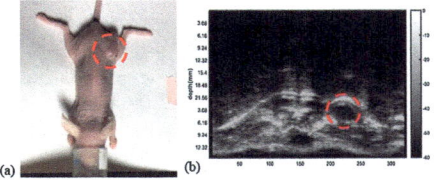

Fig. 6. Nude mice and its ultrasound structural image

The FolateRSense™ 680 (targeted fluorescence imaging agent, Perkin Elmer) fluorescent molecules were injected into the mice through the tail vein injection for systemic circulation. FR680 can be targeted on Folate Receptor alpha (FRA) for monitoring and quantifying tumor growth; the purpose of this experiment was to observe the metabolic process of the drug in nude mice and the accumulation at the tumor site. Small animals were anesthetized with 2% air and anesthesia during the experiment, and angiography was performed at 0 h, 2 h, 6 h, and 8 h after the drug was injected. After scanning with the ultrasound transducer and the stepper motor, a cross-sectional structural image of the nude mouse can be obtained, as shown in Fig. 6(b). There are many strong reflexes in the nude mice, which are presumed to be caused by the spine and bones; the nude mice are about 1 cm thick, and the black circular area at the middle bottom should be the bladder position of the mouse, and the tumor position and shape can be clearly seen on the upper right.

Figure 7(a) shows the diffusion of fluorescence in nude mice at different time points. This is the reconstruction result after adding the prior information provided by the ultrasound image, which can accurately locate the tumor at the same time and provide the drug circulation metabolism. It can be observed from Fig. 7(b) that the FR680 fluorescent molecule is most effective 2–6 h after injection and the increment of 0 hr–6 h is about linear growth.

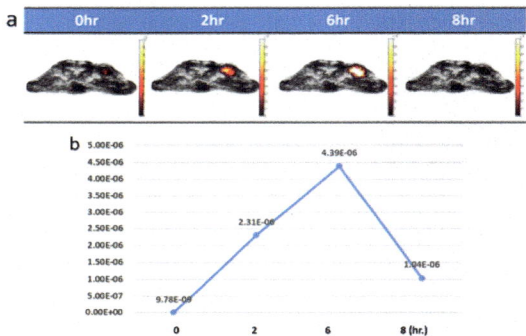

Fig. 7. (a) FDOT reconstruction results at various time points (b) Fluorescence concentration trend graph at each time point

4   Conclusions

In this study, we have presented a combined fluorescence/US imaging system. The fluorescence tomography subsystem was used to explore fluorescence emission; the US subsystem was used to provide a structural image to constraint the fluorescence reconstruction. Experiment results showed that the fluorescence reconstruction image could be significantly improved by using the structural priors. Also, the US images could help to interpret the reconstructed functional images at different sections compared with no prior reconstruction. Figures 5 and 7 demonstrated the tumor fluorophore distribution could be accurately reconstructed by the FDOT system. To do further validation, in vivo molecular imaging would be the next step.

Conflict of Interest. The authors declare that they have no conflict of interest.

References

1. Jiang, H.: Frequency-domain fluorescent diffusion tomography: a finite-element-based algorithm and simulations. Appl. Opt. **37**(22), 5337–5343 (1998)
2. Leblond, F., Davis, S.C., Valdés, P.A., Pogue, B.W.: Pre-clinical whole-body fluorescence imaging: review of instruments, methods and applications. J. Photochem. Photobiol., B **98** (1), 77–94 (2010)
3. Davis, S.C., et al.: Magnetic resonance–coupled fluorescence tomography scanner for molecular imaging of tissue. Rev. Sci. Instrum. **79**(6), 064302 (2008)
4. Brooksby, B.A., et al.: Near-infrared (NIR) tomography breast image reconstruction with a priori structural information from MRI: Algorithm development for reconstructing heterogeneities. IEEE J Sel. Topics Quantum Electron. **9**(2), 199–209 (2003)
5. Lin, Y., et al.: A photo-multiplier tube-based hybrid MRI and frequency domain fluorescence tomography system for small animal imaging. Phys. Med. Biol. **56**(15), 4731–4747 (2011)
6. Ale, A., et al.: FMT-XCT: in vivo animal studies with hybrid fluorescence molecular tomography-X-ray computed tomography. Nat. Methods **9**(6), 615–620 (2012)
7. Deng, Z., et al.: Design of a rotational ultrasound guided diffuse optical tomography system for whole breast imaging. In: Proceedings SPIE 8581, Photons Plus Ultrasound: Imaging and Sensing, 85813 p (2013)
8. Li, B., et al.: Low-cost three-dimensional imaging system combining fluorescence and ultrasound. J. Biomed. Opt. **16**(12), 126010 (2011)
9. Li, B., et al.: Ultrasound guided fluorescence molecular tomography with improved quantification by an attenuation compensated Born-normalization and in vivo preclinical study of cancer. Rev. Sci. Instrum. **85**(5), 053703 (2014)
10. Kruse, D.E., Silverman, R.H., Fornaris, R.J., Coleman, D.J., Ferrara, K.W.: A swept-scanning mode for estimation of blood velocity in the microvasculature. IEEE Trans. Ultrasound Ferroelectrics Frequency Control **45**(6), 1437–1440 (1998)
11. Kruse, D., et al.: High resolution blood flow mapping in the anterior segment of the eye. In: Proceedings of the IEEE Ultrasonics Symposium, vol. 2, pp. 1477–1480 (1999)
12. Kruse, D.E., Ferrara, K.W.: A new high resolution color flow system using an eigendecompsition-based adaptive filter for clutter rejection. IEEE Trans. Ultrasound Ferroelectrics Frequency Control **49**(10), 1384–1399 (2002)

Main Barriers and Needs to Support Clinical Cancer Research via Health Informatics

Laura Lopez-Perez[1]([✉]), Silvana Canevari[2], Leandro Pecchia[3],
Maria Teresa Arredondo[1], Lisa Licitra[2], and Giuseppe Fico[1]

[1] Universidad Politécnica de Madrid, Madrid, Spain
llopez@lst.tfo.upm.es
[2] Fondazione IRCCS Istituto Nazionale dei Tumori, Milan, Italy
[3] School of Engineering, University of Warwick, Coventry, UK

Abstract. Cancer is the second leading cause of death worldwide. In order to reduce this burden, new strategies need to be implemented. With the evolution of computational techniques, the amount of clinical data available has increased considerably. However, these data are not always easily accessible, with some barriers of different nature preventing their retrieval and analysis. With the aim of better understanding these barriers and eventually support decision making through digital tools, a literature search has been conducted and, according to the analysis of the resulting bibliography, a survey to validate the literature findings has been distributed to clinical and computer science experts who work on cancer research in different countries. The answers received allow us to identify the main issues that need to be addressed, which are analyzed and presented in this paper. This work is carried out in the context of *BD2Decide* European Research project.

Keywords: Cancer · Clinical research · Translational research · Data accessibility · Biomedical informatics

1 Introduction

Cancer is the second leading cause of death worldwide [1]. Nowadays, thanks to the rapid technological evolution in the medical and computational domains, it is possible to collect large amounts of clinical data [2]. The analysis of these data can contribute to the generation of evidence for new prevention, diagnosis and treatment strategies, hence reducing cancer mortality rate. However, these data are not always publicly available or easily accessible.

With the purpose of identifying the main issues that clinical researchers face during their work when dealing with clinical data, we conducted a literature review on this topic. With the outcomes obtained through the review, a survey has been designed and distributed among different clinical centers, to verify and understand these limitations.

The results of this survey will be used as guidelines in the implementation of a Visual Analytic Tool developed in the framework of BD2Decide (Big Data and Models for Personalized Head and Neck Cancer Decision Support), a European research project that aims to improve the Head and Neck Cancer prognosis, integrating

K.-P. Lin et al. (Eds.): ICBHI 2019, IFMBE Proceedings 74, pp. 174–182, 2020.
https://doi.org/10.1007/978-3-030-30636-6_25

multiscale data (clinical, genomics, images, radiomics and population) and providing statistical models and big data techniques via representation suites for research purposes.

2   Materials and Methods

2.1   Literature Review

In our analysis we used PubMed, a resource that provide access to the National Library of Medicine database (Sep–Nov 2018), to search the following terms:

Cancer (Malignant neoplasm): Uncontrolled growth of abnormal cells with potential for metastatic spread.

Cancer research: Investigation into cancer causes and development of strategies for prevention, diagnosis, treatment.

Translational research: Study designed to translate basic science findings into clinically useful tools.

Clinical Researcher: A health professional who works and uses clinical and translational data from patients.

Barrier: Something that blocks, prevents or limits.

Unmet: A need or request not fulfilled.

Resource: Facility, and material available for research.

Need: Anything that is necessary but lacking.

These terms were used to create four different entries, as illustrated in Fig. 1.

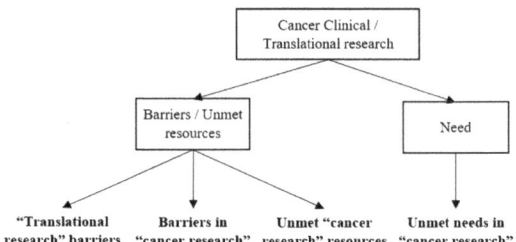

Fig. 1.   Strategy followed to identify the entry terms used for the search

The inclusion criteria for the selection of articles were: articles related to *human specimens* and *published* in the last 5 years. We excluded *non-English* publications, duplicated papers and those which do not have *full-text* availability.

2.2   Survey Design

A survey was designed with the results obtained through the literature search.

The target group of the survey includes: clinicians specialized in medical oncology, surgery, radiotherapy and molecular biology, distributed among international research groups coming from collaborations with the *Istituto Nationale dei Tumori* that work on cancer research in different countries and from the partnership within the BD2Decide project. Also from these centers, participants with expertise on biostatistics and computational science are invited to answer the questionnaire, due to their involvement on the analysis of patients' data.

The survey was structured as follows: (i) participants were presented with a brief explanation of the goal and methodology; (ii) they were asked to confirm if they agree on the barriers and needs identified in literature analysis, and they were also allowed to propose additional issues according to their experience; (iii) they were asked to rate the impact of each barrier in limiting their current research work by ranking a set of statements from 1 (not relevant) to 5 (most relevant).

3   Results

3.1   Literature Analysis

Using the entry terms presented in Fig. 1 and the inclusion criteria, more than 300 records were identified. Then, a manual assessment of the articles was carried out, discarding the least relevant ones as they were not specifically focused on data retrieval and analysis. Figure 2 shows the detailed strategy followed with the number of articles resulting from each step. Around the 70% of the excluded articles discussed about the barriers affecting the participation in clinical trials, not specifying any limitations on the research itself. 12% of the works discussed about specific research outcomes, such as the result of applying a new treatment, consequently not discussing about any barrier during their research; and the remaining 18% dealt with next generation sequencing for genomics and the need to have cheaper solutions to create data, but not on the analysis of the resulted data. After excluding all these papers that do not fulfill the requirements of this work, we looked over similar cases of the ones that were selected, finding 30 eligible publications.

From this sample, we identified the barriers and needs (classified in three main categories) summarized in Table 1:

Data-related issues: (i) Barriers: large amounts of data are not easily available in terms of accessibility and interoperability, and lack of networks to share resources, limiting exchange of information; *(ii) Needs*: to carry out translational research, data integration, and high-quality data collection and appropriate reporting.

Resources-related issues: (i) Barriers: tools to access data are limited in volume and usability (i.e. steep learning curves), required analytics experience for exploitation of large datasets, and accessibility to existing tools; *(ii) Needs*: resources for systematic analysis to identify new biomarkers, specially tailored tools need to be available to maximize the value of data.

Knowledge generation-related issues: (i) Barriers: regulatory processes for evidence validation, and standardization of terminology with the aim of facilitating collaborative research; *(ii) Needs*: well-defined semantic models to support data analysis and linking to external resources, and supporting knowledge transfer process.

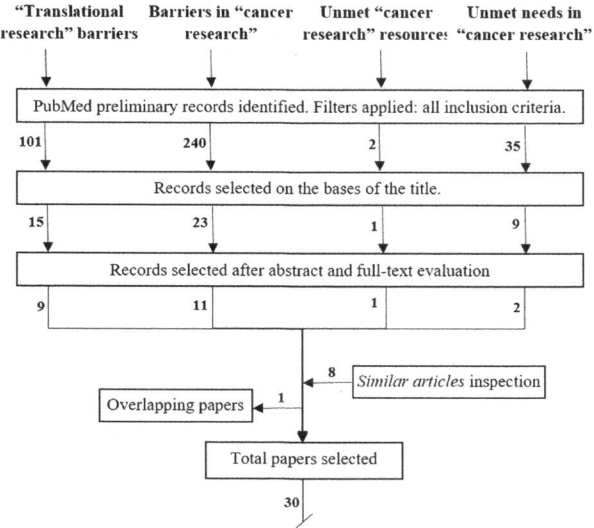

Fig. 2. Flowchart of the literature review

3.2   Survey Outcomes

To confirm the identified barriers and needs, a survey was sent electronically to the target group. 37 responses were received from 9 different countries, 5 different specializations (Fig. 3), and different experience (68% more than 10 years).

3.2.1   Issues Identification

Among all the *Data-related issues* the most accepted (86%) was the need of *High-quality data collection with the appropriate reporting*. Analyzing the answers based on the participants' specialty we find discrepancies: all medical oncologists and molecular biologists coincided also on the *High quality data collection*, whereas the 100% of surgeons concur on the barrier of data availability; on the other hand, the biostatisticians considered data integration a relevant issue. And radiologists agreed similarly (67%) to the lack of networks and *High quality data collection*.

In addition to the issues identified, some participants included their own needs: *Harmonized data sharing, data protection and other legal framework*; and *Standards for data exchange and integration* and barriers: *Sparse data available (clinical, genomics) often collected without any structured criteria*; and *Individual patient data meta-analysis of institutional trials is feasible but time consuming*. However, these issues are closely related to knowledge generation.

Concerning *resources-related issues*, 68% of participants agreed with the need of *Dedicated resources for systematic analysis to get new indicators*.

Contrary to *Data-related issues*, any group of experts coincide (100%) with the same issue. It is worth to highlight, however, that 64% of medical oncologist and 80% of surgeons concur on the barrier of resources accessibility, whereas other disciplines (also surgeons) agreed (67–83%) on the need of dedicated resources for systematic analysis.

Table 1. Literature results (* indicates papers duplicated in other issues)

Issues	Number of papers	References
Data availability (resources to access data)	7 (2*)	T. Milan et al. (2017); C. Fitzmaurice (2017); T.E. Yankeelov et al. (2016); X. Sun et al. (2018); R. Lau et al. (2016); C. Rolfo et al. (2016); M.H. Oushy et al. (2015)
High quality collection & report	2 (1*)	R.E. Jensen et al. (2014); S. Gamulin (2016)
Data integration	3 (3*)	S. Gamulin (2016); A. Esteban-Gil (2017); M. Mohaimenul et al. (2018)
Data sharing	3 (1*)	D.J. Vis et al. (2017); M.A. Turner et al. (2017); M. Mohaimenul et al. (2018)
Collect and process data	3 (2*)	N.J. Caixeiro et al. (2016); A.R. Gagliardi (2016); C. Rolfo et al. (2016)
Analyze and exploit the data	4 (2*)	A. Esteban-Gil (2017); X. Sun et al. (2018); F. Zhang et al. (2018); S.S. Mohapatra et al. (2018)
Regulatory process improvement	4 (2*)	S. Gamulin (2016); J.M. De La Torre et al. (2017); N. Silva-Illanes et al. (2018); A. Badakhshan et al. (2018)
Standardized and well-defined processes	5 (2*)	S.M. Czajkowski et al. (2016); A. Pasipoularides (2017); T.H. Ciesielski et al. (2017); A. Esteban-Gil (2017); C. Matovina et al. (2017)
Interdisciplinary collaboration	5 (2*)	T.H. Ciesielski et al. (2017); J.C. Long et al. (2014); S. Gamulin (2016); H.D. Dao et al. (2015); A.Y. Hwang et al. (2017)
Evidence-based knowledge generation support	5 (2*)	J.M. De La Torre et al. (2017); J. Bryant et al. (2014); D. Howell et al. (2014); A.R. Gagliardi (2016); L.C. Stetson et al. (2014)

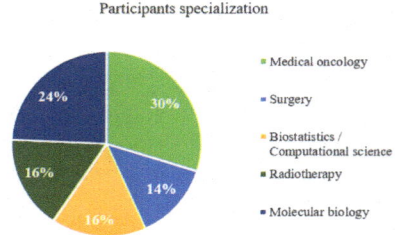

Fig. 3. Participants distribution by specialization

Participants added the specific need of *resources to the validation process*, which we find again strictly related to the knowledge generation category.

In the matter of *knowledge generation*, the most accepted (69%) was the need of *Interdisciplinary collaborations*, but considering the specialization of participants only a total consensus was reached among surgeons in the barriers of *Terminology consistency to facilitate the collaborative research*. 73% of the medical oncologists agreed on the need of *Support on knowledge transfer process* and molecular biologists' distributes their opinion on relevant issues among all of the possible options. All these results are summarized in Table 2.

Table 2. Survey results - Issues confirmed (in %)

Issues	Medical oncology (n = 11)	Surgery (n = 5)	Radiotherapy (n = 6)	Molecular biology (n = 9)	Biostatistics/ Computational science (n = 6)	Total (n = 37)
Large amounts of data exist but not easily available	64	100	50	78	50	71
Lack of networks to share resources to exchange patient information	73	40	67	44	67	63
Data integration	45	40	33	33	83	49
High-quality data collection with the appropriate reporting	100	60	67	100	67	86
Resources to access data are limited in amount and usability	64	80	33	67	33	62
Exploitation of large amount of data depends on analytics experience	55	60	50	44	50	56
Dedicated resources for systematic analysis to get new indicators	55	80	83	44	67	68
To maximize the value of data	36	20	67	22	17	35
Regulatory processes for evidence validation	55	60	50	33	67	54
Terminology consistency to facilitate the collaborative research	45	100	50	67	0	54
Well-defined semantic models to support data analysis and linking to external resources	45	40	50	44	33	51
Interdisciplinary collaborations	64	80	50	67	50	69
Support on knowledge transfer process	73	40	50	33	0	49

3.2.2 Issues Rating

The results of prioritizing the issues are available on Figs. 4, 5 and 6 (1: less-critical; 2: low-critical; 3: medium-critical; 4: moderately-critical; 5: high-critical). In summary, the four *Data-related issues* were evaluated as moderately critical by the participants (35–38% of participants agreed on that); and the *High quality (collection and reporting)* was the most relevant for all participants (41%) with the highest criticality. Dissecting the results by specialization, *Data sharing* was categorized by moderately critical for 64% of medical oncologists and 50% of biostatisticians; whereas the 60% of surgeons and 50% of radiologists, assign this level of priority to *High quality* issue (67% of molecular biologists also gives the high level to this issue but ranking as high-critical).

In the *Resources-related issues*, the high and moderately critical issue (with consensus of 30–35% of participants) was to *Collect and process data. Analyze and exploit the data* was the most accepted for all participants as medium-critical rating (45% of medical oncologists, 60% surgeon and 44% of radiologists).

In terms of *knowledge generation-related issues*, the high-critical rating was distributed among all the options, whereas the needs of *Standardized and well-defined processes* and *Interdisciplinary collaboration* were the most concurrent for all participants (43%). Considering participants expertise, medical oncologists (45%) gives the high-critical rating to the *Evidence-based knowledge generation support* whereas molecular biologists (56%) set as medium-critical the same issue.

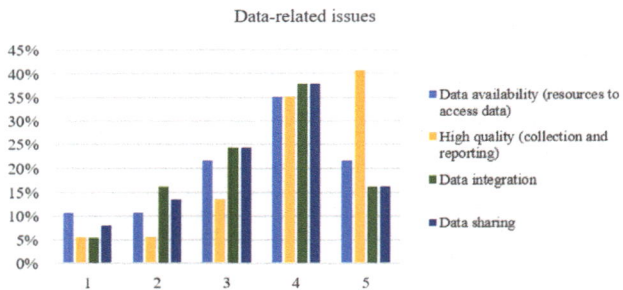

Fig. 4. *Data-related issues* prioritization

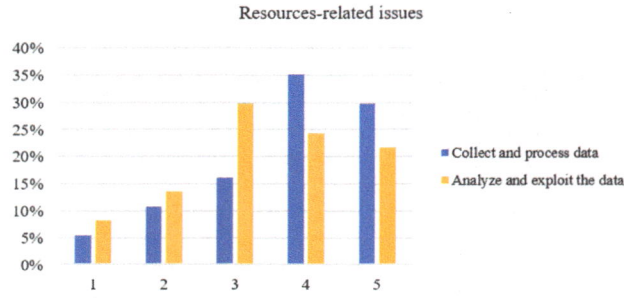

Fig. 5. *Resources-related issues* prioritization

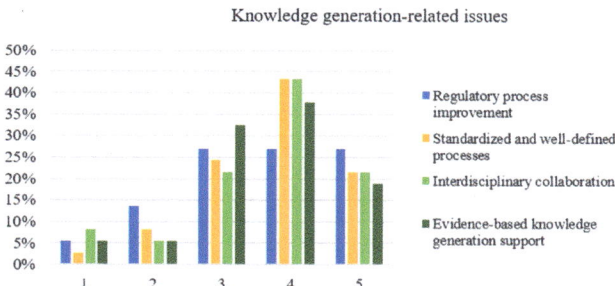

Fig. 6. *Knowledge generation-related issues* prioritization

4 Discussion and Conclusions

This work investigates the main barriers and needs that clinical researchers face when dealing with cancer clinical data. Based on our literature search, we identified three types of issues: data-related, resources-related and knowledge management-related. Moreover, we found that the number of publications about clinical cancer research barriers and needs is scarce, with most of the available literature focused on the recruiting of patients for clinical trials. Therefore, the survey outcomes support us on the understanding of the real needs that researchers face nowadays. The most accepted issue for all participants was the high-quality data collection with the consensus of the 86% of all participants. However, participants by specialization have group consensus, such as, the confirmation of the need of large amounts of data and of the terminology consistency regards *knowledge generation*. In terms of *resources-related* issues the most rating for all participants was the need of collecting and processing data. A huge interest was presented by all participants in the *knowledge generation-related issues* as they included in the survey specific issues about harmonization and standardization processes, but also on the need of resources for validation.

In conclusion, in order to develop new evidence for clinical practices, it is of paramount importance to focus on interdisciplinary collaborative research that tackles user needs such as the high quality data collection and dedicated resources to process the data and validate the analysis results.

Translating this into the development of innovative tools and applications may ensure that new treatments and research knowledge could reach the patients or populations for whom they are designed. Within BD2Decide, we intend to tackle these issues through an integrated mechanism that enables precision medicine.

Acknowledgment. The authors wish to acknowledge the BD2Decide consortium (www.bd2decide.eu), funded from the EU's Horizon 2020 program, grant agreement No. 689715.

Conflict of Interest. The authors declare that they have no conflict of interest.

References

1. You, W., et al.: Greater family size is associated with less cancer risk: an ecological analysis of 178 countries. BMC Cancer **18**(1), 924 (2018)
2. Kayyali, B., et al.: The Big-Data Revolution in US Health Care: Accelerating Value and Innovation, pp. 1–13. McKinsey & Company, New York (2013)

Stability Evaluation of a Tissue Oxygen Saturation Measurement System

Shao-Hung Lu[1]([✉]), Tieh-Cheng Fu[2], Wei-Cheng Lu[1],
Po-Hung Chang[1], Kang-Ping Lin[3,4], and Cheng-Lun Tsai[1,4]

[1] Biomedical Engineering Department,
Chung Yuan Christian University, Taoyuan, Taiwan
how998l@gmail.com, clt@cycu.edu.tw
[2] Department of Internal Medicine, Heart Failure Center,
Chang Gung Memorial Hospital, Keelung, Keelung, Taiwan
[3] Electrical Engineering Department,
Chung Yuan Christian University, Taoyuan, Taiwan
[4] Technology Translation Center for Medical Device,
Chung Yuan Christian University,
200, Chung-Pei Road, Taoyuan 32023, Taiwan

Abstract. Peripheral arterial occlusive disease has a high risk to occur in the lower extremity which causes low oxygen saturation level in muscle tissue, especially after exercise. A muscle tissue oxygen saturation measurement system was developed to detect the insufficient blood supply to lower limb.

The diffusive reflectance travelled though deep tissue is measured at two separated distance from the light sources. The individual differences in skin tissue would be cancelled out between these two measurements. Three near–infrared wavelengths are used to measure and calculate the oxygen saturation in deep muscle tissue. The stability of *in vivo* measurement is tested at different body postures in this study. The detection of the change in oxygen saturation was also tested by an artery occlusion experiment at the lower extremity. The results match the general physiological condition and the reliability of the system is confirmed.

Keywords: Peripheral arterial occlusive disease · Near-infrared spectroscopy · Muscle tissue oxygen saturation

1 Introduction

Peripheral arterial occlusive disease (PAOD) is a general term for stenosis or obstruction of major arteries other than the coronary arteries. Arteries and veins of leg generally withstand great blood static pressure that accelerate the degradation of blood vessels. The atherosclerosis on the blood vessel of the lower extremity is susceptible to rupture due to shear force changes in blood flow which in turn form artery occlusion [1].

Although Doppler ultrasound can be used to measure blood flow velocity of vessel, it requires an experienced physician to accurately identify the location of blockage or narrowing in small vessels. Both MRI and PET can obtain complete vascular

© Springer Nature Switzerland AG 2020
K.-P. Lin et al. (Eds.): ICBHI 2019, IFMBE Proceedings 74, pp. 183–190, 2020.
https://doi.org/10.1007/978-3-030-30636-6_26

information, but there are also some restrictions on their usages. Firstly, the equipment is expensive. Secondly, the cost of detection is high, and the measuring time is long. It could take over a month from the first outpatient appointment to finally get the inspection result. Even in a hospital with these expensive instruments, only emergency or critical ill patients will be examined by these instrument. Nowadays, the standard way to detect POAD is the Ankle–Brachial pressure index from a static measurement.

Most patients will wait until they feel pain or have difficulty in lower limb movements before they go to hospital for examination. The slight lameness of the patient is often mistaken for exercise pain, and miss the timing of early treatment. Especially for the patients with a high risk of high blood pressure, diabetes, and smoking, their artery occlusion should be examined and treated as early as possible. Their recurrence rate of artery occlusion is very high, therefore it needs to be traced for a long time after treatment. If arterial occlusion can be easily detected at the early stage, patient can receive more effective treatment, and the patient will suffer less by following the doctor's instructions.

Some research and clinical reports have used near-infrared spectroscopy equipment to measure muscle oxygen saturation for detecting PAOD, the results indicate some differences between normal persons and patients [2, 3]. Since exercise will greatly increase the oxygen consumption by muscle tissue, the lowering of oxygen saturation in muscle under an exercise stress test might be used as an early identification of PAOD.

In this study, an optical non-invasive wireless lower extremity arterial occlusion assessment system was developed to measure muscle tissue oxygen saturation to estimate the severity of arteries occlusion.

2   Methods and Materials

2.1   Near-Infrared Spectroscopy (NIRS)

NIRS is frequently used to analyze the light absorbance and concentration of substances. Biologic tissue has relatively low absorption to near-infrared light, so light can penetrate through skin and fat tissues to reach the underneath muscle tissue. An optical probe was designed to detect muscle oxygen saturation in this study. It has two light sources with two different light pathway to cancel the effect of individual difference in skin tissue, as shown in Fig. 1. The R_n received by the photodetector is from the near light source that travels through the skin and fat layers and into the muscle tissue. The R_f received by the photodetector is from the far light source that travels thought the similar path but passes through a slightly more in muscle tissue, ΔL.

$$A_{\Delta L} \approx \log \frac{R_n}{R_f} \tag{1}$$

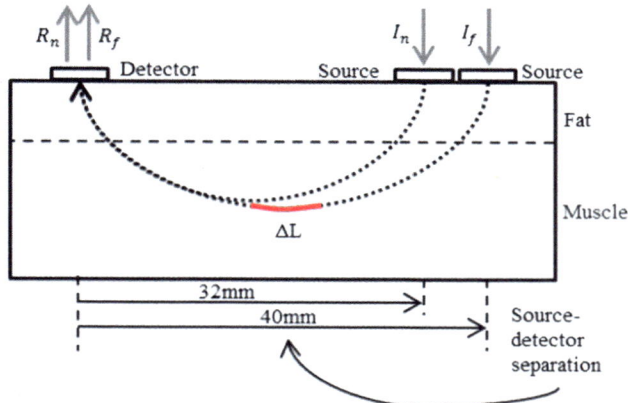

Fig. 1. Average transmission paths of light from two light sources travel through similar tissue regions are captured by the detector.

2.2 Calculate of Muscle Tissue Oxygen Saturation

According to Eq. (1), the back reflectance R_n, from the near source is treated as the incident light and the reflectance, R_n, from the far source is treated as the transmission through the different path, ΔL, in muscle tissue. The difference in intensity between these two reflectance is contributed by the absorption of hemoglobin in blood, myoglobin is muscle, and scattering in tissue. Since myoglobin has an affinity with oxygen much stronger than that of hemoglobin, the change in absorbance with deoxygenation is mostly caused by hemoglobin rather than myoglobin. Equation (2) formulates the intensity difference as an absorbance, $A_{\Delta L}$, where a_{HbO_2} is the absorption coefficient of oxygenated hemoglobin. a_{Hb} is the absorption coefficient of hemoglobin, and s_m is the scattering coefficient of tissue on the whole. Unless the oxygen saturation of blood drops to a very low level, myoglobin can be generally treated as totally saturated. The contribution of myoglobin oxygen saturation on the change in light absorbance is trivial. Δl_{HbO_2} is the average path length in oxygenated hemoglobin, Δl_{Hb} is the average path length in hemoglobin, and Δl_s is the average path length that is not affected by oxygen concentration. The scattering term is a baseline shift similar to the constant term generally added in the modified Beer's law equation.

$$A_{\Delta L} = a_{HbO_2} \cdot \Delta l_{HbO_2} + a_{Hb} \cdot \Delta l_{Hb} + s_m \cdot \Delta l_s \tag{2}$$

$$S_{mo}\% = \frac{\Delta l_{HbO_2}}{\Delta l_{HbO_2} + \Delta l_{Hb}} \times 100\% \tag{3}$$

$$\Delta S_{mo}\%(t) = S_{mo}\%(t) - S_{mo}\%(t_0) \tag{4}$$

The oxygen saturation in muscle tissue can be calculated as $S_{mo}\%$ in Eq. (3). If the oxygen saturation of tissue changes during exercise with insufficient artery blood supply, The change in tissue saturation from the initial value before exercise can be calculated using in Eq. (4).

2.3   Measurement System

The optical probe uses LEDs with three different wavelengths as the light sources (740 nm, 808 nm, 850 nm). The LEDs are driven by constant current sources and packaged in a standard 5050 package. The operational amplifier converts the detected intensity of light into a voltage signal. This signal is digitized by a System-on-a-Chip processor using a 24 bits sigma-to-delta AD converter. The digital signal is finally transmitted to a computer through Bluetooth for further analysis and recording. The traces of signal can be displayed and monitored on the computer screen. The structure of the measurement system is shown in Fig. 2.

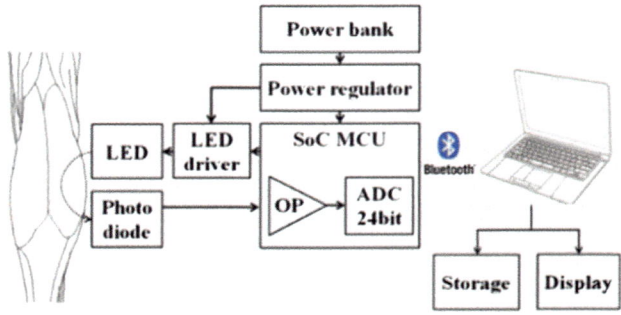

Fig. 2. Block diagram of the NIRS system

2.4   System Stability Test

The stability test of this study includes two parts: the optical stability of measurement system and the physiological signal measured on a human subject.

The optical evaluation is done by continuously measuring the diffusive reflectance intensity of light from an empty light diffusing chamber with 60 cm of height and 20 cm of diameter for eight hours.

During the supine posture measurement, the subject lay still on a bed and the optical probe is bonded at about one-third on the upper side of the gastrocnemius muscle using medical tape. Before starting the measurement, the subject was asked to lie still for at least five minutes. This is to wait for blood pressure and blood oxygen concentration to go back to stable after the posture change. The muscles of leg were relaxed, and the measurement continuously recorded for 30 min.

During the standing experiment, the subject stood still with body weight evenly distributed between two feet. The subject was also asked to stand still and rest for five minutes before starting measurement. The measurement period of this experiment was set to be ten minutes.

Finally, artery occlusion test was used to change the oxygen saturation in the muscle tissue of the lower extremity. Since it is difficult to really cause an arterial occlusion during an experiment, it was done by using a high pressure air cuff to compress the artery in the leg.

The subjects were asked to lie still for five minutes to stabilize the body condition. Then, a pressure cuff was put on the upper leg and pumped up to 250 mmHg within fifteen seconds to completely block the blood flow in the arteries and veins. The pressure was quickly released after maintaining the pressure for three minutes. The recovery signal was continuously measured for ten minutes after the pressure was released.

3   Result

3.1   Optical Evaluation System Stability

Figure 3 shows the light intensity signals of the six light-emitting diodes measured by the photodiode of the optical probe reflected from the light diffusing box. N represents the near light source and F represents the far light source. The measurement results show the reflected intensities are all very stable. The only variation of light source intensity is the slight drift within the first ten minutes after the measurement device was turned on. Once the system reaches the thermal balance stage, the signals also become stable.

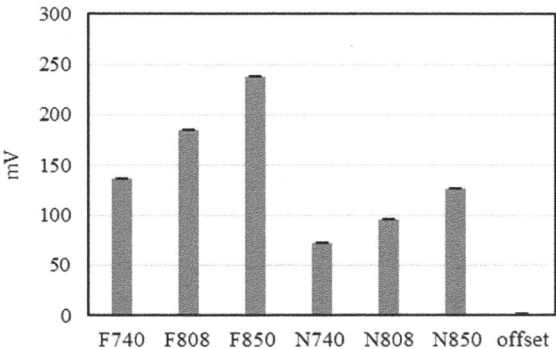

Fig. 3. Stability of LED light sources continuously measured in a light diffusion chamber for eight hours.

3.2   Measurement at Supine and Standing Postures

Figure 4 shows the stabilities of tissue oxygen saturation of calf muscle measured under supine and standing postures. With the body lay down and kept relax, the tissue oxygen saturation level was nearly at the same level throughout the experiment. The standard deviation of tissue oxygen saturation at standing posture was slightly larger than the supine posture. This is because the muscles were under certain tension and kept on adjusting to balance the body. The stretch of muscles apply forces on vessels that caused larger drift level at standing. But, the average of tissue oxygen saturation still remains at the same level as the initial value.

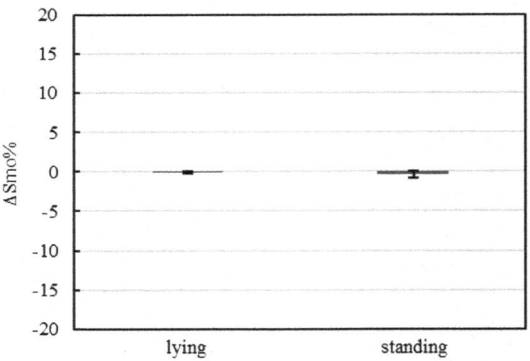

Fig. 4. Stability of tissue oxygen saturation continuously measured at supine and standing postures.

3.3   Artery Occlusion Experiment

When the blood flow of arteries were totally occluded by the air cuff, oxygen amount in blood and muscle constantly decrease as time passed. The curve of muscle tissue oxygen saturation in Fig. 5 started to drop when arteries are occluded. Before the occlusion, oxygen saturation remained at the same level at the first minute of resting period. Then, oxygen saturation decrease linearly during the entire occlusion period until it reached about -20% at the end of occlusion. When the cuff pressure was released at minute four, the tissue oxygen saturation value quickly recovered to the starting level within 15 s. The oxygen saturation value kept on bouncing to a level about 3% higher than the initial value. After two minutes of recovery, the oxygen saturation returned to the initial level. The fast recovering speed indicates the change in tissue oxygen saturation is most likely caused by hemoglobin in the blood rather than myoglobin in the tissue. Under normal condition, the hemoglobin in the blood is almost totally saturated by oxygen. The oxygen saturation of myoglobin is at the level around 70% for normal people. The measured tissue oxygen saturation is the combination of oxygen saturation of both hemoglobin and myoglobin. This value is higher than that of myoglobin but lower than that of hemoglobin. This is why the measured value could exceed the initial value and the compensatory time lasts about three minutes.

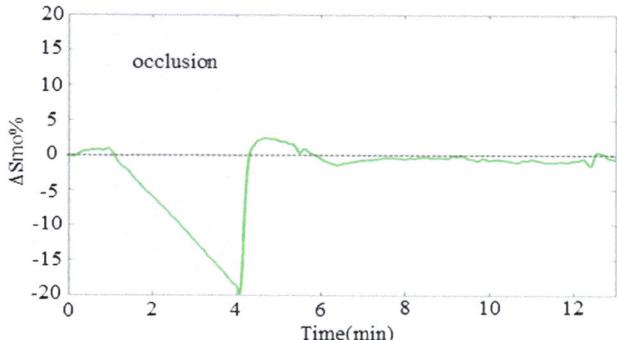

Fig. 5. The change in tissue oxygen saturation measured on calf muscle during the artery occlusion experiment.

4   Discussion

The optical probe developed in this study for measuring muscle tissue oxygen saturation was proved to be reliable. Muscle oxygen concentration has a low frequency of irregular variation in both standing and supine posture. The variation is more obvious at standing posture because the skeletal muscle is not completely dilated or contracted while standing. The varying muscle tension would squeeze on blood vessels and change the total blood content in tissue. This will affect the calculation of oxygen saturation and local muscle relaxation because the equation is based on the assumption that blood volume is a constant.

The measurement result of the artery occlusion experiment is in consistent with physiological phenomena. When blood flow is stopped by the pressure cuff, the supply of oxygen is also blocked. With the cells kept on consuming the oxygen stored in blood and tissue, the tissue oxygen saturation gradually decreases. Since the 250 mmHg of high cuff pressure caused great discomfort of the subject, the occlusion can only last for three minutes. Once the blood circulation is recovered with the release of cuff pressure, tissue oxygen concentration value quickly returned. The fast recovery of tissue oxygen saturation is a sign that hemoglobin in blood cells is in responsible of the change in oxygen saturation rather than myoglobin in muscle fibers. The swinging of curve during the three minutes of recovery period is mostly possibly caused by the change in total blood volume in the tissue.

5   Conclusions

A wireless muscle tissue oxygen saturation measurement system is developed in this study. The proof of its stability allow us to continue the future clinical study. The system is able to continuously measure the change in oxygen saturation before and after the exercise challenge. If arteries were narrowed, the oxygen saturation might decrease faster or recover slower. This is possible to use it for evaluating the degree of obstruction, and detect peripheral arterial occlusive disease at the early stage.

Acknowledgment. This research was supported by the Ministry of Science and Technology of Taiwan (MOST 106-2221-E-033-014- and MOST 107-2221-E-033-008).

Conflict of Interest. The authors declare that they have no conflict of interest.

References

1. Giswold, E.M., Landry, G.J., Sexton, G.J., Yeager, R.A., Edwards, J.M., Taylor, L.M., Moneta, G.L.: Modifiable patient factors are associated with reverse vein graft occlusion in the era of duplex scan surveillance. J. Vas. Surg. **37**, 47–53 (2003)
2. Comerota, A.J., Throm, R.C., Kelly, P., Jaff, M.: Tissue (muscle) oxygen saturation (StO2): a new measure of symptomatic lower-extremity arterial disease. J. Vas. Surg. **38**(4), 724–729 (2003)
3. Yu, G., Durduran, T., Lech, G., Zhou, C., Chance, B., Mohlers, E.R., Yodh, A.G.: Time-dependent blood flow and oxygenation in human skeletal muscles measured with noninvasive near-infrared diffuse optical spectroscopies. J. Biomed. Opt. **10**(2), 024–027 (2005)

Liquid Phantom for Calibrating Tissue Oxygen Saturation Measurement

Po-Hung Chang[1(✉)], Shao-Hung Lu[1], Tieh-Cheng Fu[3],
Kang-Ping Lin[2,4], and Cheng-Lun Tsai[1,4]

[1] Biomedical Engineering Department, Chung Yuan Christian University,
Taoyuan, Taiwan
allen121415@gmail.com, clt@cycu.edu.tw
[2] Electrical Engineering Department, Chung Yuan Christian University,
Taoyuan, Taiwan
[3] Department of Internal Medicine, Heart Failure Center,
Chang Gung Memorial Hospital, Keelung, Keelung, Taiwan
[4] Technology Translation Center for Medical Device,
Chung Yuan Christian University,
200, Chung-Pei Road, Taoyuan 32023, Taiwan

Abstract. In recent years, the prevalence of peripheral arterial disease (PAD) has increased. This disease is related to arterial occlusion in the heart and brain. Many researches mentioned, measurement of muscle tissue oxygen saturation by near-infrared spectroscopy (NIRS) has a different phenomenon for normal people and patients. In order to quantify the muscle oxygen saturation measured by near-infrared spectroscopy. In this research, we use a in-house made multi-wavelength and two light-detector distances to measure the liquid phantom with adjustable oxygen saturation. LED polarizer wavelength is 740 nm, 808 nm and 850 nm. Two light-detector distances are 32 mm and 40 mm. Liquid phantom using purified red blood cell from pig blood and intralipid to mix the blood cell solution. The liquid phantom simulated lower limbs muscles optical properties. Use yeast and oxygen to change oxygen saturation in the liquid phantom and continuous measurement at the same time. Measurement result show, absorbance at 740 nm and 850 nm will change with oxygen saturation, but absorbance at 808 nm will not. In the other side, between two light-detector distances the trend of change is small. This result is consistent with the absorption spectrum of hemoglobin to calculate a calibration curve for muscle oxygen saturation quantification in a in-house made machine. In the future, it will be embedded in the signal of clinical measurement to help PAD patient's classification. This classification will become one of the indicators for doctor diagnosis.

Keywords: Peripheral arterial occlusion · Near-infrared spectroscopy · Muscle oxygen saturation · Muscle tissue phantom

1 Introduction

Near-infrared spectroscopy (NIRS) is a non-invasive detection method commonly used today. It uses materials different absorptions for near-infrared light of different wavelengths. The absorbance of the emitted light can be analyzed for different

© Springer Nature Switzerland AG 2020
K.-P. Lin et al. (Eds.): ICBHI 2019, IFMBE Proceedings 74, pp. 191–197, 2020.
https://doi.org/10.1007/978-3-030-30636-6_27

concentrations of substances in the testing sample. Especially in the near-infrared light of 700 nm–1000 nm, have low absorption of biological tissue, which is called the "tissue window". Light can travel through the skin and fat to deep tissues, and is absorbed by the oxymyoglobin and deoxymyoglobin in the muscle tissue.

Recently, there are many studies using NIRS to measure tissue oxygen concentration in human tissues for different diseases, such as calf tissue and brain. However, many literatures compare different NIRS in the market. It is found that due to the lack of standardization of algorithms, wavelengths and photodiode configurations, it is difficult to compare them under different machines [1].

NIRS continuously measures the oxygen concentration of muscle tissue in peripheral arterial disease (PAD) patients and normal people under exercise conditions. The PAD patients have different characteristics in after exercise [2]. But there is no way to quantify the severity of the blockage. This study is to make a phantom that conforms to the optical characteristics of the human calf muscle tissue, regulate the oxygen concentration change of the prosthesis, simulate the oxygenation and hypoxia of the calf muscle tissue, and use the self-made NIRS to measure and correct the tissue oxygen concentration.

2   Methods and Materials

Human muscle tissue is mainly composed of myoglobin. Oxygen diffuses from capillary's oxyhemoglobin of red blood cells into the muscle tissue and combines with myoglobin to form oxymyoglobin. In order to let light to penetrates deep under skin to measure change of muscle tissue oxygen saturation.

We choose myoglobin and hemoglobin isosbestic point (808 nm) spectral for measurement, near isosbestic point wavelength light-emitting diode as light source (740 nm and 850 nm), in order to reduce difference of light scatter that influence measurement accuracy. And then, we use two long led-photodiode distance (40 mm, 32 mm) to insure light to penetrate deep into muscle tissue and two light sources can eliminate skin scattering effects [3]. In this research, the homemade NIRS optical probe configuration shows in Fig. 1.

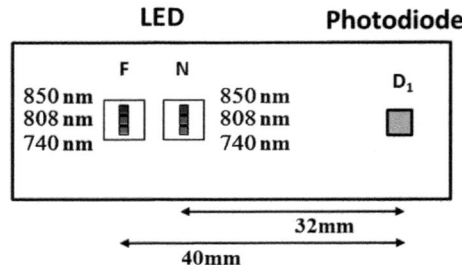

Fig. 1. Photodiode and LED configuration

The liquid phantom consisted of phosphate-buffered saline (PBS, pH = 7.4, volume in phantom = 750 ml), red blood cells purified from pig blood (volume in phantom = 11 ml), intralipid 20% (volume in phantom = 30 ml) and glucose 50% (volume in phantom = 2.7 ml). Purificatory red blood cells solution is formulated to adjust the absorbance ingredient with oxygen saturation. Optical properties of the liquid phantom are as same as lower limbs muscles optical properties [4].

In order to insure the liquid phantom blood oxygen capacity, using dissolved oxygen meter (D.O. meter, Kai-Yuan, ODO-BTA) to monitor the oxygen dissolved concentration in the liquid phantom. In a container that is closed at room temperature and is sealed, the molar of a gas dissolved in a solvent is proportional to the partial pressure of the gas that is balanced with the solution; this is called Henry's law:

$$p = kc \tag{1}$$

where p is the gas of partial pressure, c is the molar of dissolved in the solvent, k is henry's constant. Henry's constant will have different values because of temperature and gas, so use dissolved oxygen concentration to calculate the partial pressure in the solution. When phantom partial pressure increases, oxyhemoglobin proportion and tissue oxygen saturation is also increase. Conversely, phantom partial pressure decrease, oxyhemoglobin proportion and tissue oxygen saturation will decrease. So, k value can be derived from the known oxygen partial pressure.

However, there is no linear relationship between the ratio of hemoglobin to oxygen bonding and the partial pressure of oxygen dissolved in the solution. The corresponding relationship between two ratios is called Hill's equation:

$$\delta = \frac{\left(\frac{P}{P_{50}}\right)^n}{1 + \left(\frac{P}{P_{50}}\right)^n} \times 100\% \tag{2}$$

where δ is red blood cell solution oxygen saturation (%), P is partial oxygen pressure in phantom, P50 and n is constant.

The calibration experiment is designed a can change oxygen saturation and consist the solution simulated lower limbs muscle optical properties. Using a plastic thin-shell container to hold this solution and can attached optical probe to the outer wall for measurement. Figure 3 shows calibration experiment frame diagram (Fig. 2).

In order to maintain the phantom's temperature at 37 °C, uniform oxygen saturation and tunable dissolved oxygen concentration. Use hot plate and magnetic stirrer to maintain temperature and slowly stirring the phantom. The oxygen supply system uses mass flow controller (Protec, PC-540). Table 1 shows whole experimental steps.

Data processing was performed using Matlab for signal analysis. The self-made NIR spectrometer used a low-pass digital filter to calculate the ratio of the three wavelengths of near and far light. The dissolved oxygen meter is recorded at a sampling rate of 10 Hz, and is resampled to 6 Hz. The dissolved oxygen amount is converted into the oxygen content of the prosthesis tissue by the above-mentioned conversion method. Finally, the logarithmic regression of the prosthetic tissue oxygen content and the near-far light ratio was carried out to obtain the calibration curve of this study.

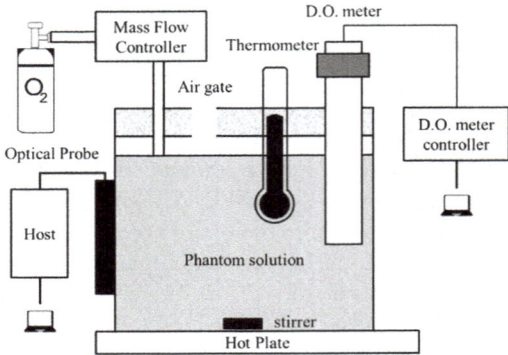

Fig. 2. Calibration experiment frame diagram

Table 1. NIRS calibration experiment step

Step	Content
1	Prepare mixture phantom as mentioned above
2	Maintain temperature at 37 °C and start stirring (50 rpm)
2	Start measurement (D.O. meter and NIRS)
3	Add 1.5 g yeast then Sealed the phantom
4	Wait until pO2 reaches low point
5	Continue to add 20% O2 in to the phantom
6	Wait until pO2 reaches high point then stop measurement

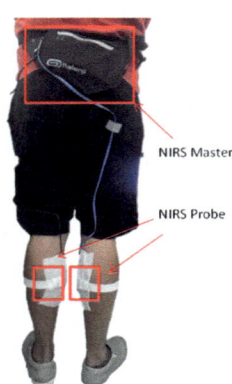

Fig. 3. Schematic diagram of optical probe wearing on the gastrocnemius muscle

In order to prove that the calibration curve can be applied to measure the tissue oxygen concentration in human body, this study recruited a 23-year-old male with a BMI of 25.7. The muscle tissue oxygen concentration of the gastrocnemius muscle was measured under static standing, and a 10-min data was continuously measured for calculation. And observe whether the value is within the normal range. The experimental probe configuration is shown in Fig. 3.

3   Result and Discussion

Figure 4 shows optical probe measure absorbance in the process of experiment. It seems absorbance stable before adding yeast. When oxygen saturation start decreasing, the measurement absorbance start changing and between two light-detector distances have consistent change response in different wavelength.

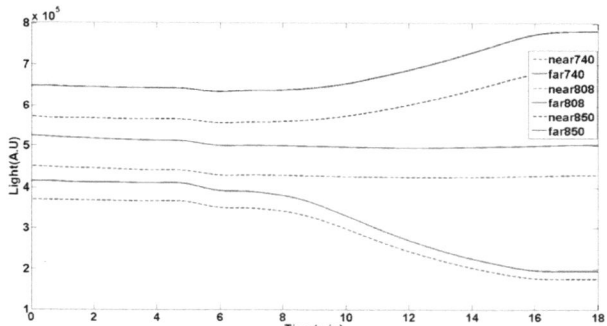

Fig. 4. Photometric changes of different wavelengths measured by optical probes when changing the oxygen concentration of the phantom

The ratio of the near 740 to the near 850 in the measured luminosity is compared with the tissue oxygen concentration measured by the D.O meter, and the result is as shown in Fig. 5. The red line represents the oxygen concentration measured by the dissolved oxygen meter. The change, the green line represents the calibration curve after regression analysis. The curve formula is as shown in Eq. 4, where StO2 represents the converted tissue oxygen concentration, R_{740850} represents the ratio of the wavelength 740 and 850, abcd is the calculation constant, and the determination coefficient of the calibration curve (R^2) Is 0.9956.

$$StO2(\%) = a\exp(bR_{740850}) + c\exp(dR_{740850}) \tag{4}$$

Finally, the calibration curve is brought into the static standing experiment. The result is shown in Fig. 6. The average of 10 min is 78.96%, the standard deviation is 0.3485, and the difference is quite small. The calculated StO2 (%) is within the normal range. The study indicated that in 42 normal subjects, the pre-exercise leg StO2 (%) ranged from 47% to 85% [5].

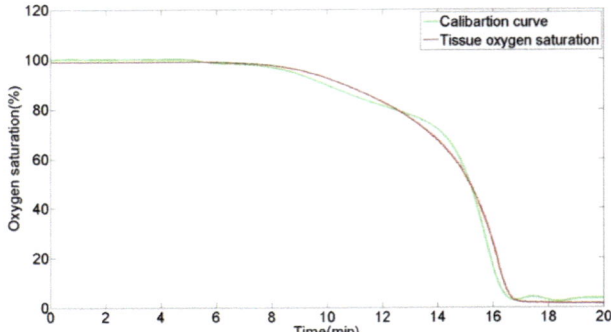

Fig. 5. Second order exponential calibration curve and D.O meter experiment data

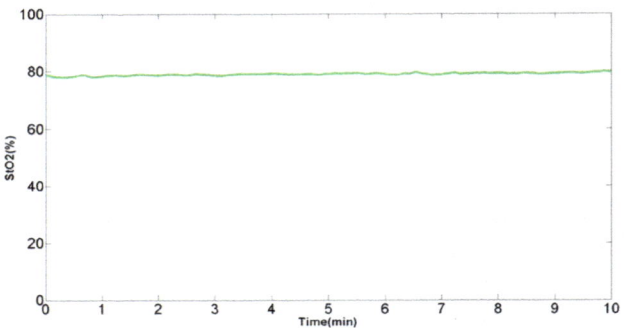

Fig. 6. In vivo measurement in ten minutes standing experiment(%)

4   Conclusions

In the calibration experiment, using purificatory red blood cell from pig blood and intralipid to simulate the phantom that optical properties similar with lower limbs muscles. By changing the oxygen saturation of the phantom, this research make calibration curve with D.O. meter measure dissolved oxygen saturation to calculate phantom tissue oxygen saturation (Hill's equation) as a standard reference and homemade optical probe measure tissue absorbance. In the future, use this calibration curve to homemade NIRS perform actual measurement of tissue oxygen saturation. It made our homemade NIRS measurement of tissue oxygen saturation more physiologically significant in clinical.

Acknowledgment.   This research was supported by the Ministry of Science and Technology of Taiwan (MOST 106-2221-E-033-014-).

Conflict of Interest.   The authors declare that they have no conflict of interest.

References

1. Ferrari, N., Quaresima, V.: Near infrared brain and muscle oximetry: from the discovery to current applications. J. Near Infrared Spectroscopy **20**, 1–14 (2012). https://doi.org/10.1255/jnirs.973
2. Yu, G., Durduran, T., Lech, G., Zhou, C., Chance, B., Mohler, E.R., Yodh, A.G.: Time-dependent blood flow and oxygenation in human skeletal muscles measured with noninvasive near-infrared diffuse optical spectroscopies. J. Biomed. Opt. **10**(2), 024–027 (2005). https://doi.org/10.1117/1.1884603
3. Lu, W.-C., Lu, S.-H., Chen, M.-F., Fu, T.-C., Lin, K.-P., Tsai, C.-L.: Portable near-infrared spectroscopy for detecting peripheral arterial occlusion. In: IFMBE Proceedings. International Conference on Bio and Health Informatics. Precision Med. Powered by pHealth and Connected Health, Thessaloniki, vol. 66, pp. 109–113 (2018)
4. Nasseri, N., Kleiser, S., Ostojic, D., Karen, T., Wolf, M.: Quantifying the effect of adipose tissue in muscle oximetry by near infrared spectroscopy. Biomed. Opt. Express **7**(11), 4605–4619 (2016). https://doi.org/10.1364/BOE.7.004605
5. Barker, T., Spencer, P., Kirkman, E., Lamber, A., Midwinter, M.: An evaluation of the normal range of StO2 measurements at rest and following a mixed exercise protocol. J. R. Army Med. Corps **161**(4), 327–331 (2015). https://doi.org/10.1136/jramc-2014-000312

Instantaneous Respiratory Phase Response of Individual with Internet Gaming Disorder During Watching Game Video

Hong-Ming Ji[1] and Tzu-Chien Hsiao[2,3(✉)]

[1] Institute of Computer Science and Engineering, College of Computer Science, National Chiao Tung University, 1001 University Road, Hsinchu, Taiwan
jhm0006023.cs00g@g2.nctu.edu.tw
[2] Department of Computer Science, College of Computer Science, National Chiao Tung University, Hsinchu, Taiwan
[3] Institute of Biomedical Engineering, College of Electrical and Computer Engineering, National Chiao Tung University, Hsinchu, Taiwan
labview@cs.nctu.edu.tw

Abstract. Users play games because of fun and relaxation. But some users engage in the online game world, and they give up their educational or work opportunity and neglect their duties. These persons have the symptoms of Internet gaming disorder (IGD). Individual with IGD plays different online game scenes with dynamically psychophysiological control for a long period of time. However, the empirical studies focus on the long period of playing experiences or the short period of physiological responses for investigating the psychophysiological properties of IGD. Few studies discuss the instantaneous psychophysiological responses of persons with IGD. Moreover, individual differences in reaction time may influence the time-variate properties of IGD. It makes investigation of instantaneous psychophysiological responses more difficult. On the basis of the concept of multi-modal pressure-flow method, we propose an index of instantaneous phase delay (IPD) as a modulation of time for observing the instantaneous coordination of respiratory wall movement during watching game video. 19 and 21 persons with high-risk IGD (HIGD) and low-risk IGD (LIGD) were participant in this study, respectively. Preliminary result shows the negative correlation between the IGD questionnaires and IPD (within 3 cycles). Our finding indicated that individuals with HIGD may rapidly modulate psychophysiological response during negative game stimuli compared with individuals with LIGD. We suggested that IPD may be an potential index to assess IGD within 3 cycles. The findings should make an important contribution to advance the understanding of instantaneous regulation mechanism for IGD. Recruiting more participles is needed to verify this finding in the near future.

Keywords: Internet gaming disorder · Instantaneous phase delay · Game video stimuli

K.-P. Lin et al. (Eds.): ICBHI 2019, IFMBE Proceedings 74, pp. 198–203, 2020.
https://doi.org/10.1007/978-3-030-30636-6_28

1 Introduction

To date, playing online games has been become the most engaging form of entertainment in campus life. There are some benefits of playing online games, however, some gamers always overuse and obsess games that may cause them to addict. Persons with game addiction may decline recreational activities, social activities, and sleep time due to overusing games, which affect them daily life and psychophysiological development. The phenomenon of game addiction occurs not only in students but also in employees. Students always disregard studies and feel fatigue in the daytime due to overusing games. Employees neglect assignment and reduce work performances due to overusing games. Regardless of negative consequences, persons with game addiction still spend a lot of time for playing games. In 2013, American psychiatric association announced that Internet gaming disorder was included in the Diagnostic and Statistical Manual of Mental Disorders, 5 Edition (DSM-5) and discussed that whether IGD be a mental disorder [1]. The World Health Organization declared, in 2018, the gaming disorder has been further included in the International Statistical Classification of Diseases 11th Revision [2].

Which psychophysiological properties result gamer in addiction that is an important issue. Researchers designed questionnaires to assess psychological properties of persons with IGD for long period of experiences, such as 6 months [3]. Researchers measured physiological signals of persons with IGD to assess their physiological properties for short periods of physiological responses, such as 5 min [4]. One of important psychophysiological properties of IGD is that individual with IGD stay with dynamically psychophysiological control in the online game for a long period of time. However, the empirical studies were no investigated instantaneously psychophysiological responses [3, 4]. So those studies can't assess real-time psychophysiological properties and explore underlying regulation mechanism for IGD.

Our previous study had proposed the empirical mode decomposition method to decompose instantaneous respiratory oscillation. The result showed that respiratory amplitude and frequency can be treated as a real-time psychophysiological property of persons with IGD [5]. We also investigated the instantaneous change of respiratory amplitude and frequency among subjects. In this paper, we combined one method of multimodal pressure-flow (MMPF) with our previous approach. The MMPF was proposed to improve the time difference of respiratory modulation between subjects in continued blood pressure signal and was derived an index of instantaneous phase was introduced to observe the coordination between continued blood pressure and cerebral blood flow [6]. The research purpose is to explorer the oscillatory phase responses of the respiratory modulation of individuals with IGD during watching game video. This is the first study to investigate the relationship between the IGD symptoms and instantaneous phase responses of respiratory modulation during audio-visual stimuli of game. We hoped that this study will contribute to provide a new physiological index to assess IGD, and a deep understanding of psychophysiological regulation mechanism of persons with IGD.

2   Material and Method

In this study, IGD questionnaire (IGDQ) from DSM-5 [1] was used to assess IGD symptoms of participants. IGDQ contains 9 items, and each item is 2-point Likert scale (disagreement = 0 and agreement = 1). We also adopted Chen Internet addiction scale (CIAS) [7] to assess Internet addiction symptoms of participants. CIAS contains 26 items, and each item is 4-point Likert scale (from very disagreement to very agreement). We recruited participants from National Chiao Tung University (NCTU), Taiwan. Initially, each participant was asked to sit in a comfortable chair and sign informed consent document. Participant was also asked to execute 10 min abdominal breathing exercise (6 cycles/min) to relax body. Next, participant executed experiment. The experimental procedure consisted of the 2 min rest status (relaxing psychophysiological responses), 2 min stimuli status (watching the game video of Resident Evil), and self-report status (Self-Assessment Manikin for emotional valence and arousal, 9-point Likert scale [8]). During rest and stimuli statuses, participant's abdominal wall movement signals were acquired by using RIPmate inductance belts (Respiratory Inductance Plethysmography, Abdomen Kit, Adult, Alice 5, Ambu Inc., Denmark), 1000 samples/sec.

The procedures of signal processing are (1) reducing the sampling rate form 1000 Hz to 50 Hz, (2) adopting the ensemble empirical mode decomposition method [9] to decompose into 6 ordering oscillatory modes (intrinsic mode function, IMF, from high to low frequencies), (3) calculating the power of each IMF [10], (4) defining the maximal power value as dominant frequency component (IMF_{DF}), (5) treating the latter IMF as lower frequency component (IMF_{LF}), (6) calculating the instantaneous amplitude and phase of IMF_{LF} by using normalized direct quadrature [11], (7) defining the starting point and turning point, and (8) transforming to phase domain and calculating the difference between these two points, and the difference was called instantaneous phase delay (IPD). The condition of turning point is defined as the first point which slope of the instantaneous amplitude was reversed. All of data management and analysis performance were done under LabVIEW environment (v.2016, National Instruments, Austin, US). Figure 1 demonstrates the distribution of IMF amplitude and phase of individual with low-risk IGD (LIGD).

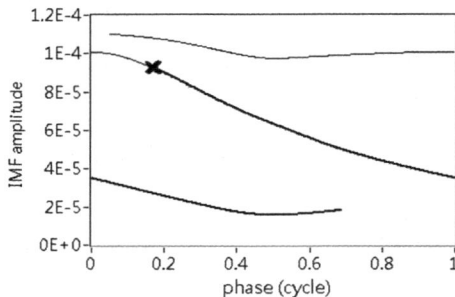

Fig. 1. The distribution of IMF amplitude value and phase of individual with LIGD. The thin line and the thick line are denoted IMF amplitude during rest status and during stimuli status, respectively. The cross mark is denoted transition from rest status to stimuli status.

3   Preliminary Result

There are 50 participants (36 men and 14 women, 23 ± 4 years old) were recruited from NCTU campus. We considered individual with IGD who must be an Internet addition, and individual with non-IGD who is not an Internet addition. Therefore, participants based on the cut-off score for IGDQ and CIAS were group into 21 LIGD (IGDQ score < 5 and CIAS score < 64) and 19 high-risk IGD (HIGD, IGDQ score ≥ 5 and CIAS score ≥ 64). Table 1 displays the statistical result (mean ± SD) of age, questionnaire score (IGDQ and CIAS), Self-Assessment Manikin rating (valence and arousal), and IPD value for individuals with HIGD and LIGD. On the basis of the valence score, the game video of Resident Evil for individuals with LIGD and HIGD was a negatively emotional stimuli. The difference between the IPD value of individuals with HIGD and individuals with LIGD exhibited statistical significance ($p < 0.05$). Figure 2 indicates those results of IGDQ score, CIAS score, and corresponding IPD values. We also used the logarithmic curve fit for evaluating the correlation coefficient. The results show that IPD value is negative correlative with IGDQ ($r = -0.389$) and CIAS ($r = -0.435$).

Table 1. The statistical result (mean ± SD) of age, IGDQ and CIAS score, valence and arousal rating, and IPD value for individuals with HIGD and LIGD. M: men; W: women.

	HIGD (15 M, 4 W)	LIGD (12 M, 9 W)
Age	24 ± 5	23 ± 2
IGDQ score	6.58 ± 1.5	1.48 ± 1.25
CIAS score	79.26 ± 8.63	52.10 ± 8.03
Video valence	3.68 ± 1.20	3.81 ± 1.97
Video arousal	5.37 ± 1.92	5.67 ± 2.13
IPD (cycle)	0.51 ± 0.29[a]	1.11 ± 0.84

[a]Statistically significant differences between IPD value of HIGD group and IPD value of LIGD group ($p < 0.05$) according to a t-test.

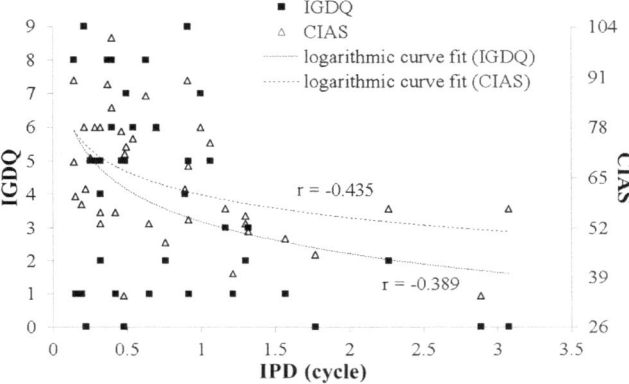

Fig. 2. Scatter plot of IGDQ score and CIAS score with IPD value.

4   Discussion

Instantaneous physiological responses are critical indexes for exploring psychophysiological regulation mechanism of persons with IGD. We had been proposed that respiratory amplitude and frequency for real-time psychophysiological property is value physiological response [5]. In this study, we based on MMPF [6] reduced the time difference of respiratory modulation between subjects and investigated the instantaneous phase responses of the respiratory modulation during game-related material stimuli for individuals with HIGD and LIGD.

To preliminary result, the valence and arousal rating of individuals with HIGD was lower than those with individuals with LIGD. It implied that HIGD group perceived more negative stimuli and were induced lower emotional intensity during watching game video of Resident Evil than those of LIGD group. The possible inference is that individuals of HIGD conceal their emotional intensity. Another explanation for this is that the abdominal breathing exercises effect emotional responses of individuals of HIGD. The breathing exercises have been used to relieve emotion for patients with IGD [12].

In this study, we also found that the IPD value of individuals of HIGD during watching negative game video was significantly lower than those of individuals with LIGD. Moreover, the severity of IGD was negative associated with IPD value. It is likely that modulation of respiratory wall movement during negatively emotional stimuli in persons with HIGD was faster than those of persons with LIGD. Fast modulation of psychophysiological responses may help persons with HIGD staying online games for a lengthy period of time. We suggested IPD may be a psychophysiological index to assess IGD.

The further study must recruit more participants to verify our finding. Second, the different type of games, e.g., action, strategy, role-playing, or puzzle video games, should be selected as game-related stimuli to observe corresponding instantaneous phase responses of IGD people. The IGD group plays more time on strategy and role-playing games [13]. Third, regarding the oscillatory physiological responses of respiratory modulation, we can observe cardiovascular responses of individuals with IGD, and then we can investigate autonomic nervous system responses. The instantaneous phase had been observed the coordination between blood pressure and cerebral blood flow [6].

5   Conclusions

The aim of the present research was to investigate the instantaneous respiratory phase responses of individuals with IGD during watching game video. One of the more significant findings from this study is that the IPD value is negative associated with the IGD symptoms. The current data may be highlighted that the index of Instantaneous phase not only observes instantaneous psychophysiological modulation, but also improves the effect of individual differences. Investigating the link between instantaneous phase responses and IGD level may help researchers to understand the respiratory regulation of persons with IGD. Further studies need to collect more sample size and select different type of games as stimuli to validate our finding.

Acknowledgment. This study was supported by the Taiwan Ministry of Science and Technology (MOST 105-2221-E-009-159, MOST 105-2634-E-009-003, and MOST 107-2221-E-009-153). Ethical approval was obtained from REC for Human Subject Protection, NCTU, Taiwan (NCTU-REC-102-009-e).

Conflict of Interest. The authors declare that they have no conflict of interest.

References

1. American Psychiatric Association: Diagnostic and statistical manual of mental disorders, 5th (DSM-5). American Psychiatric Association Press Inc., Arlington (2013)
2. Hans-Jürgen, R., Achab, S., Billieux, J., et al.: Including gaming disorder in ICD-11: the need to do so from a clinical and public health perspective. J. Behav. Addict. **7**, 556–561 (2018)
3. Petry, N., Rehbein, F., Gentile, D.A., et al.: An international consensus for assessing internet gaming disorder using the new DSM-5 approach. Addiction **109**(9), 1399–1406 (2014)
4. Chang, J.-S., Kim, E.-Y., Jung, D., et al.: Altered cardiorespiratory coupling in young male adults with excessive online gaming. Biol. Psychol. **110**, 159–166 (2015)
5. Hsieh, D.-L., Ji, H.-M., Hsiao, T.-C., et al.: Respiratory feature extraction in emotion of internet addiction addicts using complementary ensemble empirical mode decomposition. J. Med. Imaging Health Inform. **5**, 391–399 (2015)
6. Novak, V., Yang, A.C.C., Lepicovsky, L., et al.: Multimodal pressure-flow method to assess dynamics of cerebral autoregulation in stroke and hypertension. Biomed. Eng. Online **3**, 39 (2004)
7. Chen, S.-H., Weng, L.-J., Su, Y.-J., et al.: Development of a Chinese Internet addiction scale and its psychometric study. Chin. J. Psychol. **45**, 279–294 (2003)
8. Lang, P.J.: Behavioral treatment and bio-behavioral assessment: computer applications. In: Sidowski, J.B., Johnson, J.H., Williams, T.A. (eds.) Technology in Mental Health Care Delivery Systems, pp. 119–137 (1980)
9. Wu, Z., Huang, N.-E.: Ensemble empirical mode decomposition: a noise-assisted data analysis method. Adv. Adapt. Data Anal. **1**(1), 1–41 (2009)
10. Wu, Z., Huang, N.E.: A study of the characteristic of white noise using the empirical mode decomposition method. Proc. R. Soc. A Math. Phys. Eng. Sci. **460**, 1597–1611 (2004)
11. Huang, N.E., Wu, Z., Long, S.-R., et al.: On instantaneous frequency. Adv. Adapt. Data Anal. **1**, 177–229 (2009)
12. Li, W., Garland, E.L., OBrien, J.E., et al.: Mindfulness-oriented recovery enhancement for video game addiction in emerging adults: preliminary findings from case reports. Int. J. Ment. Health Addict. **16**, 928–945 (2017)
13. Adam, E., Kattner, F., Bradford, D., et al.: Role-playing and real-time strategy games associated with greater probability of Internet gaming disorder. Cyberpsychol. Behav. Soc. Netw. **18**(8), 480–485 (2015)

Photoplethysmographic Signals Measured at the Nose

Pin-Lu Li[1(✉)], Shao-Hung Lu[1], Kang-Ping Lin[2,3],
and Cheng-Lun Tsai[1,3]

[1] Biomedical Engineering Department, Chung-Yuan Christian University,
200, Chung-Bei Road, Taoyuan 32023, Taiwan
tony3204203@gmail.com, clt@cycu.edu.tw
[2] Electrical Engineering Department, Chung-Yuan Christian University,
Taoyuan, Taiwan
[3] Technology Translation Center for Medical Device,
Chung Yuan Christian University, Taoyuan, Taiwan

Abstract. Polysomnography is the main diagnostic instrument for sleep apnea, but it is not convenient for patient to take frequent measurements at home. An in-home sleep test is a solution to help physicians to collect more information. Sleep medicine societies suggest that a home sleep-apnea testing device should measure at least oxygen saturation and breathing signals. To reduce the discomfort of measurement during sleep, the device should be also as small as possible. One possible measuring site for both signals is at the nose. The accuracy of oxygen saturation measurement relies on the quality of photoplethysmographic signals (PPG). PPG signals of red and near-infrared light measured at the nasal septum and nasal wing were compared. PPG signals were also measured at different body postures includes standing, sitting and supine.

Although nasal septum and wing are both thin layer of tissue, the perfusion index is greater and has a larger variation at nasal septum than at nasal wing. Although the PPG at nasal wing is relatively stable and not greatly affected by the autonomic nervous regulation, the change in signals with oxygen saturation is also small. Therefore, the nasal septum is a better position for measuring oxygen saturation at the nose.

Keywords: Photo-plethysmography · Perfusion index · Oxygen saturation · Sleep apnea

1 Introduction

Patients with sleep apnea have sleep disorders that might stop breathing for several times during sleep. Recent studies show that sleep apnea could also increase the risk of cardiovascular disease and other chronic diseases.

The main diagnostic apparatus of sleep apnea is polysomnography. The measurement is generally carried out at a sleep diagnostic center, and it takes a whole night to measure. With the entangled wires and strange environment, some people even have difficulty to really fall asleep during the test. These factors often affect the quality of evaluation result.

© Springer Nature Switzerland AG 2020
K.-P. Lin et al. (Eds.): ICBHI 2019, IFMBE Proceedings 74, pp. 204–211, 2020.
https://doi.org/10.1007/978-3-030-30636-6_29

Therefore, many researchers and companies are still seeking for a better home sleep apnea testing device that people can do the test at home in a familiar environment.

To find the most suitable place at nose for measuring blood oxygen concentration, this study designed a continuous measuring system to detect the penetrating intensity of red and near-infrared light through different parts of nose tissue. The quantity of PPG detected at different positions were compared to determine the best measuring site.

2 Materials and Methods

2.1 Measurement Sites and System

The lower part of nose has abundant of blood supply, and close to the surface level of upper lip. In order to find the best position of oxygen saturation measurement for device put on the upper lip, measurement were taken at nasal septum and nasal wing, as shown in Fig. 1. Optical probe could be designed to take measurement at both positions without using an extension cable. There are no nasal bones at these two places to interfere the penetration of light. Nasal wing is only composed of soft tissue, but nasal septum has a septal cartridge that could cause strong scattering of light. To reduce the interference of environment light, the photo-detector was put on the cavity side of nasal wing. Nasal septum at nostril is very close to the Kiesselbach's plexus that is highly perfused. Arteries in this area of septum includes anterior and posterior ethmoidal arteries, sphenopalatine and greater palatine arteries and superior labial artery. The arteries run through nasal wings are anterior ethmoidal artery at the inner lateral wall and the angular branch of facial artery at the outer wall.

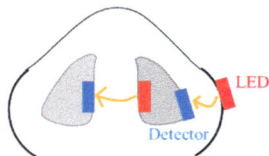

Fig. 1. Measurement sites at nasal septum and nasal wing.

Figure 2 shows the block diagram of the optical measurement system built in this study. A System-on-a-Chip (SoC H16F3981, Hycon) with a 24-bits resolution ADC is used to control the flashing sequences of a red LED (660 nm) and a near-infrared LED (940 nm). The SoC minimizes the circuit board, and the high resolution ADC provides a very large dynamic range of measurement. The transmitting light picked up by the photodiode is digitized and sent to a computer. The measured data is stored in the computer for further process (Fig. 3).

PPG signal is a time varying transmission of light through a living tissue. It includes a small and fast pulsatile variation (AC_H) caused by beating heart, a slow drifting with breathing (AC_L) and muscle tone of vessel, and a large shift of base line (DC). The accuracy of oxygen saturation measurement depends on a high resolution of

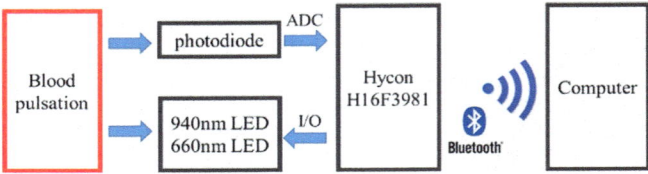

Fig. 2. Block diagram of the PPG measurement system.

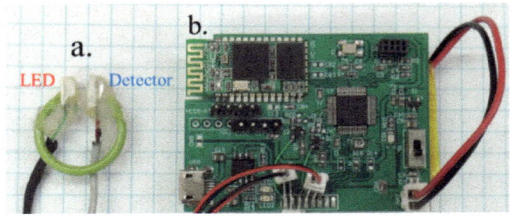

Fig. 3. (a) Optical probe and (b) system board.

the pulsatile signal. The amplitude of pulsatile signal is determined by the amount of blood perfused, therefore, tissue with a higher perfusion rate will have a larger change in light absorption. However, the amplitude of PPG signal also change with light source intensity. To accurately evaluate the perfusion rate of tissue, the pulsatile amplitude should normalize to the intensity of light source. The most common way of doing this is to divide the peak-to-peak value of signal pulse by the drifting baseline amplitude. This perfusion index is ratio of the reduced intensity of light by increasing blood volume with pulse related to the stable light transmittance through the rest of tissue. The PI value also varies with the total blood volume changing in time, and it is formulated as Eq. (1). The PI value was reported to range from 0.02% to 20%. The larger the PI value is, the higher the gain can be used at the first stage without signal saturation.

$$PI(t) = \frac{|AC_H|}{DC + AC_L} \times 100\% \tag{1}$$

2.2   Experiments

To make sure the optical probe can detect the similar signal when it is attached despite of the displacement in measuring site. PPG signal of both red and near-infrared light were measured on a young healthy subject. Measurements were also taken at different body positions with the probe being put on and taken down repeatedly.

The signal was measured for one minute with the subject staying still during normal breathing. Five measurements were taken at each measuring site at nose before changing body position.

To study how the PPG varies with the subject changing body posture, PPG signal of both red and near-infrared light were continuously measured for five minutes at standing, sitting, and supine postures.

Since the blockage of breath during sleep apnea can affect the baseline drift of PPG signal, a breath-holding experiment was performed to simulate the apnea condition. Subjects were asked to breathe under normal breathing rate for 30 s, then held the breath for 30 s, and finally resume normal breathing rate for 1 min during the recovery period.

A signal processing program detected the maximum and minimum points of each pulse. The AC_H amplitude was calculated by using cubic spine interpolation to find the $AC_L + DC$ value at the same time with the peak. PI value of each pulse was calculated, and their average and standard variation were calculated for final comparison.

3 Results and Discussion

3.1 PPG Signal Variations

The perfusion indices measured at nasal septum and nasal wing under different body postures are compared in Fig. 4. Because the light absorption coefficient of hemoglobin is larger in near-infrared range than in red region, the transmission of red light is generally higher than the near-infrared.

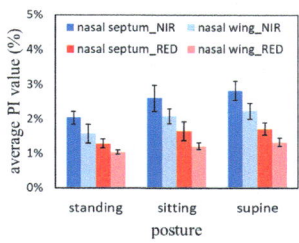

Fig. 4. Averages of PI of red and near-infrared measured at nasal septum and nasal wing in different postures.

Since the transmission intensity could be caused by a higher light source intensity, the pulse amplitude is normalized to the total transmission as perfusion index for comparison. The perfusion index falls roughly at the range between 1% and 3%. The greater values at nasal septum than at nasal wing is most possibly caused by higher blood perfusion rate. The results also show the PI values of measurement are very consistent.

3.2 Continuous Measurement with Posture Changes

Figure 5 show the continuous recording of PPG measured at nasal septum and nasal wing during posture changes. Both red and near-infrared have higher variation in

baseline at nasal septum. The baselines look like more stable in the nasal wing measurement. The transmission of red light is only a half of the intensity of near-infrared.

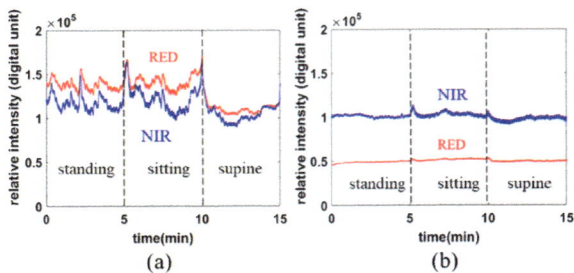

Fig. 5. PPG signals of red and near-infrared measured at (a) nasal septum and (b) nasal wing
during posture changes.

By taking the perfusion indexes of the signals in Fig. 5, the results of red and near-
infrared are very consistent as shown in Figs. 6 and 7. The trends of PI variation with
posture changes are quite similar at nasal septum and nasal wing for red and near-
infrared. The main difference is the PI value of red light is about two-thirds of the value
of near-infrared. The PI at nasal septum became lower when the subject lay down,
whereas the PI at nasal wing became higher. The PI measured at nasal septum also has
a larger variation than that measured at nasal wing. The statistics of the PI values of red
and near-infrared at different postures are plotted in Fig. 8 for comparison. The average
of PI value at the nasal septum is highest during the sitting posture, and the average PI
value at the nasal wing is highest during the supine posture. The variation of PI value
represents the variation in blood perfusion at different body postures.

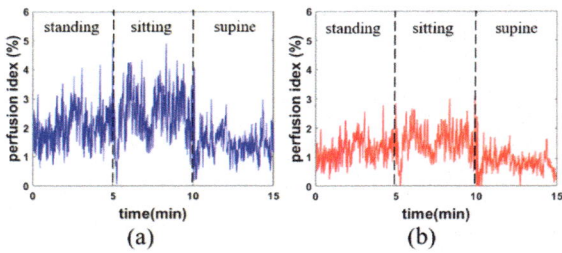

Fig. 6. Continuous PI curves of (a) near-infrared and (b) red measured at nasal septum during
posture changes.

3.3   Breath-Holding Experiment

The change in light absorption coefficient of hemoglobin with oxygen saturation is much
greater in red region than in near-infrared region. Curves in Fig. 9 are the continuous
recording of PPG signals at nasal septum and nasal wing during the breath-holding

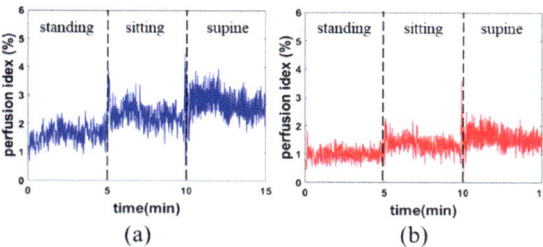

Fig. 7. Continuous PI curves of (a) near-infrared and (b) red measured at nasal wing during posture changes.

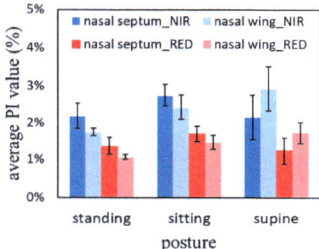

Fig. 8. Averages of PI of red and near-infrared continuously measured at nasal septum and nasal wing in different postures.

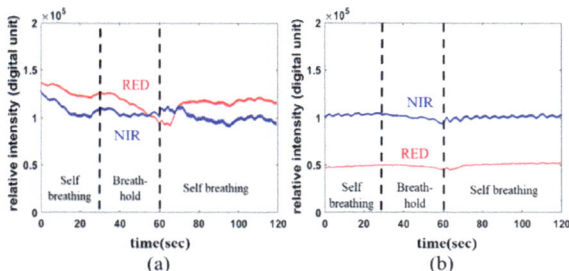

Fig. 9. PPG signals of red and near-infrared measured at (a) nasal septum and (b) nasal wing during the breath-holding experiment.

experiment. The transmission intensity of red light at nasal septum did not have a great change within the first 30 s of breath-hold. After 30 s, the oxygen combined with hemoglobin was greatly consumed, the spectrum of hemoglobin started to change and the transmission of red light showed an obvious drop, as seen in Fig. 9(a).

Figure 9(a) also shows the blood perfusion at nasal septum had a great variation through the breath-holding experiment. Both the baselines of both near-infrared and red transmission through the nasal wing are very stable, as shown in Fig. 9(b). The ripple on the near-infrared transmission during self-breathing period is caused by the change in blood perfusion with breathing. The breathing signal disappeared when breath was hold, but the regulation of vessel tone still caused change in blood volume that resulted in the baseline drift.

Figures 10 and 11 show the changes in PI value during the breath-holding experiment at two measuring sites of the nose. The breathing signal is very clear when the subject was under normal and self-breathing periods. They also show clear deeper breath right after the breath-holding period.

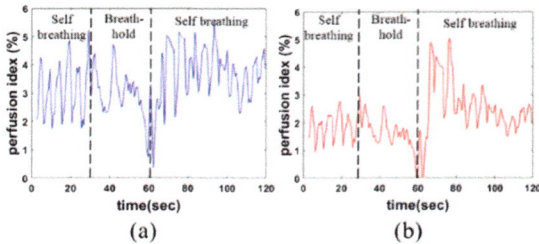

Fig. 10. PI curves of (a) near-infrared and (b) red measured at nasal septum during the breath-holding experiment.

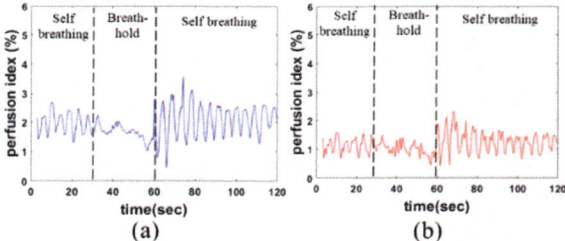

Fig. 11. PI curves of (a) near-infrared and (b) red measured at nasal wing during the breath-holding experiment.

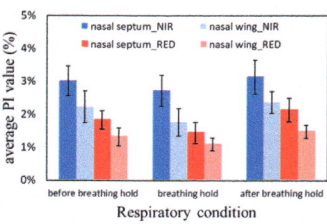

Fig. 12. Averages of PI at different periods during the breath-holding experiment.

The averages of PI values during different periods of the breath-holding experiment are plotted in Fig. 12. The subject was in a sitting position and the average of PI values are relatively the same during the whole experiment.

4   Conclusions

The continuous recording of PPG signals show great influence by the change in body postures and breath-holding experiment. The measurement taken at nasal wing are relatively stable which is good for detecting heart rate and respiratory rate. On the other hand, the signal measured at nasal septum is susceptible to the influence of the autonomic nervous system. The change in PI value with breath-holding is much greater at the nasal septum which is important to the calculation of oxygen saturation.

Acknowledgment. This research was supported by the Ministry of Science and Technology of Taiwan (MOST 106-2221-E-033-014- and MOST 107-2221-E-033-008-).

Conflict of Interest. The authors declare that they have no conflict of interest.

References

1. Comerota, A.J., Throm, R.C., Kelly, P., Jaff, M.: Tissue (muscle) oxygen saturation (StO2): a new measure of symptomatic lower-extremity arterial disease. J. Vasc. Surg. **38**(4), 724–729 (2003)
2. Giswold, M.E., Landry, G.J., Sexton, G.J., Yeager, R.A., Edwards, J.M., Taylor Jr., L.M., Moneta, G.L.: Modifiable patient factors are associated with reverse vein graft occlusion in the era of duplex scan surveillance. J. Vasc. Surg. **37**, 47–53 (2003)
3. Yu, G., Durduran, T., Gwen, L., Zhou, C., Chance, B., Mohler, E.R., Yodh, A.G.: Time-dependent blood flow and oxygenation in human skeletal muscles measured with noninvasive near-infrared diffuse optical spectroscopies. J. Biomed. Opt. **10**(2), 024–027 (2005)
4. De Felice, C., Latini, G., Vacca, P.: The pulse oximeter perfusion index as a predictor for high illness severity in neonates. Eur. J. Pediatr. **161**, 561–562 (2002)
5. McCully, K.K., Hamaoka, T.: Near-infrared spectroscopy: what can it tell us about oxygen saturation in skeletal muscle? Exerc. Sport Sci. Rev. **28**(3), 123–127 (2000)

Correlation Between Time-Domain Features of Electrohysterogram Data of Pregnant Women and Gestational Age

Chomkansak Hemthanon and Suparerk Janjarasjitt[✉]

Department of Electrical and Electronic Engineering, Ubon Ratchathani
University, Ubon Ratchathani, Thailand
suparerk.j@ubu.ac.th

Abstract. Electrohysterography (EHG) has been recently applied as one of diagnostic tools for pregnant women. In this study, six time-domain features commonly applied to EMG data, namely, the root mean square, the mean absolute value, the v-order, the average amplitude change, the difference absolute standard deviation value and the zero crossing, are applied to EHG data recorded from pregnant women who delivered at term or prematurely. The correlation between the time-domain features of EHG data and their corresponding time of recordings are examined using Pearson's correlation coefficients. From the computational results, it is shown that the mean absolute value, the v-order, the zero crossing, and the difference absolute standard deviation value are the time-domain features of EHG data that exhibit the strongest linear correlation with the time of recordings for each class of EHG data. Furthermore, the characteristics of time-domain features of EHG data associated with preterm and term births are shown to be different according to their correlation with the time of recordings.

Keywords: Uterine electromyogram · Time-domain features · Preterm birth · Pearson's correlation coefficient

1 Introduction

Electromyography (EMG) that measures an electrical signal corresponding to activity of muscles have been one of the most common biomedical signals. EMG data recorded from electrodes placed on abdominal around uterine, called uterine EMG or electrohysterography (EHG), for measuring the activity of uterine muscles [1] are recently applied for term and preterm labor assessments [1–3]. Prematurity is one of major health concerns as a preterm birth gives the baby less time to develop in the womb [4]. An estimated 15 million babies are born preterm every year [5]. Prematurity is the leading cause of death among children under 5 years of age [5, 6] where it can cause several health problems to babies including short-term complications and also long-term complications [4].

Characteristics of EHG data have been examined using various digital signal processing techniques. Quantitative measures obtained using both linear techniques (the root mean square, the peak frequency, the median frequency and the

© Springer Nature Switzerland AG 2020
K.-P. Lin et al. (Eds.): ICBHI 2019, IFMBE Proceedings 74, pp. 212–218, 2020.
https://doi.org/10.1007/978-3-030-30636-6_30

autocorrelation zero crossing) and nonlinear techniques (the maximal Lyapunov exponent, the correlation dimension and the sample entropy) [1] of EHG data publicly available on PhysioNet [7] called the Term-Preterm EHG Database (TPEHGDB) (available online at https://www.physionet.org/physiobank/database/tpehgdb/) are examined for dissimilarity. The median frequency and the sample entropy of EHG recording associated with the preterm birth and those with the term birth are shown to be noticeably different [1]. The discrete wavelet transform is another computational tool applied to the EHG data. The wavelet-based quantitative measures extracted from EHG data were applied for examining their potential on term and preterm birth classification [8, 9].

In this study, six time-domain features that are commonly applied to EMG signals for various applications are selected and applied to EHG data contained in the TPEHGDB. The characteristics of EHG data quantified from those six common time-domain features are examined. Rather than examining on their potential on classification or discrimination between the subject groups, i.e., term and preterm births, like in many of previous studies, the correlations between those six common time-domain features of EHG and corresponding time of recordings are examined.

2 Methods

2.1 Subjects and EHG Data

The Term-Preterm EHG Database (TPEHGDB) contains a total of 300 recordings of EHG data. Those recordings are divided into 2 subject groups: preterm birth (38 subjects) and term birth (262 subjects). Furthermore, the recordings can be divided 2 recording periods: early period (obtained before the 26th week of gestation) and later period (obtained during or after the 26th week of gestation). For the preterm birth group, there are 19 recordings obtained in the early period and 19 recordings obtained in the later period; while there are 143 recordings obtained in the early period and 119 recordings obtained in the later period for the term birth group [1, 7]. The EHG recordings are therefore categorized into 4 classes: PE (EHG recordings obtained from preterm birth subjects in the early period), PL (EHG recordings obtained from preterm birth subjects in the later period), TE (EHG recordings obtained from term birth subjects in the early period), and TL (EHG recordings obtained from term birth subjects in the later period).

The EHG data were recorded using the sampling frequency of 20 Hz [1, 7]. Each EHG recording is composed of 3 channels, referred to as s_1, s_2, and s_3 [1, 7]. In addition, the original 3-channel EHG data were filtered with 3 different bandpass frequencies including (a) from 0.08 Hz and 4 Hz; (b) from 0.3 Hz to 3 Hz; and (c) 0.3 Hz to 4 Hz [1, 7]. The first, second, and third subbands of EHG channels s_1, s_2, and s_3 are, respectively, referred to as s_{1a}, s_{1b} and s_{1c}, s_{2a}, s_{2b} and s_{2c}, and s_{3a}, s_{3b} and s_{3c}. A middle segment of each EHG signal with length of 8192 samples is examined.

2.2 Time-Domain Features of EMG Signals

Six distinct time-domain features [10] including the root mean square (RMS), the mean absolute value (MAV), the v-order, the average amplitude change (AAC), the difference absolute standard deviation value (DASDV), and the zero crossing (ZC) are applied to EHG segments. The RMS, MAV, v-order, AAC, DASDV, and ZC referred to as F_1, F_2, F_3, F_4, F_5, and F_6, respectively, can be given by

RMS:

$$F_1 = \sqrt{\frac{1}{N}\sum_{n=0}^{N-1} x^2[n]}, \tag{1}$$

MAV:

$$F_2 = \frac{1}{N}\sum_{n=0}^{N-1} |x[n]|, \tag{2}$$

v-order:

$$F_3 = \left(\frac{1}{N}\sum_{n=0}^{N-1} x^v[n]\right)^{1/v}, \tag{3}$$

AAC:

$$F_4 = \frac{1}{N}\sum_{n=0}^{N-1} |x[n+1] - x[n]|, \tag{4}$$

DASDV:

$$F_5 = \sqrt{\frac{1}{N-1}\sum_{n=0}^{N-1} (x[n+1] - x[n])^2}, \text{ and} \tag{5}$$

ZC:

$$F_6 = \sum_{n=1}^{N-1} [\mathrm{sgn}(x[n] \cdot x[n-1]) \cup |x[n] - x[n-1]| \geq 0] \tag{6}$$

where

$$\mathrm{sgn}(\alpha) = \begin{cases} 1 & \alpha \geq 0 \\ 0 & \text{otherwise.} \end{cases}$$

2.3   Data Analysis

All six time-domain features, i.e., F_1, F_2, F_3, F_4, F_5, and F_6, are extracted from all channels of EHG segment including their subbands. The statistically significant difference test, i.e., two-sample t-test, is applied to determine whether there is a significant difference between the mean of time-domain features of a channel of EHG segments associated with the PE (or TE) class and the mean of time-domain features of a channel of EHG segments associated with the PL (or TL) class with the significance level of 0.01.

Furthermore, the linear correlation between the time-domain features of a channel of EHG segments and their corresponding time of recordings is assessed using the Pearson's correlation coefficient defined as [11]

$$R(i) = \frac{\text{cov}(x_i, Y)}{\sqrt{\text{var}(x_i) \cdot \text{var}(Y)}}$$

where x_i is the ith variable, Y is the corresponding class, and $\text{cov}(\cdot)$ and $\text{var}(\cdot)$ denote, respectively, the covariance and the variance.

3   Results

3.1   Difference of the Time-Domain Features of EHG Segments

The results obtained from the two-sample t-tests performed on the time-domain features of EHG segments associated with the PE class and those of EHG segments associated with the PL class are summarized in Table 1. The results obtained from the two-sample t-tests performed on the time-domain features of EHG segments associated with the TE class and those of EHG segments associated with the TL class are also summarized in Table 1. The value of h that is equal to 1 denotes that the null hypothesis of corresponding t-test can be rejected while the value of h that is equal to 0 denotes the opposite.

The distributions of AAC of s_{1a}, s_{1b}, and s_{1c} of EHG segments associated with the TE and TL classes that are implied to be significantly different are, respectively, compared in Fig. 1(a)–(c). Likewise, the distributions of ZC of s_{1b}, s_{1c}, and s_{3b} of EHG segments associated with the TE and TL classes that are implied to be significantly different are compared in Fig. 2(a)–(c), respectively.

3.2   Correlation of the Time-Domain Features of EHG Segments

The maximum absolute values of Pearson's correlation coefficients between the time-domain features of EHG segments and the time of recordings among each class, i.e., PE, PL, TE, and TL, are summarized in Table 2. In addition, in Table 2, the corresponding time-domain features of EHG segments for each class are included. A line that is a best fit in a least-squares sense for the corresponding time-domain features of EHG segments associated with the PE, PL, TE, and TL classes shown in Figs. 3(a)–(d) is plotted in magenta.

Table 1. Results of two-sample t-tests

EHG segment	Preterm birth						Term birth					
	F_1	F_2	F_3	F_4	F_5	F_6	F_1	F_2	F_3	F_4	F_5	F_6
s_1	0	0	0	0	0	0	0	0	0	0	0	0
s_{1a}	0	0	0	0	0	0	0	0	0	1	0	0
s_{1b}	0	0	0	0	0	0	0	0	0	1	0	1
s_{1c}	0	0	0	0	0	0	0	0	0	1	0	1
s_2	0	0	0	0	0	0	0	0	0	0	0	0
s_{2a}	0	0	0	0	0	0	0	0	0	0	0	0
s_{2b}	0	0	0	0	0	0	0	0	0	0	0	0
s_{2c}	0	0	0	0	0	0	0	0	0	0	0	0
s_3	0	0	0	0	0	0	0	0	0	0	0	0
s_{3a}	0	0	0	0	0	0	0	0	0	0	0	0
s_{3b}	0	0	0	0	0	0	0	0	0	0	0	1
s_{3c}	0	0	0	0	0	0	0	0	0	0	0	0

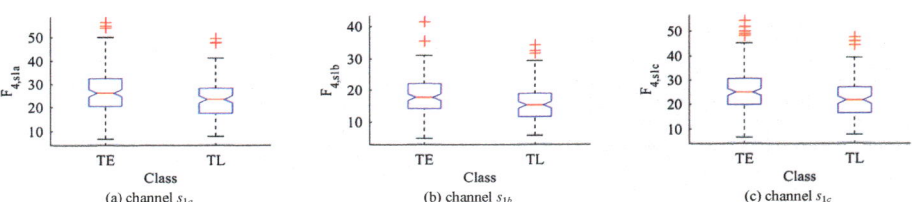

Fig. 1. Box plots of the average amplitude change (AAC) of EHG segments

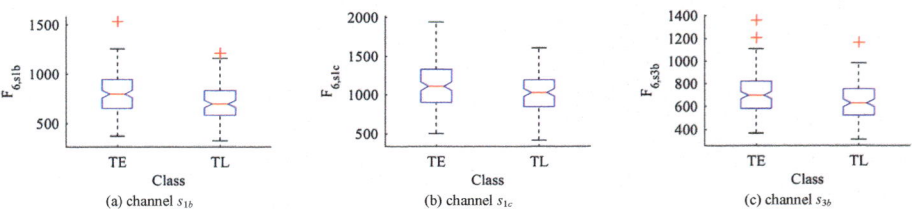

Fig. 2. Box plots of the zero crossing (ZC) of EHG segments

Table 2. Results of Pearson's correlation coefficients

Class	Pearson's correlation coefficient	EHG segment	Time-domain feature
PE	0.4548	s_3	F_2
PL	0.3324	s_{2a}	F_3
TE	0.2423	s_{2a}	F_6
TL	−0.2358	s_3	F_5

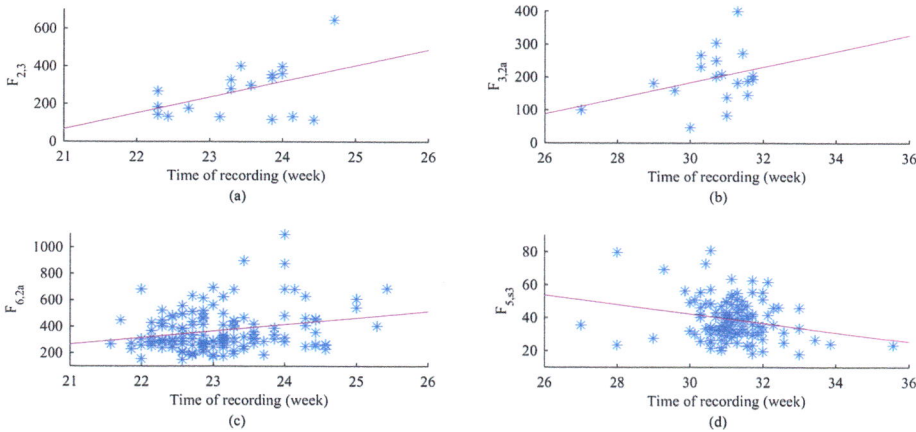

Fig. 3. Time-domain features of EHG segments corresponding to each class

The models of linear correlation between the time-domain features of EHG segments and the time of recordings are given, respectively, for the classes

PE:

$$F_{2,S_3}(t) = 84.142t - 1702.10,$$

PL:

$$F_{3,S_{2a}}(t) = 23.767t - 531.61,$$

TE:

$$F_{6,S_{2a}}(t) = 49.442t - 775.27, \text{ and}$$

TL:

$$F_{5,S_3}(t) = -2.863t + 127.84$$

where t denotes the time of recordings.

4   Conclusions

From the computational results, it is shown that two time-domain features, i.e., AAC and ZC, of EHG segments recorded from pregnant women who delivered at term in the early period (i.e., the TE class) are significantly different from those of EHG segments recorded from pregnant women who delivered at term in the later period (i.e., the TL class). On the contrary, the results obtained from the two-sample t-tests imply that there are no significant differences between the time-domain features of EHG segments recorded from pregnant women who delivered prematurely in the early and later periods (i.e., the PE and PL classes). This suggests that the characteristics of EHG signals considerably change when the gestational age increases for only the pregnant women who delivered at term. Also, such dissimilarity can be further applied for discriminating between term and preterm subjects.

In addition, the mean absolute value (MAV), the v-order, the zero crossing (ZC), and the difference absolute standard deviation value (DASDV) of EHG segments associated with, respectively, the PE, PL, TE, and TL classes are shown to have the strongest linear correlation with the time of recordings (or the gestational age). The MAV, the v-order, and the ZC of the corresponding EHG segments tend to increase as the gestational age increases while the DASDV of the corresponding EHG segments tend to decrease as the gestational age increases.

Acknowledgments. This work is supported by a TRF Research Career Development Grant, jointly funded by the Thailand Research Fund (TRF) and the Ubon Ratchathani University, under the Contract No. RSA6180041.

Conflict of Interest. The authors declare that they have no conflict of interest.

References

1. Fele-Zorz, G., Kavsek, G., Novak-Antolic, Z., Jager, F.: A comparison of various linear and non-linear signal processing techniques to separate uterine EMG records of term and preterm delivery groups. Med. Biol. Eng. Comput. **46**, 911–922 (2008)
2. Maner, W.L., Garfield, R.E.: Identification of human term and preterm labor using artificial neural networks on uterine electromyography data. Ann. Biomed. Eng. **35**, 465–473 (2007)
3. Leman, H., Marque, C., Gondry, J.: Use of the electrohysterogram signal for characterization of contractions during pregnancy. IEEE Trans. Biomed. Eng. **46**, 1222–1229 (1999)
4. Premature Birth at https://www.mayoclinic.org/diseases-conditions/premature-birth/symptoms-causes/syc-20376730
5. Preterm Birth at http://www.who.int/mediacentre/factsheets/fs363/en/
6. World Health Organization: Born too soon: the global action report on preterm birth. Geneva (2012)
7. Goldberger, A.L., et al.: PhysioBank, PhysioToolkit, and PhysioNet: components of a new research resource for complex physiologic signals. Circulation **101**, e215–e220 (2000)
8. Janjarasjitt, S.: Examination of single wavelet-based features of EHG signals for preterm birth classification. IAENG Int. J. Comput. Sci. **44**, 212–218 (2017)
9. Janjarasjitt, S.: Evaluation of performance on preterm birth classification using single wavelet-based features of EHG signals. In: Proceedings of the 2017 Biomedical Engineering International Conference, Hokkaido, Japan (2017). https://doi.org/10.1109/bmeicon.2017. 8229118
10. Phinyomark, A., Phukpattaranont, P., Limsakul, C.: Feature reduction and selection for EMG signal classification. Expert Syst. Appl. **39**, 7420–7431 (2012)
11. Chandrashekar, G., Sahin, F.: A survey on feature selection methods. Comput. Electr. Eng. **40**(1), 16–28 (2014)

A Study of Speech Phase in Dysarthria Voice Conversion System

Ko-Chiang Chen, Ji-Yan Han, Sin-Hua Jhang, and Ying-Hui Lai[✉]

Department of Biomedical Engineering, National Yang-Ming University,
Taipei, Taiwan
yh.lai@gm.ym.edu.tw

Abstract. Dysarthria is a communication disorder common in people with damaged neuro-muscular apparatus resulting from events such as stroke. For a dysarthric speaker, voice conversion (VC) is one of the well-known approaches to improve speech intelligibility for a dysarthric speaker. Most of the well-known VC methods focus on converting amplitude features without phase information. Previous studies indicated that phase is an important factor in the speech signal. Therefore, we are interested in adding the correct phase information to VC for dysarthria speech. The results of automatic speech recognition and spectrum analysis show that intelligibility is improved by replacing the dysarthria phase with the normal phase during the synthesis step. It implies that the correct phase information must be considered for the dysarthria VC system.

Keywords: Voice conversion · Speech phase · Dysarthria

1 Introduction

Approximately 40 million Americans have communication disorders, costing the U.S. approximately \$154–186 billion annually [1]. Among them, dysarthria is a speech disorder caused by muscle weakness resulting from a brain injury, and it is present in many neurologic developments such as stroke, traumatic brain injury, and Parkinson's disease. People who communicate with a dysarthric speaker may have difficulties in understanding their speech. Therefore, voice conversion (VC) technology, an approach to convert dysarthria speech into normal speech, could be one of the potential approaches to improve the intelligibility and quality of speech for dysarthric speakers [2].

The purpose of VC is to convert a source speaker's speech into the target speaker's one based on a nonlinear model. More specifically, it extracts acoustic features (e.g., fundamental frequency, band aperiodic components, Mel-cepstral coefficients) from the source speech. Then, these features are mapped toward the target speech features by a conversion model. Many VC methods have been proposed in the past few decades. One of the popular VC models is based on a Gaussian mixture model (GMM) [3, 4], and comes from a clustering algorithm. Another well-known VC model is the non-negative matrix factorization (NMF) [5, 6], which focuses on spectral conversion using a dictionary matrix. More recently, a joint dictionary learning-based NMF (JD_NMF) VC algorithm was proposed in [7], which has shown higher performance than the conventional NMF-based VC method for oral surgery patients.

K.-P. Lin et al. (Eds.): ICBHI 2019, IFMBE Proceedings 74, pp. 219–226, 2020.
https://doi.org/10.1007/978-3-030-30636-6_31

In addition, a neural network (NN)-based model is used for VC in cases such as [8–11]. The aforementioned models have been used for a normal speaker VC task, their focus being on converting acoustic features; however, there still is room for improvement for dysarthric speakers. Meanwhile, issues still exist with the phase information of the converted speech, which need studying.

There are many uncertainties in the contribution of speech intelligibility in the phase information. For example, Ohm [12] observed that the human auditory system is "phase-deaf," which means that humans only use the amplitude spectrum for speech perception but ignore the phase spectrum; furthermore, Helmholtz [13] confirmed the observation of Ohm by simulating the same magnitude spectrum but synthesized with different phase spectra. The results indicated that the auditory differences between these simulations were not heard. Nevertheless, recent studies indicate that phase plays an important role in intelligibility [14]. In the application of speech synthesis, phase spectra have been shown to have a considerable impact on the quality and naturalness of the synthesized speech [15]. In other words, a suitable approach for phase-converting could benefit the VC task regarding dysarthria. The purpose of this study is to investigate whether the phase information is helpful in improving the intelligibility of dysarthria VC. Moreover, three standard NN-based models are used in this study.

2   The Typical Voice Conversion System

The typical VC system included training and conversion stages; the architecture is displayed in Fig. 1. Detailed descriptions are presented in the following sections.

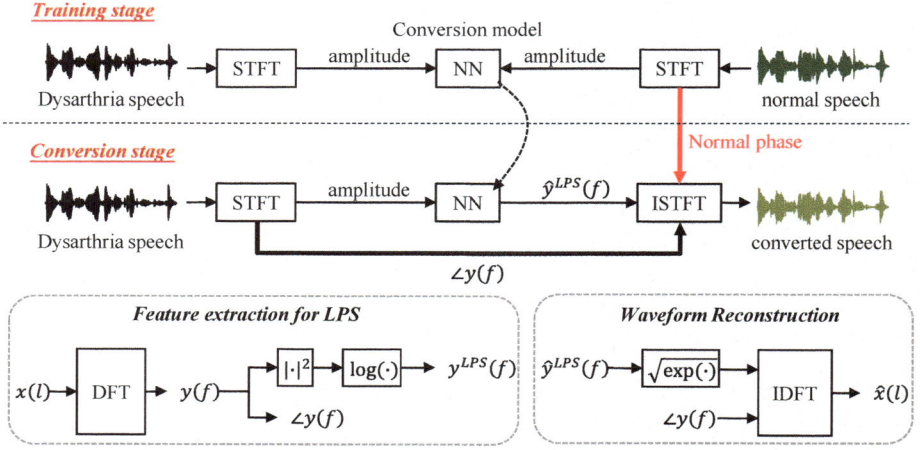

Fig. 1. Structure of dysarthria voice conversion with STFT.

2.1 Training Stage

First, the parallel utterances between the source and the target were prepared based on aligned technology (e.g., dynamic time warping, DTW [16]). log-power spectrum (LPS) were then extracted from the utterances according to the following equation. We apply a discrete Fourier transform (DFT) to achieve a short-time Fourier transform (STFT) analysis of the input signal of each overlapping windowed frame. More specifically, when a frame, with length (L), of speech (x) is obtained. The following equation be used to transfer speech signal from time domain to frequency domain

$$y(f) = \sum_{l=0}^{L-1} x(l)h(l)e^{-j2\pi f l/L}, \, l = 0, 1, \cdots, L-1 \tag{1}$$

where f is the frequency index, l is the time domain sample index, and $h(l)$ denotes the Hamming window function. Then log-power spectra are calculated by

$$y^{LPS}(f) = log|y(f)|^2, f = 0, 1, \cdots, F-1 \tag{2}$$

$$\angle y(f) = tan^{-1}\left(\frac{\Im(y(f))}{\Re(y(f))}\right), f = 0, 1, \cdots, F-1 \tag{3}$$

where $F = L/2 + 1$, because the negative part of the frequency index is ignored. $\Im(y(f))$ and $\Re(y(f))$ are the imaginary and the real part of $y(f)$, respectively. Relations among $x(l), y(f), y^{LPS}(f)$, and phase information $\angle y(f)$ are shown in the feature extraction module in Fig. 1.

In training stage, the conversion model was trained with these features (i.e., LPS), which were extracted by aligned utterances. In addition, three common NN-based architectures, namely deep neural network (DNN) [9], convolution neural network (CNN) [17], and bidirectional gated recurrent unit (GRU) [10, 11], were used as conversion models in this study. For detailed information on the training method and network settings, refer to [9–11, 17] and Table 1.

2.2 Conversion Stage

In the conversion stages, a well-trained model was used to directly convert the source speech into target speech. A detailed description can be found in [18]. The converted LPS, $\hat{y}^{LPS}(f)$, was then obtained from each VC model. The reconstructed spectrum $\hat{y}(f)$ is given by

$$\hat{y}(f) = e^{\hat{y}^{LPS}(f)/2}e^{j\angle y(f)}, f = 0, 1, \cdots, F-1 \tag{4}$$

where the phase information $\angle y(f)$ is derived from the source speech. Then, a frame of the speech signal is reconstructed by computing the inverse DFT (IDFT) of the current frame of the spectrum as follows:

Table 1. Model setting

DNN
Input shape: (129)
Layer 1: 500 hidden units, shape (129, 500), by PReLU
Layer 2: 500 hidden units, shape (500, 500), by PReLU
Layer 3: 500 hidden units, shape (500, 500), by PReLU
Layer 4: 129 hidden units, shape (500, 129), by Linear

CNN
Input shape: (10, 129, 1) with ten time step
Layer 1: 16 filters, receptive field (3, 3), by (2, 2) strided, by PReLU
Layer 2: 32 filters, receptive field (3, 3), by (2, 2) strided, by PReLU
Layer 3: 64 filters, receptive field (3, 3), by (2, 2) strided, by PReLU
Layer 4: 128 filters, receptive field (3, 3), by (2, 2) strided, by PReLU
Layer 5: 256 filters, receptive field (3, 3), by (2, 2) strided, by PReLU
Layer 6: 129 filters, receptive field (1, 1), by (1, 1) strided, by PReLU
Layer 7: 129 hidden units, shape (387, 129), by Linear

GRU
Input shape: (10, 129, 1) *with 10-time step*
Layer 1: Bidirectional GRU, units: 200, activation: tanh, recurrent_activation: hard_sigmoid
Layer 2: Bidirectional GRU, units: 200, activation: tanh, recurrent_activation: hard_sigmoid
Layer 3: 200 hidden units, shape (400, 200), by Linear
Layer 4: 129 hidden units, shape (200, 129), by Linear

$$\hat{x}(l) = \frac{1}{L}\sum_{f=0}^{L-1}\hat{y}(f)e^{j2\pi fl/L}, f = 0, 1, \cdots, F - 1 \qquad (5)$$

The waveform for the whole utterance can then be synthesized through a traditional overlap-add procedure as described in [19]; meanwhile, a Hamming window similar to that in the speech analysis step is used for waveform synthesis.

3 Methods and Results

3.1 Materials and Evaluation Methods

In this study, 249 dysarthria-normal-paired utterances were collected, with corpus text adopted from the list of Taiwan Mandarin hearing in noise test [20]. The corpus was recorded with a 16 kHz sampling rate and 16-bit resolution. The dysarthric and clear utterances were spoken by a stroke patient and a normal speaker, respectively. In the experiment, 249 dysarthria-normal-paired utterances were used as the training set, and close-set testing was conducted with the same 249 utterances. The dysarthria-normal-paired utterances were aligned through dynamic time warping approach before feature extraction [21]. First we need to do the STFT with a frame size of 256 sample and frameshift of 16 in this study.

In the objective evaluation part, we conducted an intelligibility test on Google Auto Speech Recognition (ASR), which is a computer process for recognizing and translating spoken language into text. The test process used 249 sentences. The text generated from the ASR was compared with the corpus text to assess word accuracy.

For another objective evaluation, we used log-spectral distortion (LSD) to analyze the performance of conversion. The methods are as follows:

$$L = \frac{1}{N} \sum\nolimits_{m=1}^{N} \sqrt{\frac{1}{M} \sum\nolimits_{j=1}^{M} \left[log(d_j) - log(y_j) \right]^2} \qquad (6)$$

N is the total number of frames. M is the spectrum dimension. d_j and y_j denote j-th dimension of LPS for converted and target speech, respectively. We use dB as a unit. The lower the LSD value, the more similar the voice. The minimum is 0, which means the spectrum of the two speeches is the same.

3.2   Cross-Test of Dysarthric and Normal Phase

To confirm that replacing the dysarthria phase by a normal phase is helpful for intelligibility, we performed cross-tests and exchanged amplitude and phase for dysarthria speech and normal speech. A total of four permutations (i.e., dysarthric amplitude + dysarthric phase, dysarthric amplitude + normal phase, normal amplitude + dysarthric phase, normal amplitude + normal phase) were combined. We reconstructed the speech with amplitude and phase spectrum by inverse STFT (ISTFT); Fig. 2 displays the results for the ASR evaluation system. It is worth noting that a higher accuracy implies that the processed method provided better speech intelligibility performance. The results indicate that when the same dysarthric (or normal) amplitude is reconstructed with a normal phase, it can achieve better intelligibility performance

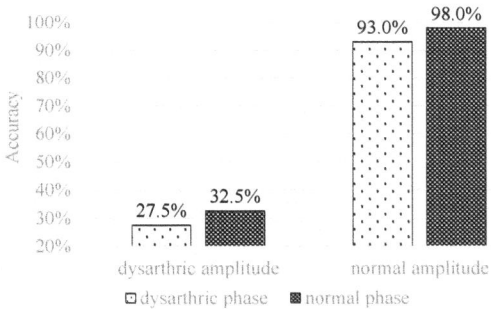

Fig. 2. The ASR accuracy of cross test on amplitude and phase of dysarthria speech and normal speech. The x-axis represents the type of amplitude spectrum and the y-axis represents the accuracy of ASR.

than using dysarthric phase. In addition, the normal speech amplitude is reconstructed with the dysarthric phase; hence, accuracy will be reduced. This implies that the dysarthric phase will affect intelligibility. On average, the correct phase information could increase by approximately 5% intelligibility of the ASR system.

3.3   Objective Tests of Three Simple NN Models

After confirming that the correct phase has an impact on the recognition rate of ASR, we test whether it is desirable in the actual VC operation. The features extracted from STFT contain two components: amplitude spectrum and phase spectrum. The amplitude spectrum is converted into a typical VC model. The dysarthric phase spectrum is delivered to the synthesis step without any processing, as indicated in Fig. 1. In this test, we replace the dysarthria phase spectrum in the synthesis step with a normal

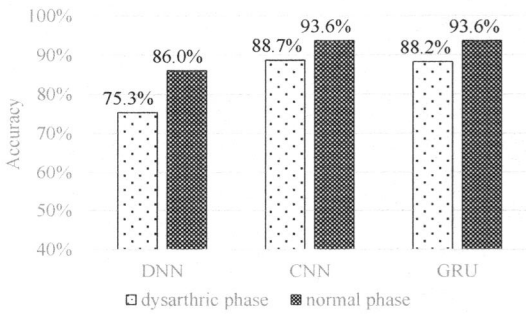

Fig. 3. The ASR accuracy of the test to change the phase of the speech converted through different simple models. The x-axis represents the type of model, and the y-axis represents the accuracy of the ASR.

speech phase spectrum, as indicated by the red arrow in Fig. 1, to observe the impact on performance.

The three types of NN models (DNN, CNN, and GRU) are used to test the influence of phase in dysarthria VC, as per Fig. 3. The results for ASR show that the speech synthesized through normal phase spectrum has a higher accuracy (4–6%) than that synthesized through dysarthria phase spectrum in each of these three models.

The LSD assessment is based on speech amplitude. The Fig. 4 show that although the same amplitude is used to synthesize speech, the amplitude of the converted speech is not consistent and is greatly affected by the phase. Noted, correct phase information achieves lower LSD score. It follows that the correct phase information could help the VC system to provide better conversion benefits (a lower LSD).

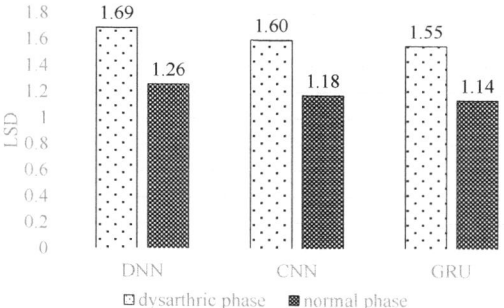

Fig. 4. Comparison of LSD between three simple models. The x-axis represents the type of model, and the y-axis represents the LSD.

4   Conclusions

The results showed that the phase information plays an important role in synthesizing dysarthria speech. The correct phase information in the dysarthria VC system could improve the intelligibility of the converted speech evaluated by an ASR system; meanwhile, a lower LSD can be obtained. Our results suggest that the correct phase will improve the intelligibility and the quality of the converted speech for listeners.

Acknowledgment. This work was supported by the Ministry of Science and Technology, Taiwan, under Grant MOST 107-2218-E-010-006.

Conflict of Interest. The authors declare that they have no conflict of interest.

References

1. Quick Facts About ASHA: American Speech-Language-Hearing Association (n.d.). https://www.asha.org/about/news/quick-facts/. Accessed 1 Feb 2019
2. Hosom, J.-P., Kain, A.B., Mishra, T., Van Santen, J.P., Fried-Oken, M., Staehely, J.: Intelligibility of modifications to dysarthric speech. In: Proceedings of Acoustics, Speech, and Signal Processing, p. I (2003)
3. Hwang, H.-T., Tsao, Y., Wang, H.-M., Wang, Y.-R., Chen, S.-H.: Alleviating the over-smoothing problem in GMM-based voice conversion with discriminative training. In: Proceedings of Interspeech, pp. 3062–3066 (2013)
4. Toda, T., Black, A.W., Tokuda, K.: Voice conversion based on maximum-likelihood estimation of spectral parameter trajectory. IEEE Trans. Audio Speech Lang. Process. **15**(8), 2222–2235 (2007)
5. Virtanen, T.: Monaural sound source separation by nonnegative matrix factorization with temporal continuity and sparseness criteria. IEEE Trans. Audio Speech Lang. Process. **15**(3), 1066–1074 (2007)
6. Zhang, Q., Tao, L., Zhou, J., Wang, H.: The voice conversion method based on sparse convolutive non-negative matrix factorization. In: Proceedings of International Conference on Electrical and Information Technologies for Rail Transportation, pp. 259–267 (2016)

7. Fu, S.-W., Li, P.-C., Lai, Y.-H., Yang, C.-C., Hsieh, L.-C., Tsao, Y.: Joint dictionary learning-based non-negative matrix factorization for voice conversion to improve speech intelligibility after oral surgery. IEEE Trans. Biomed. Eng. **64**(11), 2584–2594 (2017)

8. Narendranath, M., Murthy, H.A., Rajendran, S., Yegnanarayana, B.: Transformation of formants for voice conversion using artificial neural networks. Speech Commun. **16**(2), 207–216 (1995)

9. Chen, L.-H., Ling, Z.-H., Liu, L.-J., Dai, L.-R.: Voice conversion using deep neural networks with layer-wise generative training. IEEE/ACM Trans. Audio Speech Lang. Process. **22**(12), 1859–1872 (2014)

10. Zhou, C., Horgan, M., Kumar, V., Vasco, C., Darcy, D.: Voice conversion with conditional sampleRNN. arXiv preprint arXiv:1808.08311 (2018)

11. Chorowski, J., Weiss, R.J., Saurous, R.A., Bengio, S.: On using backpropagation for speech texture generation and voice conversion. In: Proceedings of Acoustics, Speech and Signal Processing, pp. 2256–2260 (2018)

12. Ohm, G.S.: Über die Definition des Tones, nebst daran geknüpfter Theorie der Sirene und ähnlicher tonbildender Vorrichtungen. Ann. Phys. **135**(8), 513–565 (1843)

13. Helmholtz, H.: On the sensations of tone. Courier Corporation (2013)

14. Kim, D.-S.: Perceptual phase redundancy in speech. In: Proceedings of Acoustics, Speech, and Signal Processing, pp. 1383–1386 (2000)

15. Pobloth, H., Kleijn, W.B.: On phase perception in speech. In: Proceedings of Acoustics, Speech, and Signal Processing, pp. 29–32 (1999)

16. Keogh, E., Ratanamahatana, C.A.: Exact indexing of dynamic time warping. Knowl. Inf. Syst. **7**(3), 358–386 (2005)

17. Salamon, J., Bello, J.P.: Deep convolutional neural networks and data augmentation for environmental sound classification. IEEE Signal Process. Lett. **24**(3), 279–283 (2017). https://doi.org/10.1109/LSP.2017.2657381

18. Mohammadi, S.H., Kain, A.: An overview of voice conversion systems. Speech Commun. **88**, 65–82 (2017)

19. Griffin, D.W.: Signal estimation from modified short-time Fourier transfrom. IEEE ASSP **32**, 2 (1984)

20. Wong, L.L., Soli, S.D., Liu, S., Han, N., Huang, M.-W.: Development of the Mandarin hearing in noise test (MHINT). Ear Hear. **28**(2), 70S–74S (2007)

21. Muda, L., Begam, M., Elamvazuthi, I.: Voice recognition algorithms using mel frequency cepstral coefficient (MFCC) and dynamic time warping (DTW) techniques. arXiv preprint arXiv:1003.4083 (2010)

Toward the Precision Medicine for a Psychiatric Disorder: Light Therapy for Major Depressive Disorder with Neuroimaging Validation

Fan-pei Gloria Yang[1]([✉]), Wei-cheng Chao[2], Sung-wei Chen[3,4], Ernie Du[5], Chi-chin Yang[2], Li-chi Su[2], and Mu-tao Chu[2]

[1] Center for Cognition and Mind Science, National Tsing Hua University, Hsinchu, Taiwan, R.O.C.
fpyang@cnrl.fl.nthu.edu.tw
[2] Electronic and Optoelectronic System Research Laboratory, Industrial Technology Research Institute, Hsinchu, Taiwan, R.O.C.
[3] Department of General Psychiatry, Taoyuan Psychiatric Center, Ministry of Health and Welfare, Taoyuan, Taiwan, R.O.C.
[4] Department of Medical Humanities, School of Medicine, College of Medicine, Taipei Medical University, Taipei, Taiwan, R.O.C.
[5] Keelung Chang Gung Memorial Hospital, Keelung, Taiwan, R.O.C.

Abstract. In recent therapeutic studies, light therapy has been used to treat seasonal depression disorder in countries where there is insufficient daylight during winter. Previous light therapy studies have used one treatment for all patients, irrespective of individual differences and drug control. Although light therapy has been extended to uses in a few psychiatric treatment programs for major depressive disorder (MDD), there is a lack of consistent research and conclusion regarding its effects of different combinations of lights and the neural mechanism underlying the improvement after therapy. The present study intends to propose several combinations of lights using the beneficial physical properties in prior research and validate the efficacy of the therapies with neurophysiological techniques.

Twelve patients suffering from major depressive disorder were enrolled in the study. Five were in the experimental group who will receive the two-month light therapy, with 1 female and 4 males, aged from 38 to 63 years old (mean = 49, SD = 8.51). Seven were in the control group, with 5 females and 2 males, aged from 32 to 53 years old (mean = 42.71, SD = 8.56). All participants were scanned when they were enrolled in the program, a month after pure drug treatment. The control group were scanned a month after their light therapy, and the last time after the light therapy were completed. Results revealed that the default mode network and the salience network were altered after the therapy. The self-report of life quality was better after the therapy. The conclusion is that light therapy could have a lasting effect on the brain by changing the neural connectivity, which led to the improvement in patients with MDD.

Keywords: Light therapy · Light equipment · Major Depressive Disorder (MDD) · Depression · fMRI · EEG

© Springer Nature Switzerland AG 2020
K.-P. Lin et al. (Eds.): ICBHI 2019, IFMBE Proceedings 74, pp. 227–234, 2020.
https://doi.org/10.1007/978-3-030-30636-6_32

1   Introduction

There are many researches on the visual effects of medical environment lighting, but there is a lack of therapeutic application as studies on its physiological, psychological and biological effects are relatively lacking as well. Light therapy has always been considered to treat sleep disorders and seasonal affective disorder (SAD), however, the causes of depression among local patients vary from each other, it cannot be resolved with light therapy by only considering the seasonal factors. This study is aimed to design customized light therapy sessions for patients diagnosed with major depressive disorder (MDD) according to their symptoms and mood, and the advantages of this development are as follows: (1) light therapy is non-invasive and is able to assist in current treatment of any unit, (2) long-term light therapy helps regulating brain's response, and it can be measured by using functional Magnetic Resonance Imaging (fMRI), (3) equipment needed for light therapy is user-friendly for medical staff to operate easily. Therefore, our study aims to create suitable light therapy sessions for patients according to their psychological symptoms, measured using fMRI and psychological tests.

Past studies on light therapy and its effect on managing depression are mostly based on self-report inventory such as Beck Depression Inventory (BDI) and sleep records are stated as dependent variables after the treatment. Such sept-reported dependent variables often fail to record the emotional changes during the light therapy session, thus the results of light therapy may be affected by other confounding variables. In consideration of such distortion, we combine fMRI with EEG techniques used by Industrial Technology Research Institute (ITRI), to study biomedical brain signals and to plan appropriate treatments according to the outcomes.

There are many different research results in past studies on correlation between light therapy and emotion, that is about which kind of light source is effective on boosting positive emotions of the patients. Some studies believe that, although red light is not as effective as blue light on adjusting body clock, it has the effect of boosting positive emotions and anti-depression. Therefore, unlike past studies which focused only on blue light's effect on treating depression, we work with hospitals to develop a variety of light sources to create customized light therapy sessions for patients.

There are currently no products similar to this therapeutic lighting on the market, as the system becomes massively produced, it can be used not only to prevent depression and relieve emotions, it is also expected to be applied on lighting systems in hospital ward, to improve the recovery effect by soothing the patient's mood and sleep quality, which as well reduces the burden of medical staff and family members of the patients.

2   Method

2.1   Participants

Twelve patients suffering from major depression order were recruited at the psychiatric clinics at National Taiwan University Hospital Hsinchu Branch. Five were in the experimental group, with 1 female and 4 males, aged from 38 to 63 years old (mean = 49, SD = 8.51). Seven were in the control group, with 5 females and 2 males, aged from 32 to 53 years old (mean = 42.71, SD = 8.56). The experimental group received light therapy for two months while taking prescribed drugs whereas the control group only took the prescribed drugs.

2.2   Experimental Procedure

When the participants were enrolled, they were scanned to establish the baseline of the resting state of the brain. They were scanned a month later to find out the change after taking the prescribed drug for a month. At this time, the experimental group were tested with different light therapy options, including blue (λmax 470, 460–480 nm, 4 lx, 40 μW/cm^2), green (λmax 530 nm, 520–540 nm, 4 lx, 40 μW/cm^2), amber (λmax 591 nm, 580–600 nm, 10 lx, 40 μW/cm^2) and red (λmax 627 nm, 620–640 nm, 10 lx, 40 μW/cm^2) with EEG recordings. By means of their brain wave response, we selected the optimal light therapy option for each patient. We had four types of therapy options (Fig. 1):

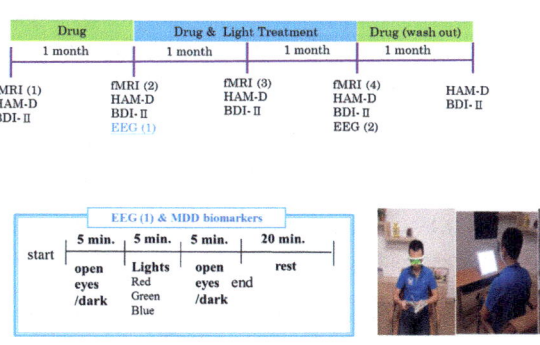

Fig. 1. Experimental procedure

The EEG recordings were conducted using BR32S. it provides the function to derive the high-quality EEG data for BCI applications. BR32S transmits the real-time EEG data via Bluetooth and outputs the raw data with easy-to-apply formats like txt/edf/cnt.

The resting state connectivity of the participants were analyzed with the CONN TOOLBOX, which was developed by the NITRC. CONN is an open-source Matlab/SPM-based cross-platform software for the computation, display, and analysis of functional connectivity Magnetic Resonance Imaging (fcMRI). CONN is used to analyze resting state data (rsfMRI) as well as task-related designs. Using this tool, images were preprocessed, such as registration, segmentation and smoothing, with motion correction control. Various connectivity calculations were performed, including Seed-Based Correlations (SBC), ROI-to-ROI analyses.

3   Results and Discussion

We selected two neural network systems, Salience Network (SN) and Default-mode Network (DMN), and performed the Second-Level analysis of all patients using Matlab's Toolbox-CONN.

Salience Network (SN) is involved in detecting and filtering salient stimuli, as well as in recruiting relevant functional networks. The network also contributes to a variety of complex functions, including communication, social behavior, and self-awareness through the integration of sensory, emotional, and cognitive information. While Default-mode Network (DMN) is most commonly active when a person is not focused on the outside world and the brain is at wakeful rest, such as during daydreaming and mind-wandering. Both neural networks are representative of the brain's functions in rest, cognition and emotion, and are also the origin of the change in depression.

We conducted connectivity analysis for the following brain areas, the brain areas of the pictures below are important brain areas of SN and DMN, they are all located in the prefrontal lobe, and regardless of which part of the brain is selected, the signification correlation results presented are related to the Cingulate Gyrus.

The 4th fMRI radiography (a month after the end of light therapy) was compared with the first fMRI radiography (before light treatment was started), and the results were the most significant. Brain areas that exhibit significant responses include Anterior Cingulate Cortex (ACC), Insula (L) 和 Rostral Prefrontal Cortex (RPFC), which are all involved in regulating emotions and cognition.

Anterior Cingulate Cortex, ACC, appears to play a role in a wide variety of autonomic functions, such as regulating blood pressure and heart rate. It is also involved in certain higher-level functions, such as attention allocation, reward anticipation, decision-making, ethics and morality, impulse control and emotion (Fig. 2).

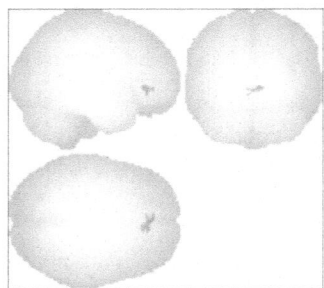

Fig. 2. Anterior Cingulate Cortex

Insula, involved in consciousness and play a role in diverse functions usually linked to emotion or the regulation of the body's homeostasis. These functions include compassion and empathy, perception, motor control, self-awareness, cognitive functioning, and interpersonal experience (Fig. 3).

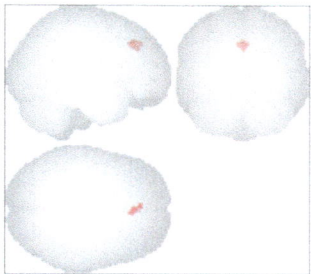

Fig. 3. Insula (L)

Rostral Prefrontal Cortex is in charge of higher-level cognition behavior, decision making and social behavior (Figs. 4 and 5).

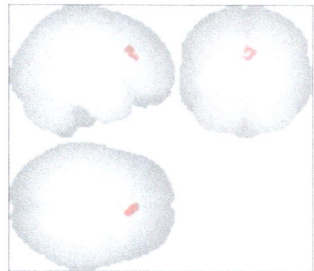

Fig. 4. Rostral Prefrontal Cortex (L)

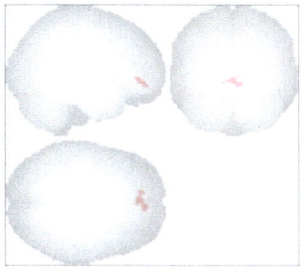

Fig. 5. Rostral Prefrontal Cortex (R)

By comparing the third fMRI radiography with the first fMRI radiography, it is shown that Frontal Pole area presented an obvious response. Frontal Pole, which belongs to Brodmann's Area 10, is one of the areas where cognitive functions are performed, and it is responsible for handling information such as perception, emotion, and memory (Fig. 6).

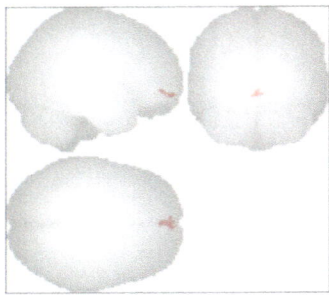

Fig. 6. Frontal Pole

In DMN, the third fMRI radiography was compared with the first fMRI radiography, and the result shows that a strong response is found in cerebellum. Cerebellum plays an important role in motor control, and is also involved in cognitive functions such as attention and language as well as in regulating fear and pleasure responses (Fig. 7).

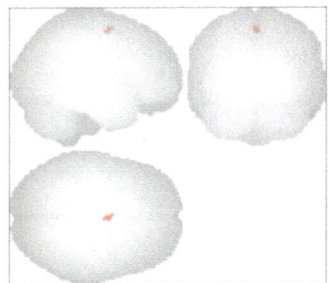

Fig. 7. Cerebellum

Also in DMN, the second fMRI radiography was compared to that of the first fMRI, and significant response occurred in Lateral Parietal Lobe (LPL). LPL plays important roles in integrating sensory information from various parts of the body, knowledge of numbers and their relations, and in the manipulation of objects. Its function also includes processing information relating to the sense of touch, and is also related to language, memory, attention and other functions (Fig. 8).

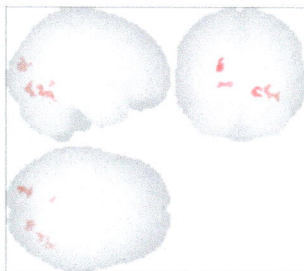

Fig. 8. Lateral Parietal Lobe

As a combination of the above results, significant responses are found in brain areas related to memory before and after the treatment. We believe that this study may bring a new direction and opportunity to the treatment of depression. Therefore, the highlight of this study is also the biggest breakthrough in the application of LED mental illness. By establishing the changing subtypes of various light therapy sessions, it is possible to design a fine-tuning scheme based on the characteristics and mood of MDD patients under the framework of light therapy treatment for depression, to achieve customization, as well as maintaining the consistency in scientific research. This development could be an option for the hospitals in the future, and with the long-term treatment and clinical observation, physicians will determine whether the light therapy can be considered as an independent treatment for specific subgroup among MDD patients.

4   Conclusion

As a radiographic study, it is shown that the main phenomenon of depression is that the activity of the prefrontal lobe of MDD patients is significantly lower than that of healthy human, which means their memory and motor functions are affected as well. The result in this study shows that light therapy helps triggering the cingulate gyrus which is related to memory function, and the motor function related areas are becoming more active as well. This phenomenon is surprising and we hope that it can be discussed in future academic or in clinical uses.

It is a shame that the number of participants who completed the whole experiment has yet to reach our expectation, we hope to invite more participants to take part in our study in the future to increase the persuasiveness and visibility of the data.

Acknowledgment. The authors thank Jeff Liu, Jesse Lee and Fangyu Kuo for assistance in data collection.

Conflict of Interest. The authors declare that they have no conflict of interest.

References

1. Crowther, A., Smoski, M.J., Minkel, J., Moore, T., Gibbs, D., Petty, C., Bizzell, J., Schiller, C.E., Sideris, J., Carl, H., Dichter, G.S.: Resting-state connectivity predictors of response to psychotherapy in major depressive disorder. Neuropsychopharmacology **40**(7), 1659 (2015)
2. Kaiser, R.H., Andrews-Hanna, J.R., Wager, T.D., Pizzagalli, D.A.: Large-scale network dysfunction in major depressive disorder: a meta-analysis of resting-state functional connectivity. JAMA Psychiatry **72**(6), 603–611 (2015)
3. Mulders, P.C., van Eijndhoven, P.F., Schene, A.H., Beckmann, C.F., Tendolkar, I.: Resting-state functional connectivity in major depressive disorder: a review. Neurosci. Biobehav. Rev. **56**, 330–344 (2015)
4. Liu, J., Ren, L., Womer, F.Y., Wang, J., Fan, G., Jiang, W., Wang, F.: Alterations in amplitude of low frequency fluctuation in treatment-naïve major depressive disorder measured with resting-state fMRI. Hum. Brain Mapp. **35**(10), 4979–4988 (2014)

Integrated RFID Aperture and Washing Chamber Shielding Design for Real-Time Cleaning Performance Monitoring in Healthcare Laundry System

Kampol Woradit[1]([✉]), Setta Sassananan[2], Sasithorn Boonjun[3],
and Amaraporn Boonpratatong[4]

[1] Department of Electrical Engineering, Faculty of Engineering,
Srinakharinwirot University, Ongkharak, Thailand
k.woradit@gmail.com
[2] Department of Civil and Environmental Engineering, Faculty of Engineering,
Srinakharinwirot University, Ongkharak, Thailand
[3] Department of Occupational Health and Environment,
HRH Princess Mahachakrisirindorn Medical Center,
Srinakharinwirot University, Ongkharak, Thailand
[4] Department of Biomedical Engineering, Faculty of Engineering,
Srinakharinwirot University, Ongkharak, Nakonnayok, Thailand

Abstract. A preliminary design of integrated RFID aperture and washing chamber shield for real-time cleaning monitoring in healthcare laundry system is proposed. The installation of RF based monitoring system includes sewing attachment of the RFID tags to the healthcare clothes and the setting up of RFID shield, aperture, and reader to the washing tub, and open area of the washing machine. During the wash, the clothes circulation was tracked by filtered RF transmission between the tags and reader. Software was designed to evaluate the circulation e.g. rotating, sinking, and floating of the various clothes in the batch and update the circulation level in real-time. Two types of conventional healthcare washing machines i.e. agitator and pulse flow were selected for the experiments. The Received Signal Strength Indicator (RSSI) was evaluated on each combination of RFID design, washing condition and clothes circulation level. The cleaning performance of each combination of washing condition and circulation was evaluated by using Microbiological (RODAC plate count) testing. Design of experiments (DOE) methodology of 2^5 was used to examine the relationship between washing circulation and cleaning performance on representative healthcare laundry machines. 5 trials were repeated at each experimental condition before the repeatability of RSSI was examined. The design providing best repetitive RSSI is presented.

Keywords: RFID aperture · Cleaning performance · Healthcare laundry · RFID tracking · Clothes circulation tracking

© Springer Nature Switzerland AG 2020
K.-P. Lin et al. (Eds.): ICBHI 2019, IFMBE Proceedings 74, pp. 235–242, 2020.
https://doi.org/10.1007/978-3-030-30636-6_33

1 Introduction

Most nursing homes, clinics, and hospitals are concerned with improving laundry infection control when the economic and reliable production is also the utmost importance. Washing a variety of items including clothes, sheets, towels, and bed pad thoroughly and consistently in one batch using properly programmed machine is one of the commonly accepted schemes [1]. Despite the popularity of the mixed wash, the investigation on its infection control quality versus the economy and speed of production has yet to be found [2].

RFID based healthcare clothing management has been widely employed by using washable RFID tags attached to the clothes and readers placement in related departments. The healthcare organization and laundry service providers perceived shared benefits in reducing staff's work load and loss of clothing assets, yet were seeking more encouragement in exchange for time and financial investment in adoption [3]. A more benefit has then been added by clothes type identification to pre-determine economic washing programs e.g. least consumption washing cycle with optimum detergent [4].

Environmental infection control is primary requirement in healthcare laundry standards [1, 2, 5]. As drying temperatures and times are dictated by materials in the fabrics, hot-air drying process may then be used to provide microbiocidal action in addition to microbial decontamination performed by the washing process. Washing process has then become the key control of environmental infection in healthcare laundry system. Microbial decontamination by using hot-water has substantial operating costs [2, 5]. Cold water (22–25 °C) wash can increase microbial decontamination with relatively low operating cost given that the clothes circulation and the type and amount of wash detergent and additive are carefully controlled [1, 5]. Given the above limitation and advantage, a simple way to improve infection control and maintain economy and reliability of the healthcare laundry production is the balance control of clothes circulation, detergent and additive. In addition to fabric identification for washing program pre-determination, the washable property of RFID tags and under-water ability of RF transmission [4, 6] can also be utilized in real-time monitoring of the clothes washing circulation which is a major key in developing real-time infection and economy washing control.

Therefore, in this research, the integrated RFID aperture, RFID washing chamber shield and evaluation software for real-time clothes circulation tracking in healthcare washing machines was developed. Two representatives of conventional washing machines i.e. agitator and pulse flow type were tested with different designs of RFID washing circulation tracking. Design of the experiments (DOE) methodology of 2^5 multiplied by 5 trials was used to examine the repeatability of Received Signal Strength Indicator (RSSI) on each RFID design and cleaning performance on the number of clothes circulation. Microbiological (RODAC plate count) testing was conducted on the washed and spin-dried sample clothes, so that the relationship between clothes circulation and cleaning performance on the representative healthcare laundry washing machines was established. The design providing best and most repetitive RSSI is proposed. Based on clothes circulation-cleaning performance relationship, the real-time cleaning performance can then be estimated on the number of clothes circulation.

This system is proposed for real-time clothes circulation control to improve environmental infection and economic control of healthcare laundry production.

2   Materials and Method

2.1   RFID Washing Circulation Tracking Designs

See Fig. 1.

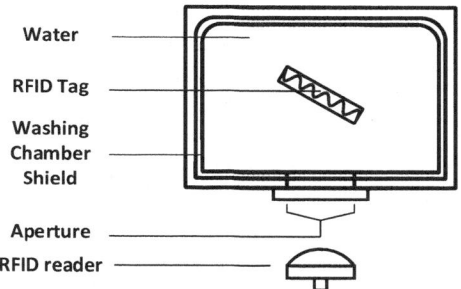

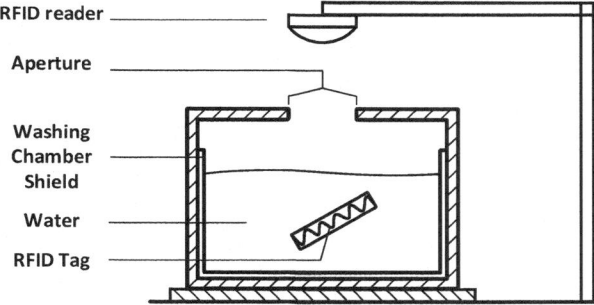

Fig. 1. Top layout of integrated RFID aperture and washing chamber shielding design in horizontal agitator (top) and side layout of pulse flow (bottom) washing machines in healthcare laundry system

2.2   Cleaning Performance Calculation

When samples of the same batch were washed in the tested washing condition and machine for a tested number of clothes circulation, the soiled area on the samples were then cut off and then collected to perform replicate organism detection and counting microbiological (RODAC plate count) test i.e. total aerobic microbial count (TAMC) to determine the hygienically cleaning performance. The calculation of RODAC based cleaning performance (c_R) for each tested washing condition and circulation can be expressed as

$$c_R = \frac{Y_t - Y_i}{Y_q - Y_i} = \frac{Y'_t}{Y'_q} \qquad (1)$$

When Y_t is the total aerobic microbial count (TAMC) after the tested no. of clothes circulation, Y_i is the total aerobic microbial count (TAMC) before washing process, Y_q is TRSA [5] acceptance criterion for microbiological quality for producing hygienically clean reusable textile (20 cfu/dm^2), Y'_t is the reduction of microbial quality due to tested washing circulation and Y'_q is the required quality of microbiological reduction according to TRSA standards.

2.3   Experimental Methods

The clothes circulation monitoring was performed in two representative healthcare washing machines: horizontal agitator type with averaged spin speed of 1500 rpm and pulse flow type with averaged water pressure of 0.5 mpa. Each machine was equipped with two different integrated designs of RFID aperture, washing chamber shield and reader placement. To examine the relationship between clothes circulation and cleaning performance on different types of washing condition and integrated designs of RFID tracking, the design of experiment (DOE) of 2^5 multiplied by 5 trials was implemented. The horizontal agitator and pulse flow type was programmed to work for the duration of 45 and 30 min, respectively with given washing condition as shown in Table 2. The sample washed clothes in horizontal agitator and pulse flow type were randomly taken out of the batch at each 75 and 50 s, respectively. Before and after each cleaning performance sampling, the margin of power used to detect the tags representing the Received Signal Strength Indicator (RSSI), was recorded. All washed clothes were then spin-dried before proceeded to replicate organism detection and counting microbiological (RODAC plate count) testing [5].

Table 1. Integrated RFID aperture and washing chamber shielding designs

Specification	Type A	Type B
Aperture size (cm) and shape	21.2, Square	15, Circle
Shielding proportion	Full	Half (porous)
Reader distance (cm)	15	10

Table 2. Washing experimental designs

Washing condition	Horizontal agitator	Pulse flow
Clothes weight (kg)	25	25
Soil type	Blood stains	
Detergent	Chlorine, Ozone	
Washing speed (rpm)	1500	–
Averaged water pressure (mpa)	–	0.5
Duration (min)	45	30
Water temperature (°C)	60,35	

3 Results

The change of margin power representing the change of received signal strength indicator (RSSI) at each sampling time during washing course is shown in Fig. 1. By using type-A design of integrated RFID system (See Table 2), the changes of margin power needed to identify the clothes tags during the washing course in agitator and pulse-flow washing machines under ozone washing condition were consistent. The summation of margin power change representing the total circulation of the clothes at each sampling time during the washing course is shown in Fig. 2. The proportional increase of the summation with the increase of washing time indicates the direct relationship between the total circulation of the clothes and the time in both types of healthcare washing machine.

The repeatability of the changes of margin power needed to indentify the clothes tags during 5-repetitive washing courses under 16 different washing conditions by using A- and B- types of integrated RFID designs is shown in Fig. 3. The comparison between the correlation coefficient representing the repeatability of RFID signal

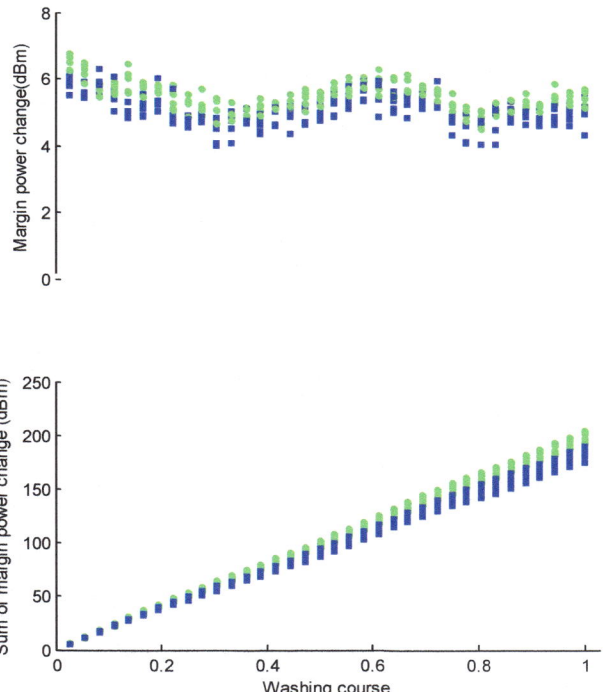

Fig. 2. The change of received signal strength indicator (RSSI) represented by margin power needed to identify clothes tags at each sampling time during the washing course in agitator (round marker) and pulse-flow (squared marker) healthcare washing machines under the condition of mixed healthcare clothes in ozone washing.

strength received by A- and B- types of integrated RFID designs (Table 1) shows that the tags circulation identified by using A-type design is more reliable in all of given washing conditions including machine type, detergent, water temperature and clothes variety (Table 2) in the batch.

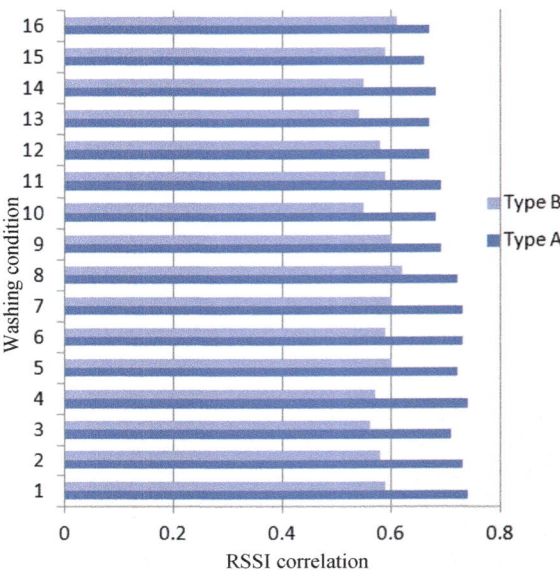

Fig. 3. The correlation coefficient of the RSSI (change of margin power needed to indentify the clothes tags) during the five repetitive washing courses under 16 washing conditions monitored by using A- and B- types of integrated RFID designs

The relationship between cleaning performance and clothes circulation level under the representative washing condition in two representative washing machines is shown in Fig. 4. The increases of cleaning performance with the increases of clothes circulation level were found in both representative washing machines. The relatively high cleaning performance of the pulse flow washing machine in the beginning of the clothes circulation course possibly represented the performance of the pulse flow water pressure in the initiation of microbial decontamination. Despite the differences in washing duration and technique, the consistent relationships between cleaning performance and clothes circulation level in horizontal agitation and pulse flow washings were found. The decreased rate of change of cleaning performance after the middle of the circulation course indicates the requirement of clothes circulation monitoring to optimize the washing course for the best cleaning performance.

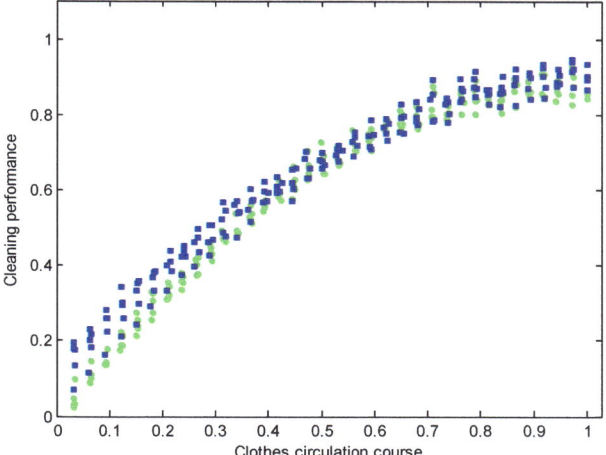

Fig. 4. The cleaning performance during the course of circulation of the mixed healthcare clothes in agitator (round marker) and pulse-flow (squared marker) washing machines under ozone washing condition identified by A-type RFID integrated design.

4   Discussions

In this research, the real-time cleaning performance monitoring in healthcare laundry system was performed by using integrated designs of RFID aperture and washing chamber shielding. The repeatability of signal strength received by the designed system indicates the reliability of clothes circulation monitoring in the various washing condition and machine. The proposed calculation of cleaning performance for healthcare laundry system provided the measures of healthcare clothes cleanliness after a specified level of clothes circulation under a given washing condition following TRSA [5] acceptance criterion for microbiological quality for producing hygienically clean reusable textile. The non-linear relationship between the cleaning performance and clothes circulation level in both of agitation and pulse flow washing machines indicates that the clothes circulation monitoring is crucial in microbial decontamination as the longer washing course does not necessarily produce the greater effect on microbial decontamination. Unlike the evaluation method of cleaning performance for household washing machines [7] considering stain removal perception as a basis, the evaluation and monitoring method of cleaning performance for healthcare laundry machines are on hygienical bases in which the microbial decontamination is the major priority followed by the microbiocidal action in drying process. The clothes circulation level will, therefore, assist in washing course determination not only for the purpose in maximizing the microbial decontamination but also minimizing the washing and drying durations or the energy costs.

Conflict of Interest. The authors declare that they have no conflict of interest.

References

1. Centre for Disease Control and Prevention: Guidelines for environmental infection control in healthcare facilities. US Department of Health & Human Service (2003)
2. Bain, J., Beton, B., Schultze, A., et al.: Reducing the environmental impact of clothes cleaning. Department for Environment, Food and Rural Affairs, London (2009)
3. Fisher, A.J., Monahan, T.: Evaluation of real-time location systems in their hospital contexts. Int. J. Med. Inform. **81**, 705–712 (2012)
4. Lock, I., Jerov, M., Scovith, S.: RFID in e-health systems: applications, challenges, and perspectives. Ann. Telecommun. **65**(9), 497–500 (2003)
5. Hygienically clean certifications: Standard for producing Hygienically clean reusable textiles for use in healthcare industry, TRSA, Australia (2018)
6. Finkenzeller, K.: RFID Handbook: Radio Frequency Identification Fundamentals and Applications. Wiley, Hoboken (2000)
7. Stamminger, R., Lambert, E., Hilgers, T.: New evaluation method of cleaning performance for washing machines. Tenside Surf. Det. **53**(5), 445–456 (2016)

Manual Wheelchair Propulsion and Joint Power Transmission Efficiency for Diagnosis of Upper-Limb Overuse

Supanat Sakunwitunthai[1(✉)], Worapol Aramrussameekul[2],
and Amaraporn Boonpratatong[1]

[1] Department of Biomedical Engineering, Faculty of Engineering,
Srinakharinwirot University, Onkharak, Nakhonnayok, Thailand
supanat4400@gmail.com
[2] Department of Rehabilitation Medicine, HRH Princess Mahachakri-sirindorn
Medical Center, Faculty of Medicine, Srinakharinwirot University,
Onkharak, Thailand

Abstract. This research paper proposed the measurement and calculation of upper-limb joint power transmission efficiency derived from propulsion efficiency and upper limb joint power efficiency during manual wheelchair propulsion. Portable measurement system was used to collect propulsion force at the push rim and inertia of each upper-limb segment (dominant limb). The relationship between upper-limb joint power transmission efficiency and the overuse of upper limbs was established on the manual wheelchair propulsion experiments in experienced, inexperienced and joint problem recovery users riding on level and slope paths. The data collected by using portable instruments were validated by that collected by using motion analysis system. The diagnosis of upper-limb overuse signifies the highest risks in inexperienced wheelchair riding group.

Keywords: Upper-limb joint power efficiency ·
Manual wheelchair propulsion efficiency ·
Upper-limb joint power transmission efficiency

1 Introduction

A number of studies have been carried out to reveal mechanics behind the mobility, power and efficiency of manual wheelchair (MW) riding [1–3]. Depending on the purpose of intervention, different instruments and methods have been presented or even specifically developed [6] to provide the measurement and analysis that help to improve the wheelchair user's ability to get around in his/her environment.

It is accepted that excessive and repetitive load during wheelchair propulsion is one of the leading causes of upper-limb pain and injuries [6]. However, there has not yet been any measurement and/or methods commonly accepted in the quantification and diagnosis of the wheelchair overuse [3]. By using wheel equipped instrument e.g. SMART wheel [3], the kinematics of push rim propulsion was measured, analyzed and used as a guide in the selection of wheelchair design, propel method and etc. The integration between torque measures using wheelchair dynamometer and mathematical

© Springer Nature Switzerland AG 2020
K.-P. Lin et al. (Eds.): ICBHI 2019, IFMBE Proceedings 74, pp. 243–251, 2020.
https://doi.org/10.1007/978-3-030-30636-6_34

problem solving using inverse dynamics [6] has been utilized to study in environmental factors that affect on upper-limb joint kinematics during manual wheelchair propulsion.

In addition to propulsion dynamics, the dynamics of upper-limb joints has been measured by using wheel equipped instruments and motion analysis system [7]. The upper-limb joint dynamic contributing to mechanical efficiency of manual wheelchair propulsion was analyzed and the quantities indicating injury risk was suggested. There is also a simple and inexpensive method that evaluated wheelchair mobility by using stopwatch and practitioner's observation [10] to measure cycle time and number and propulsion method.

However, in the above studies the analysis was restricted to physiologic and medical practitioners, although, some instruments can be used out of laboratory, the experimental or calculation results provided in time-series of mechanical quantities are not descriptive to general end users. A study of slope and friction effects on the manual wheelchair propulsion proposed a set of portable instruments and simple method for propulsion efficiency estimation [4]. The measurement and the interpretation were simple. No replacement was required on manual wheelchair and the analysis providing efficiency number between 0–1 is interpretative to end users [5]. However, it was found that the relationship between the propulsion efficiency and gravity resistance is not straightforward.

Not only easy-to-use instruments, but also a simple analysis involving all contributing factors of manual wheelchair over use is required. The existing analyses may be simplified and integrated, so that the excessive or the inefficient use of the upper-limbs during manual wheelchair propulsion can be diagnosed. Therefore, in this research, a method including the portable measurement [8, 9] and simple calculation of propulsion efficiency, joint power efficiency and joint power transmission efficiency for diagnosis of upper-limb overuse is proposed. Wearable units of contact pressure and inertia sensors and inverse dynamic calculation of manual wheelchair propulsion efficiency in Boonpratatong [5] were used. The calculation of upper-limb joint power efficiency was adopted from 3D angle analysis in Desroches [7]. The upper-limb joint power transmission efficiency as a ratio between propulsion efficiency and upper-limb joint power efficiency was calculated and analyzed. The relationship between upper-limb joint power transmission efficiency and the excessive and repetitive propulsion was established on the manual wheelchair propulsion experiments in experienced, inexperienced and joint problem recovery riding on level and slope ride ways. The data collected by using portable instruments were also validated by that collected by using motion analysis system.

2   Material and Method

2.1   The Derivation of Upper-Limb Joint Power Transmission

2.1.1   Propulsion Efficiency

Propulsion efficiency (η) proposed in Boonpratatong [5] was used. It is the ratio of tangential force (F_t) on the push rim and the resultant force due to wheelchair riding motion (F) as shown in Eqs. 1–2.

$$F = \sqrt{F_x^2 + Fy^2 + F_z^2} \tag{1}$$

$$\eta = \frac{F_t}{F} \tag{2}$$

when F_x, F_y, and F_z are the riding force components in forward, vertical and lateral direction, respectively.

2.1.2   Joint Power Efficiency

Modified from Desroches [7], joint power efficiency (μ) was determined by considering the angle (α) between the vector of joint moment (M) and joint angular velocity (ω) on local coordinate reference of volunteer's upper extremity joint during wheelchair propulsion. The joint power efficiency (μ) as shown in Eqs. 3-4 was derived based on the fact that, the smaller is the angle (α) between the vector of joint moment (M) and joint angular velocity (ω), the higher is the efficiency of joint power.

$$\alpha = \cos^{-1}\left(\frac{M \cdot \omega}{|M||\omega|}\right) \tag{3}$$

$$\mu = \frac{|\alpha - 180|}{180} \tag{4}$$

2.1.3   Power Transmission Efficiency

Representing the rate of conversion from upper-limb joint power to the forward propelling force applied on the wheelchair's push rim, the joint power transmission efficiency (φ) was, therefore, derived by the ratio of propulsion efficiency (η) and joint power efficiency (μ).

$$\varphi = \frac{\eta}{\mu} \tag{5}$$

2.2   Ramp

An adjustable ramp was used for the experiments of manual wheelchair riding on the slope of 1:8, 1:10 and 1:12 ratio of rise and run. There is a platform at the end of ride way which has dimension of 1.5×1.5 m (Fig. 1).

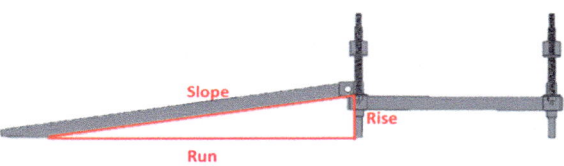

Fig. 1. Adjustable ramp and ratio of rise and run

2.3   Experimental Method

5 young healthy subjects and 5 manual wheelchair users were asked to propel manual wheelchair on the ramp of 3 different slope and 5-m level ride way with self-selected speeds.

2.3.1   Data Collection Using Inertia (IMU) and Contact Force Sensors

IMU were attached on volunteer's dominant upper limb and wheelchair's push rim while pressure measurement unit was placed on subject's dominant hand to allow the attachment of sensing unit on the thumb. All data were collected simultaneously at the 100 Hz sampling rate.

2.3.2   Data Collection Using Motion Analysis System

19 reflective markers were attached on the subject's upper extremity according to CAST markers set to include the anatomical landmarks: C7, T8, incisura jugularis (IJ), Left and right scapula-acromial edge (SAE), sternum, xiphoid process, superior part of upper arm, humerus-lateral epicondyle (HLE), ulnar and radial styloid processes, 2nd and 5th metacarpal head. One reflective marker was attached on wheelchair's center of rotation to interpret wheelchair's motion as shown in Fig. 2. Tangential force was collected from force plate at sampling rate of 100 Hz.

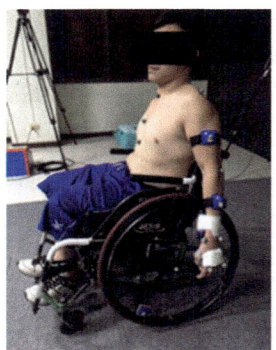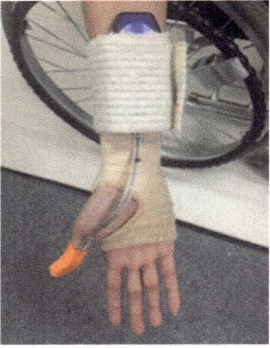

Fig. 2. Marker and sensor attachment on wheelchair and volunteers' upper limbs

2.3.3   Measurement Validation Using Inertia (IMU) and Contact Pressure Sensors and Motion Analysis System

The manual wheelchair propulsion measurement was validated by using motion analysis system see experimental method (b). The 3D angle between moment and angular velocity at the shoulder joint was measured by using portable and motion analysis system, simultaneously [11]. The correlation between two measures was calculated.

3   Result and Discussion

The repetitive and excessive propulsion was introduced, during wheelchair riding trials, by the increase of ride way slope and self-selected riding speeds. Figure 3(Top) shows the effects of normalized riding velocity on the power transmission efficiency in experienced and inexperienced wheelchair propulsion. The rapid decrease of power transmission efficiency with normalized riding velocity indicates the deficient power transmission due to relatively high frequency propulsion, especially in inexperienced riding. Figure 3(Bottom) shows the effects of slope (rise-to-run) ratio of ride way on power transmission efficiency. The power transmission efficiency was almost doubled as the combination of repetitiveness and gravitational resistance was introduced. However, it was less affected by the change in slope ratio or the gravitational resistance.

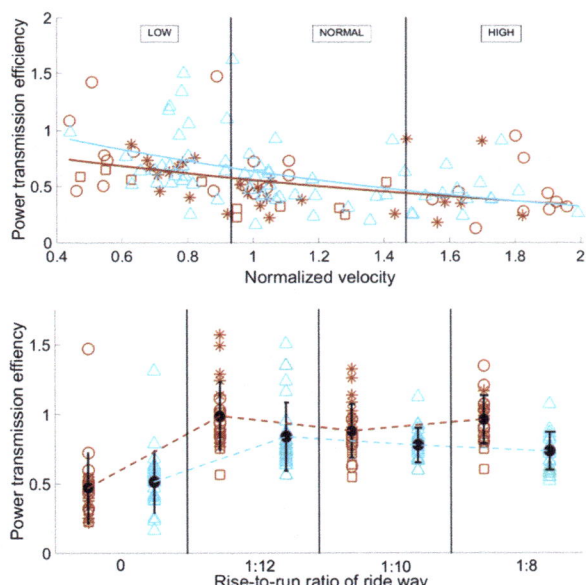

Fig. 3. Power transmission efficiency (φ) changes due to riding speeds (normalized velocity) and slope (rise-to-run) ratio of ride way in sporty experienced (o), healthy experienced (□) and post-wrist injury experienced (*) wheelchair riding compared to those in inexperienced (^) wheelchair riding

The change of propulsion efficiency and wrist joint power efficiency due to the change in slope (rise-to-run) ratio of ride way were used to analyze the effects of excessive propulsion on the power transmission efficiency. As shown in Fig. 4 the propulsion efficiency increased as the slope ratio increased from zero to 1/12 indicates the enhancement of propulsion effectiveness to overcome gravity. However, the wrist joint power efficiency maintenance as the slope ratio increased indicates the limit of motion-power transfer in both of experienced and inexperienced wheelchair propulsion with slightly higher wrist joint power efficiencies in inexperienced propulsion. It is interesting that under the limit of wrist joint power efficiency, the excessive propulsion induced by the increase of gravitational resistance contributed very slightly on the propulsion and power transmission efficiency in both of experienced and inexperienced wheelchair propulsion with higher power transmission efficiency in experienced propulsion.

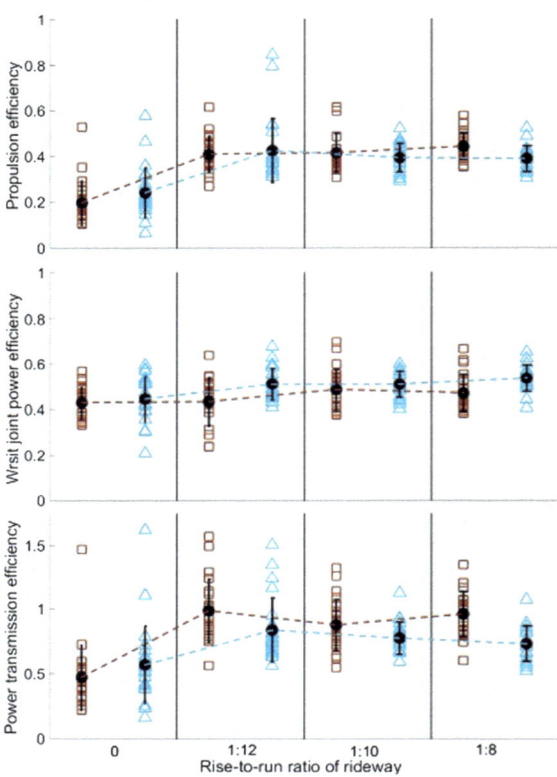

Fig. 4. Propulsion (η), wrist joint power (μ) and power transmission efficiency (φ) changes due to slope (rise-to-run) ratio of ride way in all types of experienced wheelchair riding ($\square$) compared to those in inexperienced wheelchair riding ($\wedge$)

In addition to the effects of wheelchair riding experience, the effects of post-joint injury on all types of efficiency were also investigated. The propulsion, wrist joint power and power transmission efficiencies of 2 in 5 of experienced wheelchair riding volunteers who had consecutive histories of joint injury i.e. CTS (Carpal tunnel syndrome), wrist surgery and full recovery are shown in Fig. 5. Similar to the experienced wheelchair ridings without post-wrist injury, those with post-wrist injury showed slight contribution of the increased gravitational resistance on propulsion and power transmission efficiencies. It is also interesting that, with the lower wrist joint power efficiency, the propulsion and power transmission efficiencies during experienced wheelchair propulsion with post-wrist injury were higher than that of experienced wheelchair propulsion without post-wrist injury.

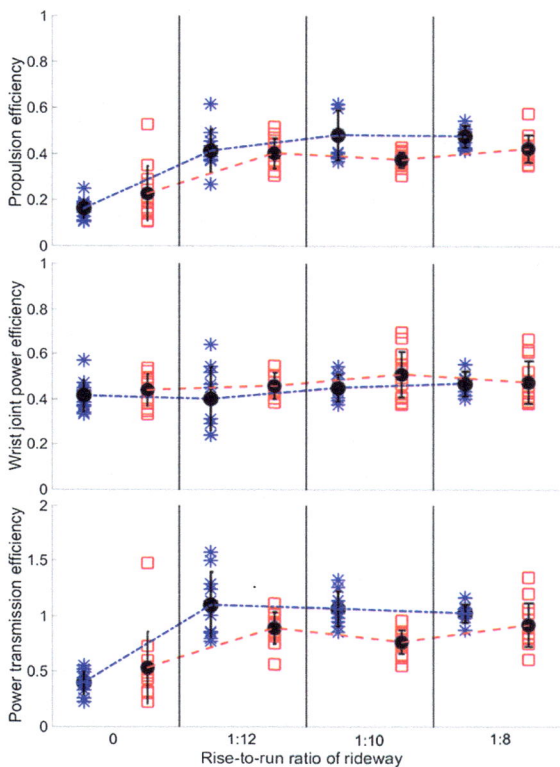

Fig. 5. Propulsion (η), wrist joint power (μ) and power transmission (φ) efficiency changes due to slope (rise-to-run) ratio of ride way in experienced wheelchair riding with (*) and without ($\square$) post-wrist injury

The validation of manual wheelchair propulsion measurement by using motion analysis system was shown in Fig. 6. The root-mean-square-error (RMSE) of 20% in percentage of averaged 3D shoulder joint angle during wheelchair propulsion measured by portable and motion analysis system indicates the close relationship between the two measures.

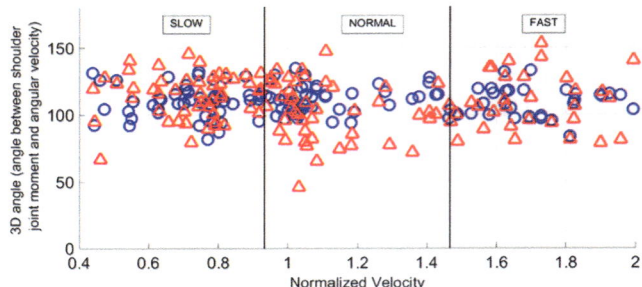

Fig. 6. The comparison of 3D angle (between moment and angular velocity at the shoulder joint) measured by using portable and motion analysis system

4   Conclusion

The upper-limb overuse diagnosis based on the analysis of the propulsion efficiency (η), joint power efficiency (μ) and joint power transmission efficiency (φ) in experienced and inexperienced wheelchair propulsion signifies that the repetitive and excessive propulsion have greater effects on inexperienced manual wheelchair riding than on experienced one. The least effects found in experienced manual wheelchair riders with post-wrist joint injury possibly signify the regulated propulsion due to joint injury experiences.

Conflict of Interest. The authors declare that they have no conflict of interest.

References

1. Sie, I., Waters, R., Adkins, R., Gellman, H.: Upper extremity pain in the postrehabilitation spinal cord injured patient. Arch. Phys. Med. Rehabil. **73**, 44–48 (1992)
2. Bayley, J.C., Cocharan, T.P., Sledge, C.B.: The weight-bearing shoulder. The impingement syndrome in paraplegics. J. Bone Joint Surg. Am. **69**, 676–678 (1987)
3. Cooper, R.A., Cooper, R., Boninger, M.L.: Trends and issues in wheelchair technologies. Assist. Technol. **20**, 61–72 (2008)
4. Viriyamatanont, T., Chotsangsri, S., Boonpratatong, A.: The effect of tilting and friction coefficients on manual wheelchair propulsion efficiency. In: Proceeding of the 14th International Symposium on 3D Analysis of Human Movement 2016, vol. P72, pp. 433–436 (2016)
5. Boonpratatong, A., Pantong, J., Kiattisaksophon, S., Senavongse, W.: Manual wheelchair propulsion efficiency on different slopes. Waset Int. J. Biomed. Biol. Eng. **3**(5), 381–384 (2016)
6. Hwang, S.H., Lee, H.Y., Kim, Y.H.: Upper limb dynamics during manual wheelchair propulsion with different resistances. In: IFBME Proceedings, vol. 31, pp. 632–635 (2010)
7. Desroches, G., Dumas, R., Oradon, D., Vaslin, P., Lopoutre, F.-X., Cheze, L.: Upper limb joint dynamics during manual wheelchair propulsion. Clin. Biomech. **25**, 299–306 (2010)

8. Lp-research, Inc.: LPMS-B reference manual version 1.2.7 life performance research. Tokyu, Japan (2014)
9. Tekscan, Inc.: Improving medical devices with force sensing technology. Massachesetts, USA (2013)
10. Askari, S., Kirby, L., Parker, K., et al.: Wheelchair propulsion test: development and measurement properties of a new test for manual wheelchair users. Arch. Phys. Med. Rehabil. **94**, 1690–1698 (2013)
11. Wells, D., Alderson, J., Camomilla, V., Donnelly, C., Elliott, B., Cereatti, A.: Elbow joint kinematics during cricket bowling using magneto-inertial sensors: a feasibility study. J. Sports Sci. (2018). https://doi.org/10.1080/02640414.2018.1512845

Individual Margins of Instantaneous Dynamic Stability: Verification in Elderly with Mobility and Balance Tests

Pattranit Kitiratchai[1]([⊠]), Waranya Mongkholhatthi[1],
Sugunya Wongbuangam[2], and Amaraporn Boonpratatong[1]

[1] Department of Biomedical Engineering, Faculty of Engineering,
Srinakharinwirot University, Nakhannayok, Thailand
kitiratchai.pattra@gmail.com
[2] Sudthavas Foundation, Nakhannayok, Thailand

Abstract. A verification of individual margins of instantaneous dynamic stability in elderly volunteers is presented. The modified condition and margins of instantaneous dynamic stability permitting the estimation in elderly are proposed. By utilizing in experimental protocols of conventional tests of mobility, i.e. Up-and-Go activity, and balance, i.e. mini-BEST, the periodic stability indices were estimated in elderly without introducing fall prone incidence. The margins of instantaneous dynamic stability or the risk of falls of each elderly volunteer was compared to the healthy young group. The accuracy of fall risk estimation by using the current method tested in fall incidences of young and healthy volunteers was presented.

Keywords: Dynamic stability · Individual margins of dynamic stability · Fall risk estimation · Elderly motion · Mobility and balance tests

1 Introduction

Falls is now accepted as an incidence of global concern as aging society has grown widely and related costs is of high maintenance. The use of interventions, e.g. strength training, hip protectors or air bags [2], to prevent falls and falling-induced injuries have been proposed. However, the effectiveness of such interventions is not yet classified as sufficient. Intelligent processing of motion signals, e.g. neural network classifier, spectral analysis, feature extraction and hidden Markov model have been used in wearable ambulatory monitoring system (WAMs) [1]. The data processing of fall and long term daily-life motion was used to estimated margins and allowances for fall identification. However, the requirement for fall motion samples limits this approach to the identification of accidental falls rather falls due to sensory deficiency or disease. In addition, these intense computational margins and allowances are not yet found to be physiologically interpretative.

Multidisciplinary approaches for fall estimation, e.g. the combination of maximum Lyapunov exponents, maximum Floquet multipliers and variability measures appear more effective than singular approaches [2]. However, the advance mathematical basis

© Springer Nature Switzerland AG 2020
K.-P. Lin et al. (Eds.): ICBHI 2019, IFMBE Proceedings 74, pp. 252–259, 2020.
https://doi.org/10.1007/978-3-030-30636-6_35

and the requirements for long time-series kinematic records of walking trails limit these approaches to individuals with dedicated time, lab accessibility and specific practitioner's diagnosis.

Fall risk estimation for the purpose of elderly intervention designs is preferable to rely on home based measurement and indicators that are interpretative to fallers, caregivers and clinicians, so that the training or protection can be deployed efficiently. A set of fall risk indicators derived from dynamic stability basis and experimental protocol developed from activity of daily-living (ADL) has been proposed to estimate individual margins of dynamic stability. Kinematics of daily-living and fall prone activities, e.g. walking, stair climbing and roller skating, of individual was measured by using inertia sensor [5]. The periodicity score of kinematic records was calculated starting from first motion cycle and then repeated at next instance of time. The individual margins of instantaneous dynamic stability were estimated from the discrimination between periodicity and fall prone scores. The preliminary criterion for the discrimination was 2-s notified time before fall hits [3]. The estimation was simple and interpretative as the lower margins signified the stronger periodic motion and the lower risk of falls. However, this fall risk estimation is limited to the fall events that last longer than 2 s before fall hits. A modified approach was proposed by introducing fall recovery indices. The individual margins of instantaneous dynamic stability were estimated from the extrapolation of indices from daily-living and fall recovery activities rather than 2-s notification rule. The quantification then allowed the fall risk notification in the activities that last shorter than 2 s and did not require the kinematic records of fall prone activities. However, fall prone motion samples were still required in validation [4] and, therefore, limit the approach to be performed on elderly or frail individuals.

Both of the intelligent processing and dynamic stability theory approaches shared a limitation due to requirement for fall motion samples. The utilizing in experimental protocols of other disciplines, e.g. balance tests from physiologic therapy, that does not require volunteers in fall prone activities may improve the practice of these instantaneous fall identifications. Therefore, in this research paper, the individual margins of instantaneous dynamic stability estimated from modified derivations of fall risk indices and the corporation with mobility and balance tests of Up-and-Go, and mini-BESTest [6, 7] were proposed. Without the requirement on fall motion samples, the experiments were safe to be conducted on elderly volunteers. The margins of instantaneous dynamic stability or the risk of falls of each elderly volunteer was presented and compared to the healthy young group.

2   Materials and Methods

2.1   Modified Condition and Margins of Instantaneous Dynamic Stability

Two indices of instantaneous dynamic stability, so called, periodic acceleration and periodic jerk indices proposed in A. Boonpratatong [3] were used in this research. However, to establish the margins of instantaneous dynamic stability without inducing fall incidence to volunteers, some modification needs to be applied to the derivation in previous work [3]. During the mobility test, i.e. Up-and-Go, and balance test, i.e. mini-Best, the volunteers were asked to wear inertia sensors (see Sect 2.2.), so that the periodic acceleration (A_n) and jerk (J_n) indices can be calculated from the kinematic measures (inertia records). The modified condition of instantaneous dynamic stability based on Up-and-Go and mini-Best tests was then defined by

$$A_n \leq A_m, \; and \; J_n \leq J_m \tag{1}$$

where A_m and J_m are the margin of instantaneous dynamic stability justified by periodic acceleration (A_n) and jerk (J_n) indices, respectively, during activities of daily-living. These margins were established on the extrapolation of the dynamic stability indices obtained during Up-and-Go and mini-BESTests under an assumption that the Up-and-Go activities is a dynamically stable motion subjected to greater perturbation than that of the mini-BESTests. Therefore, the modified derivation of margin of periodic acceleration (A_m) can be expressed by

$$A_m = \overline{Ag}_\vee + k\left(\overline{Ag}_\vee - \overline{Ab}_\vee\right) \tag{2}$$

$$\overline{A}_\vee = \left\langle A_\vee^1, A_\vee^j, \ldots, A_\vee^p \right\rangle \tag{3}$$

$$A_\vee^j = max\left(A_1^j, A_2^j, \ldots, A_n^j\right) \tag{4}$$

where A_n^j is the periodic acceleration index at step wise number n of the motion trial j. $A_\vee^j$ is the peak of the periodic acceleration index over the entire course of the jth motion trial. $\overline{A}_\vee$ is the average of the peaks of periodic acceleration index obtained from all of p motion trials. $\overline{Ab}_\vee$ is the average of the peaks of periodic acceleration index obtained from p motion trials during mini-BESTests. Similar to $\overline{Ag}_\vee$ is that obtained from p motion trials during Up-and-Go test. k is a marginal constant. The same derivation manner is applied to margin of periodic jerk (J_m).

The modified condition of instantaneous dynamic stability was established by using Eqs. (1) to (4) and the extension to define margin of periodic acceleration (A_m) and jerk (J_m). The marginal constant (k) providing least percentage of false prediction in healthy young volunteers was selected and used to establish the individual margin of periodic acceleration (A_m) and jerk (J_m) of all volunteers including non-faller elderly and faller elderly volunteers.

2.2   Experimental Method

Two healthy male and three healthy female volunteers [age 21–22 years], and seven female elderly volunteers [age 60–75 years] participated in this study. Instructions of testing processes were provided, and written consent was obtained from each subject prior to the measurement. All elderly volunteers declared independent state of daily activity. Three out of seven declared a few incidences of falls in past years (fallers). The inertia sensors [5] were affixed at 1 inch above the navel of individual volunteer. The sensor was wrapped in polyester straps of which the length can be adjusted to fit on volunteer's waist. All volunteers were asked to perform five trials of following activities.

Up-and-Go Test:

1. Stand up from a chair, walk for 3 m, turn around, walk back, and sit down on the same chair.

mini-BESTest:

1. Walk 3–5 steps at normal speed, and then increase walking speed when the cue of fast walk is heard. Continue to walk other 3–5 steps before decrease walking speed when the cue of slow walk is heard.
2. Walk 3–5 steps at normal speed, and then face left or right according to the "left" or "right" cues provided (Figs. 1 and 2).

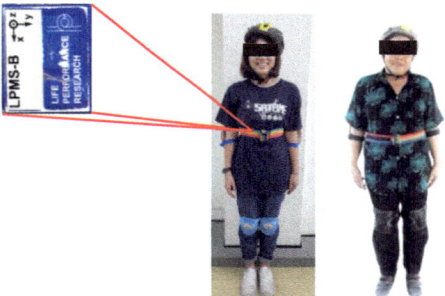

Fig. 1. Inertia sensor [5] orientation and placement on volunteers's body

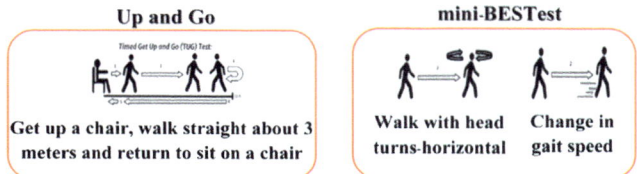

Fig. 2. The protocols for Up-and-Go and mini-BESTests.

In addition to Up-and-Go and mini-BESTests, all of healthy young volunteers who declared beginning level of roller skating were also asked to perform roller skating on a 5-m track without previous practices. The five trials of fall over motion during skating were recorded.

3   Results

The instantaneous dynamic stability indices during Up-and-Go, mini-BESTest1 and mini-BESTest2 activities of representative healthy young, non-faller and faller elderly volunteers are shown in Figs. 3 and 4. Similar to the previous studies [3, 4], the overall indices of periodic acceleration (A-index) were found to be smaller than those of periodic jerk (J-index). Both of the periodic acceleration and jerk indices were greater when obtained from Up-and-Go activity and elderly volunteers than mini-BESTests and healthy young volunteers.

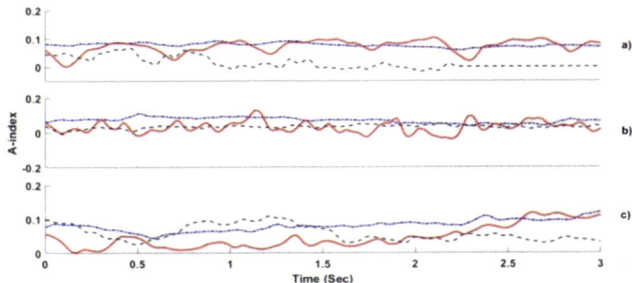

Fig. 3. The comparison between periodic acceleration indices (A-index) during mini-BEST1 (a), mini-BEST2 (b) and Up and Go activities (c) of healthy (--), faller (—) and non-faller (···) elderly volunteers

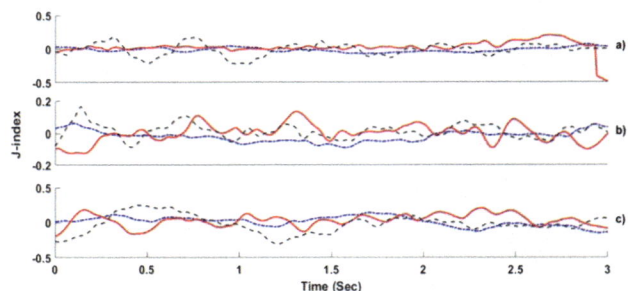

Fig. 4. The comparison between periodic jerk indices (J-index) during mini-BEST test1 (a), mini-BEST test2 (b) and Up and Go activities (c) of healthy (--), faller (—) and non-faller (···) elderly volunteers

The false prediction justified by marginal constant (k) and corresponding margin of periodic acceleration (A_m) and jerk (J_m) of all healthy young volunteers is shown in Figs. 5 and 6. It was found that the false positive prediction decreases whereas the false negative prediction increases as the marginal constant (k) is increased. By verifying one-factor-at -a time (OFAT) the margin of periodic acceleration (A_m) with marginal constant (k) of 0.2 was found to provide minimum percentage of false prediction. By following the same technique as of the periodic acceleration (a-index), the margin of periodic jerk (J_m) with marginal constant (k) of 1.0 was found to provide minimum percentage of false prediction.

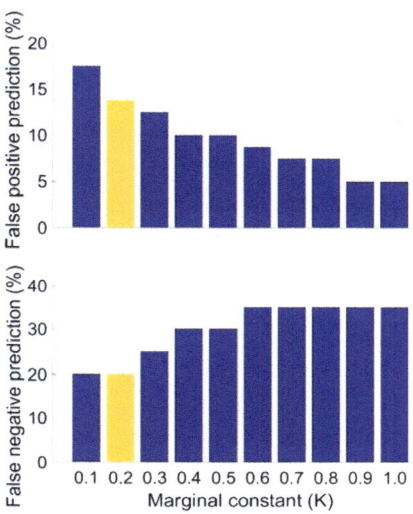

Fig. 5. The false positive and negative prediction of falls regulated by periodic acceleration indices (A-index) of young and healthy volunteers and a marginal constant (k) providing minimum total false prediction (☐).

By using the marginal constants (k) established from instantaneous dynamic stability indices during Up-and-Go, mini-BESTest1 and mini-BESTest2 activities of all healthy young volunteers, the margin of periodic acceleration (A_m) and jerk (J_m) of all elderly volunteers was established without any requirements on fall induced activities. Individual margins of dynamic stability of healthy young, non-faller elderly, and faller elderly volunteers based on modified condition and margins of instantaneous dynamic stability are shown in Table 1. The margins of instantaneous dynamic stability were higher in elderly than healthy young and highest in faller elderly volunteers.

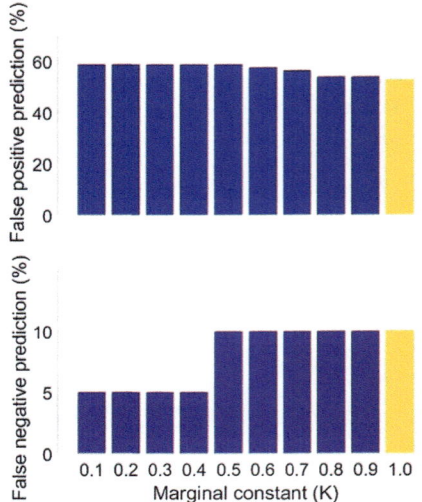

Fig. 6. The false positive and negative prediction of falls regulated by periodic jerk indices (J-index) of young and healthy volunteers and a marginal constant (k) providing minimum total false prediction (▢)

Table 1. Individual margins of dynamic stability of young and healthy, non-faller elderly, and faller elderly volunteers based on modified condition and margins of instantaneous dynamic stability.

	Volunteer no.	Am	Jm
Healthy young adult	1	0.15	0.3
	2	0.21	0.33
	3	0.17	0.34
	4	0.16	0.25
	5	0.17	0.36
Non-Faller elderly	6	0.26	0.4
	7	0.21	0.32
Faller elderly	8	0.19	0.54
	9	0.21	0.51
	10	0.27	0.63
	11	0.28	0.43
	12	0.24	0.59

4   Discussion

The margins of periodic acceleration (A_m) and jerk (J_m) from marginal constant (k) and periodic acceleration (*A-index*) and jerk (*J-index*) indices of Up-and-Go, mini-BESTest1 and mini-BESTest2 activities providing minimum false prediction on all healthy young volunteers were established. The resultance marginal constants (k) were used to establish margins of periodic acceleration (A_m) and jerk (J_m) on the individual dynamic stability indices (A and J indices) of elderly volunteers without the requirement on fall motion. The margins of instantaneous dynamic stability being lowest, moderate and highest in healthy young, non-faller elderly and faller elderly volunteers, respectively, indicate the fall risks discrimination between the three groups. Compared to the previous research [3, 4], the relatively high value of false predictive percentage indicates the overlaps between periodic indices obtained from Up-and-Go $(\overline{Ag}_\vee)$ and mini-BESTests $(\overline{Ab}_\vee)$.

5 Conclusion

This research established margins of instantaneous dynamic stability of individual elderly volunteers on the extrapolation of periodic acceleration (A-*index*) and jerk (*J-index*) indices obtained from mobility and balance tests. The fall risk discrimination between healthy young, non-faller and faller volunteers were presented, however, the alteration on mobility and balance tests for periodic stability index establishment and the additional indices obtained from foot part of the body [3, 4] may be needed to reduce the false prediction.

Conflict of Interest. The authors declare that they have no conflict of interest.

References

1. Shany, T., Redmond, S.J., Narayana, M.R., Lovell, N.H.: Sensors-based wearable systems for monitoring of human movement and falls. IEEE Sens. J. **12**, 658–670 (2012). https://doi.org/10.1109/JSEN.2011.2146246
2. Bruijin, S.M., Meijer, O.G., Beek, P.J., Dieen, J.H.: Assessing the stability of human locomotion: a review of current measures. J. Roy. Soc. Interface **10**, 20120999 (2013)
3. Amaraporn, B., Settawut, K., Jurairat, P., Piyawalee, A., Ramida, S.: Individual margins of instanteneous dynamic stability: a preliminary study on periodic and roller skating motion. In: Proceedings of the 12th IASTED International Conference on Biomedical Engineering, Innsbruck, Austria, pp. 169–175 (2016). ISBN: 978-0-88986-981-3
4. Amaraporn, B., Walaithip, P., Nutthavara, V., Kanokwan, S.: Instability predicted by instantaneous dynamic stability: a preliminary study on periodic and fall recovery motion. In: Proceedings of i-CREATe 2017 Proceedings of the 11th International Convention on Rehabilitation Engineering and Assistive Technology (2017)
5. LP-RESEARCH CORPORATION, Ichigaya Yakuouiimachi 14-4-203, Shinjuku-ku, 162-0063 Tokyo, Japan (2012). Email: info@lp-research.com. http://www.lp-research.com
6. Yingyongyudha, A., Saengsirisuwan, V., Panichaporn, W., Boonsinsukh, R.: The mini-balance evaluation systems test (Mini-BESTest) demonstrates higher accuracy in identifying older adult participants with history of falls than do the BESTest, berg balance scale, or timed up and go test. J. Geriatr. Phys. Ther. **39**(2), 64–70 (2016)
7. Mini-BESTest: Balance Evaluation Systems Test. http://www.bestest.us/files/7413/6380/7277/MiniBest_revised_final_3_8_13.pdf

Cyber-Physical Secure VLC Applications

Noriharu Miyaho[1](✉), Noriko Konno[1], Takamasa Shimada[1],
Kana Egawa[1], Kosuke Watai[1], Kotaro Murase[1], and Atsuya Yokoi[2]

[1] The School of System Design and Technology, Tokyo Denki University,
Tokyo, Japan
miyaho@mail.dendai.ac.jp
[2] Samsung R&D Institute Japan, Yokohama, Japan

Abstract. Visible light communication (VLC) can play a versatile role in future IoT (Internet of Things) - based communication services. In this paper, we first describe the latest encryption technology required to guarantee security specific to VLC and IoT to prevent eavesdropping and then the cyber-physical VLC applications of this technology.

This paper clarifies the latest communication concepts that can be implemented with the current technological level of color shift keying (CSK) communications. The CSK receiver and transmitter can identify a specific SDM frame shape, chromaticity coordinate assignment area in a color diagram, and the CSK code. After identifying both the chromaticity coordinates of CSK cells and the frame shape, the corresponding CSK cell content is paraphrased into the original data by different mapping tables. To introduce CSK communications for commercial purposes, security must be enhanced by adopting encryption technologies. It should also be noted that changing the shape of the CSK frame can significantly improve security and the error-free performance can be attained by increasing the number of CSK symbols in a frame.

We also describe new communication service concepts that can be implemented with the current technological level of CSK communication. We propose smart glasses applications using cyber-physical space by combining the VLC technology and a computer database, leading AR applications.

Keywords: VLC · CSK · Security · Smart glasses · AR

1 Introduction

Many different visible light communication (VLC) methods have been proposed and developed for commercial release. Visible light communication is characterized by freedom from the constraints of the laws governing radio transmission and allows visual inspection of data transmission/reception. Visual technology can prevent eavesdropping, a risk that is normally difficult to counter in wireless communication. Hospitals should be able to provide secret and secure communication environments in which medical electronic equipment is safe from [external] interference. All the light sources around us, such as room lighting, TV screens, traffic signals, and neon signs,

© Springer Nature Switzerland AG 2020
K.-P. Lin et al. (Eds.): ICBHI 2019, IFMBE Proceedings 74, pp. 260–267, 2020.
https://doi.org/10.1007/978-3-030-30636-6_36

have great potential to serve as visible light communication devices. This paper adopts color shift keying (CSK) for the modulation of visible light communication services and describes the latest security mechanism for CSK encryption [1]. Considering potential IoT communication services, encryption technology needs to be able to guarantee security for visible light communication.

2 Secure Communication Requirements in IOT-Based Network Applications

It is becoming increasingly important to provide communication services that are secure and that give users the assurance of safety regardless of location. The information communication environment is characterized by an effective activation of Big Data usage, based on widely distributed clouds, in addition to smartphone and IoT communication devices becoming an integral part of our daily lives. However, the current communication security levels of clouds and communication services are not sufficient to give users sufficient assurance of safety. In light of this situation, this paper focuses on CSK, a modulation method for visible light communication, and discusses the technology of CSK-based communications between smart phones and other devices. CSK is one of the modulation schemes for VLC that was adopted in the IEEE802.15.7. Substantially, a conventional OOK (On Off Keying)-VLC system, makes it possible to transmit any information by the blinking of a light source.

The CSK information is transmitted as color symbols that are generated by multi-color light sources such as RGB LEDs.

The transmitter converts the data being sent into visible light CSK color information, using a rule that is kept confidential from third parties, and shows it continuously on the display. The receiver decodes the color information as follows. It uses the built-in camera of a smartphone or a Web camera to capture the image on the display, performs signal processing on the color information, and converts it back to the original by using the pre-determined specific code conversion rule that was only specified between the transmitter and the receiver.

Because anyone can easily see the display, this information transport method should incorporate a means that ensures a high level of security. To achieve a high communication rate to broaden its potential application, it is necessary to increase the frame rate of the camera or incorporate space-division multiplexing (SDM). This paper proposes a feasible securely encrypted CSK communication service, where CSK cells are arranged in a specific frame shape. Figure 1 shows an example of CSK color symbol mapping on CIE1931 x-y color coordinates [2].

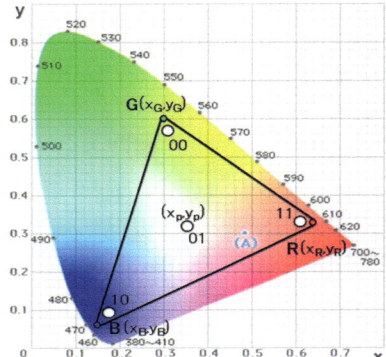

Fig. 1. CSK color symbol mapping on CIE1931 x-y color coordinate

3 Principles of CSK Communication Technology

As shown in Fig. 1, R(x_R, y_R), G(x_G, y_G), and B(x_B, y_B) are the x-y color coordinates of the RGB light sources, and (x_p, y_p) is one of the allocated color points used as CSK color symbols. When an sRGB (standard RGB color space) display is used as the light source, the coordinates are R (0.64, 0.33), G(0.30, 0.60), and B(0.15, 0.06). The outer curved boundary is the spectral locus, with wavelengths shown in nanometers. Four kinds of information (00, 01, 10, 11) are placed in the RGB triangle as CSK symbols, which means that in this case the system can send 2 bits of data per one CSK symbol. This constellation example with four color points is called 4-CSK. The IEEE standard defines 8-CSK and 16-CSK with eight and sixteen color points, respectively [1].

The information data mapped in Fig. 1 are coded into x-y values by the color mapping block, according to the color mapping rule. The x-y values are transformed into P_R, P_G, and P_B, each representing the power of the primary colors emitted by the RGB LEDs. The color of point (x_p, y_p) is determined by the relative strengths of the emitted primary colors from the three LEDs (P_R, P_G, and P_B). The relationships among (x_R, y_R), (x_G, y_G), (x_B, y_B), (x_p, y_p), P_R, P_G, and P_B are shown by the following simultaneous equations.

$$x_p = P_R \cdot x_R + P_G \cdot x_G + P_B \cdot x_B \tag{1}$$

$$y_p = P_R \cdot y_R + P_G \cdot y_G + P_B \cdot y_B \tag{2}$$

$$P_R + P_G + P_B = 1 \tag{3}$$

As Eq. (3) shows, the total power ($P_R + P_G + P_B$) is always constant. These power values are normalized to one. Therefore, the actual total power can be arbitrarily set and can even be changed during CSK communication. The x- y values on the receiver's side are calculated from the received RGB light power P_R', P_G', and P_B'. Then, the x-y values are decoded into the received data. Because it uses visible colors for communication, CSK is suitable for image sensor communications from displays to cameras.

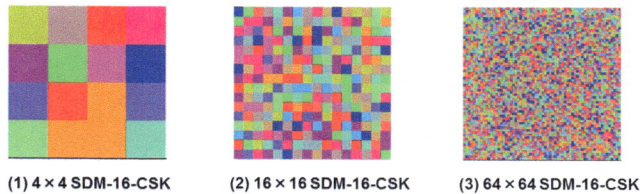

(1) 4 × 4 SDM-16-CSK   (2) 16 × 16 SDM-16-CSK   (3) 64 × 64 SDM-16-CSK

Fig. 2. Two-dimensional SDM-CSK code

Most cameras can be used as receivers of CSK without additional hardware. The capture frame rate of common cameras is 30 fps. In this case, the frame rate of CSK would have to be less than 15 frames/s assuming 2x oversampling at receivers (Fig. 2).

4   Security Technology Specific to CSK Communications and Its Applications

The proposed CSK communication system converts data into visible light color information based on a specified rule [3]. In general, a CSK code is at high risk from third-party eavesdropping. Therefore, it is essential for CSK communication to incorporate an encrypted communication function. We propose the latest secure communication service that takes advantage of the characteristics of a scheme in which CSK color symbols are arranged and displayed in a specific frame shape.

We propose a new idea that involves changing the shape of the frame arbitrarily, which is pre-determined between communication terminals in advance, thereby making secret communication feasible. One possible means of encryption is to share a conversion table that associates the correspondence between an item of data to be transmitted and its chromaticity coordinates with the shape of the frame in which the cells are arranged. Based on the correspondence (mapping table) between an item of data and its chromaticity coordinates:

(a)   The transmitter associates the item of data with a frame shape type.
(b)   The transmitter changes the frame shape type at specified time intervals.
(c)   The receiver identifies the frame shape type and selects the associated mapping table.

Using these methods, CSK code encryption can be achieved by adopting either a different frame shape or a chromaticity coordinate area as an encryption key.

Alternatively, both a frame shape and a chromaticity coordinate area can be used as encryption keys. This proposed method makes it extremely difficult to eavesdrop visible CSK code information according to the versatile shape patterns introduction.

For example, multiple mapping table types and rules for their modification are predefined for each frame shape. The transmitter changes the correspondence (mapping table) between an item of data and its chromaticity coordinates over time, and the modification rule is predefined as a color hopping pattern.

The CSK color symbols conversion method shown in Fig. 3 is based on the settings of the encryption keys. A triangular and a circular frame shape are separately predefined in mapping tables that show the correspondence between an item of data and its chromaticity coordinates. The kinds of frame shapes are not limited to a triangular or circular frame. An ellipse, a square or other intricate patterns can be adopted as well [4]. The rules are predefined such that the two color symbols (X, Y) within the triangular frame are identified as information A and B, and the same two color symbols (X, Y) within the circular frame are identified as different information C and D, respectively. This mechanism makes eavesdropping impossible.

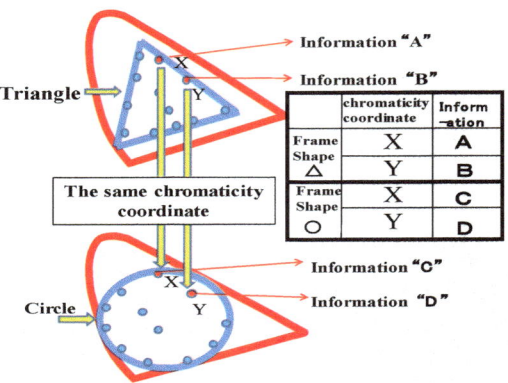

Fig. 3. CSK color symbols conversion depending on the chromaticity coordinates

The transmitter, such as a smartphone, sends data by making the color of the chromaticity coordinates blink at a specific position within the frame shape. The transmitter and receiver must use the same mapping table. The receiver can identify a CSK code using a Web camera. After identifying the displayed frame, it converts the chromaticity coordinates of the CSK code into data using a mapping table. Since existing technologies are used for this communication method, new secure CSK communication services can be implemented economically.

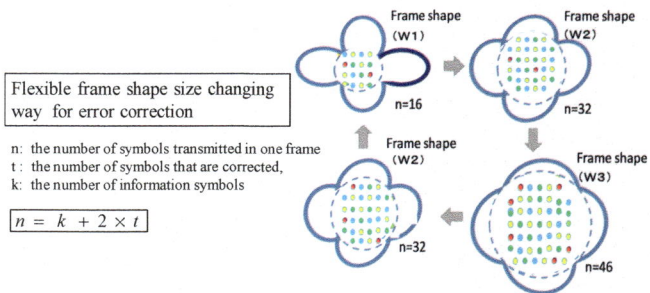

Fig. 4. Changing frame shape patterns for cell error correction

5   Secure VLC Communications

5.1   Effect of CSK Frame Pattern and Error Correction

The number of possible frame shape patterns are dependent on the number of the pixels included in a camera and the resolving power of the image sensor. Figure 4 shows one form of encrypted communication achieved by changing the frame shape of the CSK code from W1→W2→W3→W2→W1 and changing the number of CSK code cells within the frame.

The number of cells, n, contained in a frame shape varies depending on the shape, W1, W2 or W3. A frame shape can contain various cells, such as symbols for synchronization and an error correction code, in addition to the cells used to transfer information. When communication with a sufficiently high level of resolution is enabled, the amount of information and the code rate can be changed as appropriate depending on the size of the frame shape.

In cases where the Reed-Solomon code is used as the error correction code, it is known that the following Eq. (4) must be met:

$$n = k + 2 \times t \tag{4}$$

where, n is the number of symbols transmitted in one frame, t is the number of symbols that are corrected, and k is the number of information symbols. One CSK code cell represents one symbol, and the net amount of information subject to coding is $k \times 4$ bits for 16-CSK. For simplicity, let's assume the case of 4CSK and 30 frames/s. If Reed-Solomon coding is used for W2 and only 1 k bps is used for information transmission, then, at most 8 deteriorated cells are corrected and code rate efficiency is about 50%. If Reed-Solomon coding is used for W3, and 2 k bps is used for information transmission, then at most seven deteriorated cells are corrected and code rate efficiency is about 70%. By utilizing this communication method in a VLC system, it is possible to change a frame shape pattern. By making use of the Reed-Solomon code, since the number of newly required redundant symbols is 2t, the code rate becomes $(n - 2t)/n$.

It is preferable from the user's perspective if the amount of information inside the frame by using the CSK code is proportional to the size of the frame. The number of symbol error corrections should be taken into account when considering the receiver's CSK code resolution.

5.2   Cyber-Physical Secure VLC Application Using Smart Glasses

To prevent the harmful effects of a malfunction occurring in medical equipment inside a hospital, it is necessary to restrict use of radio waves. Under these circumstances, useful information still needs to be provided securely and safely to the medical staff. Figure 5 shows an example of a cyber-physical VLC application in an augmented reality (AR) space. By wearing smart glasses, VLC technology can be used effectively to realize a safe and secure communication environment.

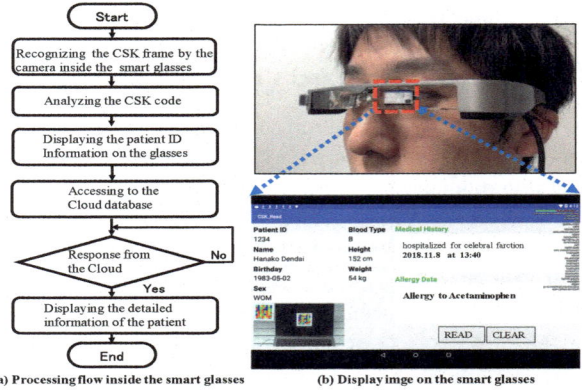

(a) Processing flow inside the smart glasses   (b) Display imge on the smart glasses

Fig. 5. Example of cyber-physical secure VLC application

Since it is possible to apply an appropriate form of the CSK encryption technology mentioned above, a secure cyber physical space can be realized. By wearing smart glasses which have VLC interfaces, a doctor can obtain, at any time, confidential personal information, such as a patient's case record stored in a locally deployed database inside the hospital or even outside such as in a cloud storage.

As for another example, it is assumed that the CSK code is utilized for identifying each patient. In this case when the doctor watches the CSK code by smart glasses, then it can immediately analyze the CSK code and displays the result on the screen of the glasses, and he recognize the patient ID and name. Thereafter, he can get the specific details information inherent to the patient disease history from the cloud database inside or outside the hospital. These procedure is shown in the Fig. 6. If a nurse registers the doctor's picture in advance, then he/she can recognize the CSK code information transmitted from the LED lighting equipment as soon as he/she enters the patient's room. The web camera continuously monitors the inside a patient's room and it notifies the message only if the registered doctors or nurses are identified using the computer. The LED devices in the VLC equipment incorporate the function of CSK code generation.

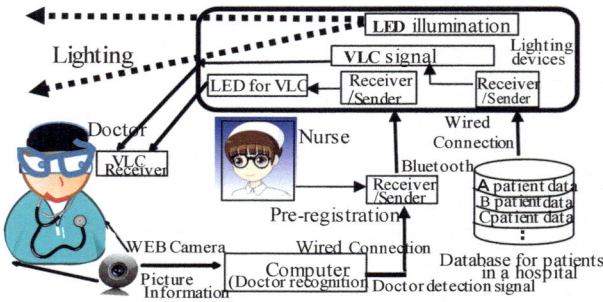

Fig. 6. Cyber-physical secure VLC application in the future

During a doctor's medical examination, he/she can continuously make use of secure smart glasses with VLC interfaces. It is often permissible for using low power Bluetooth devices with a coverage range of 10 m.

In this environment, VLC is a suitable means of providing the doctor with important information securely while at the same time avoiding interference with medical equipment.

In addition, when a nurse wants to send a secure message to the doctor without disclosing it to others, the corresponding message text information will also be shown on the doctor's smart glasses display securely. The nurse can convey the mind consciousness in the form of visible text by utilizing the smart glasses without disclosing the message to others. By installing a bone conduction microphone, it becomes possible to convert the text message to the sound that only the doctor can recognize. Thus VLC can be utilized by using the corresponding software applications and the web camera as well.

6 Conclusions

We presented the principle of CSK communication and clarified the security of VLC. To make CSK communication acceptable, advanced security must be introduced by adopting encryption technologies which enhance the advantages of CSK communication. It should also be noted that changing the shape of the CSK frame can significantly improve security and error-free performance. We proposed a cyber-physical secure VLC communication service that utilizes smart glasses for AR. VLC services can be effectively integrated with other forms of wireless communication technology.

Conflict of Interest. The authors declare that they have no conflict of interest.

References

1. Rajagopal, S., et al.: IEEE802.15.7 visible light communication: modulation schemes and dimming support. IEEE Commun. Mag. **50**(3), 72–82 (2012)
2. CIE: Commission Internationale de l'Eclairage Proceedings. Cambridge University Press, Cambridge (1932)
3. Yokoi, A., Choi, S., et al.: A new image sensor communication system using color shift keying. In: ICEVLC 2015, November Tokyo, Japan (2015)
4. Miyaho, N., et al.: Secure VLC services and practical applications, session 1-5. In: 2nd International Conference and Exhibition on Visible Light Communications 2018 (ICEVLC 2018), March, Tokyo, Japan, 2018 (2018)

Empirical Modeling of Photopolymerization for Oxygen-Mediated Anti-cancer

Kuo-Ti Chen[1], Jui-Teng Lin[2(✉)], and Hsia-Wei Liu[3(✉)]

[1] Graduate Institute of Applied Science and Engineering, Fu Jen Catholic University, New Taipei City, Taiwan, ROC
[2] New Vision Inc., Taipei, Taiwan, ROC
jtlin55@gmail.com
[3] Department of Life Science, Fu Jen Catholic University, New Taipei City, Taiwan, ROC
079336@gmail.com

Abstract. The dynamic roles of photosensitizer (PS) concentration and light intensity were measured and analyzed. The efficacy of photodynamic therapy (PDT) and cell viability (CV) are measured (in vitro) and analyzed by analytic and numerical modeling. For a fixed PS concentration, CV is a nonlinear deceasing function of light intensity and exposure time; for a fixed light intensity, higher PS concentration achieves higher efficacy or smaller CV (at steady-state), in consistent to our analytic formulas. Finally, anti-cancer efficacy may be enhanced by the resupply of PS and/or external oxygen.

Keywords: Photodynamic therapy · Oxygen-mediated · Cancer therapy · Efficacy · Cell viability

1 Introduction

Photo-polymerization has two major processes [1, 2]: (i) type-I for photodynamic therapy (PDT) using light-initiated oxygen free radical; and (ii) type-II for crosslinking (or gelation) of biomaterials using radical-substrate coupling. Photo-polymerization offers various applications in dermatology, dental, orthopedics (tissue engineering), ophthalmology, anti-cancer and anti-microbial [1–7].

Photoinitiated polymerization and crosslinking provide advantageous means over the thermal-initiated polymerization, including fast and controllable reaction rates, spatial and temporal control over the formation of the material, and without a need for high temperatures or pH conditions [4]. Tissue-engineering using scaffold-based procedures for chemical modification of polymers has been reported to improve its mechanical properties by crosslinking or polymerization with UV or visible light to produce gels or high-molecular-weight polymers [6–10]. Various crosslinking methods have been developed to stabilize collagen in aqueous solutions ex vivo, including physical inter actions, chemical reactions, or photochemical polymerization [4]. The advantages and limitations of photo crosslinking have been discussed by many researchers [4], specially for the thiol-click reactions which include Michael-addition and the thiol-ene reaction [6, 10, 11].

© Springer Nature Switzerland AG 2020
K.-P. Lin et al. (Eds.): ICBHI 2019, IFMBE Proceedings 74, pp. 268–274, 2020.
https://doi.org/10.1007/978-3-030-30636-6_37

Our previous studies presented detail of the kinetics and efficacy for type-I and type-II mechanism [1, 2]. In this study, we will focus on the type-II PDT for anti-cancer. The PDT efficacy and cell viability will be measured (in vitro) and analyzed by our analytic and numerical modeling.

2 Materials and Method

2.1 Experimental Set up

The experimental setup is shown in Fig. 1, the PS is Chlorine e6 (Ce6) solution at various concentration of 0.00312 to 0.00625%, and red LED light intensity of $I_0 = (51, 102, 203)$ mW/cm^2. The cell viability (CV) will be measured at above described various conditions to study the roles of light intensity (at a fixed Ce6 concentration), and Ce6 concentration (at a fixed light intensity). The reference initial light intensity is calibrated by its value in pure water solution, where the input light is collimated and output power is measured after a fixed aperture of 10 mm.

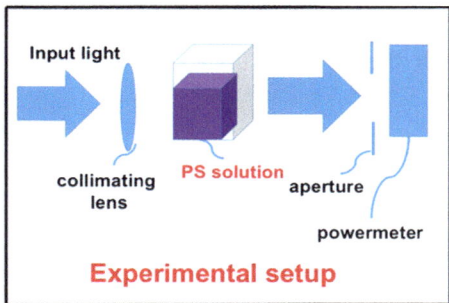

Fig. 1. Experimental setup for cells in Chlorine e6 (Ce6) solution with various concentration and exposed to LED light intensity.

It was reported that type-II, is the predominant process for anti-cancer and the efficacy related to its S-function by Eff = $1 - \exp(-S)$, where S is the accumulated singlet oxygen radicals produced by the light. S (of efficacy) reaches a steady state in time when oxygen is completely depleted.

2.2 Theory and Modeling

As shown in Fig. 2, in the type-I pathway, the excited PS triple-state (T_3) can interact directly with the substrate (A); or with the ground state oxygen (O_2) to generate a superoxide anion (O^-), which further reacts with oxygen to produce reactive radical (O^-). In comparison, in the type-II pathway, T_3 interacts with the ground state oxygen (O_2) to form a reactive singlet oxygen (O^*). In general, both type-I and type-II reactions can occur simultaneously, and the ratio between these processes depends on the types and the concentrations of PI, substrate, and oxygen, the kinetic rates involved in the process [1, 2].

Macroscopic kinetic equations was previously developed for the concentration of PS (C), oxygen (O_2), and the light intensity (I), under a so-called quasi-steady-state condition [1, 2]. Solutions of C, O_2 and I provide the anti-cancer efficacy which is related to the S-function by Ceff = 1 − exp(−S), where S1 (for type-I) and S2 (for type-II) are given by [1, 2]

$$S1 = E' \sqrt{4K'C_0 exp(A'z)/(aqI_0)} \tag{1.a}$$

$$S2 = K' \int_0^t bG(z,t)dt \tag{1.b}$$

where b = aqI (z, t), with light intensity I (z, t); g = (k_8/k_3) [A]G_0; K = 1/ (1 + C + 0.65[A]), G = CYG_0, with G_0 = Y/(Y + k), k = k_5/k_3 + (k_8/k_3) [A]; K' is an effective rate constant. and E' (z, t) = [1 − exp(−0.5Bt)], with B = a'qg, The effective coefficient A'(z, t) = 2.3[(a − b)F(m, t)C(z, t) + bC_0 + A + Q], a' = aq, with q being the quantum yield for triplet PS state; Q is the tissue absorption coefficient without PS; a and b are the extinction coefficient of the PS and the photolysis product having an concentration C(z,t) with initial value C_0; and Y and [A] are the concentration of oxygen and substrate. The fit function of A(z,t), F(m,t) = exp(−mt) was chosen to fit the numerical data by the fit parameter (m).

3   Results and Discussion

3.1   Theoretical Prediction

Figure 3 shows numerically produced typical profiles of oxygen and PS concentration, and singlet oxygen for various light intensity of 50, 100, 200 mW/cm^2, without external oxygen source (or P = 0). Figure 4 is the same as Fig. 3, but for the type-II S-function, for the case of without (A), and with (B) external oxygen source.

We note that (for the case of p = 0), higher light intensity provides higher rising rate of singlet oxygen, as shown by Fig. 5(B). However, all light intensities have the same S-function (or efficacy) at steady-state, which is defined by the time-integral (or areas covered by curves 1, 2, 3). We note that the time-accumulated singlet oxygen, or time integral of bC(z,t)G(z,t), gives the PDT efficacy in type-II process. For example, cancer cells are killed by this oxygen free radicals. The associated cell viability will be shown later in Fig. 7.

Figure 5 shows the role of PI initial concentration and external oxygen source (with p = 0 and p > 0) on cell viability (CV) in type-II dominant case. Also shown is the threshold exposure time (t') to achieve CV < 0.25%. It predicts that higher PS initial concentration and/or external oxygen source (with p > 0) kills the cancer cells more efficiently, or a less threshold time t' and dose E_0 = t'I_0, for a given light intensity. However, high PS concentration has two drawbacks: shallow crosslink depth and high cell toxicity. Therefore, an optimal concentration, with minimum cell toxicity and maximum efficacy, is desired. The optimal range of C_0 required some empirical fit for the rate constants and more details were published elsewhere [2].

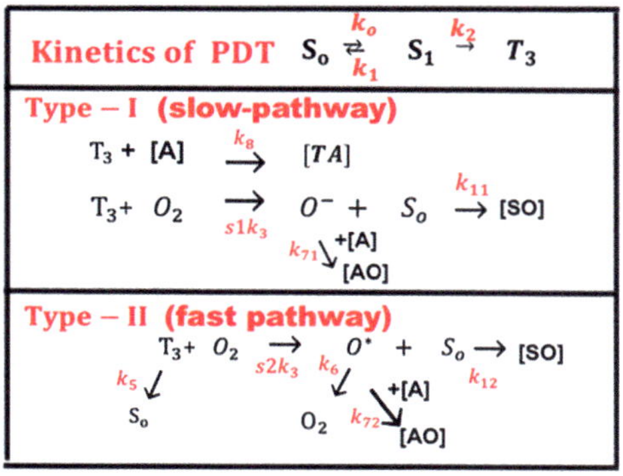

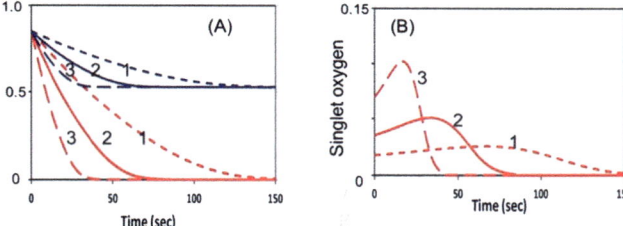

Kinetics of PDT $S_0 \underset{k_1}{\overset{k_o}{\rightleftarrows}} S_1 \overset{k_2}{\to} T_3$

Type – I (slow-pathway)

$T_3 + [A] \overset{k_8}{\to} [TA]$

$T_3 + O_2 \underset{s1k_3}{\to} O^- + S_o \overset{k_{11}}{\to} [SO]$

$\overset{k_{71}}{\searrow} \overset{+[A]}{[AO]}$

Type – II (fast pathway)

$T_3 + O_2 \underset{s2k_3}{\to} \overset{k_6}{O^\cdot} + S_o \to [SO]$

$k_5 \swarrow \qquad k_6 \swarrow \qquad \overset{+[A]}{k_{12}}$

$S_o \qquad O_2 \overset{k_{72}}{\searrow} [AO]$

Fig. 2. The kinetics of PDT, where $[S_0]$, $[S_1]$, and $[T_3]$ are the ground state, singlet excited state, and triplet excited state of PS molecules. Three pathways are shown for both the type-I and type-II processes. Ground state oxygen (O_2) may couple to T3 to form either singlet oxygen (O^*), or other reactive radical $[O^-]$. In type-I pathway, T3 can interact directly with the collagen substrate (A); or with the oxygen (O2) to generate a superoxide anion (O^-); in type-II pathway, T_3 interacts with the ground oxygen (O_2) to form a singlet oxygen (O^*) [1, 2].

Fig. 3. The numerically produced normalized temporal profiles of: (A) oxygen (red curves) and PS concentration (blue curves); (B) singlet-oxygen, for various light intensity of 50, 100, 200 mW/cm² , (for curves 1, 2, 3), without external oxygen source $(p = 0)$; $c' = 33$, $k_8[A] = 0.005$ (uM) (for type-II dominant) and for substrate $[A] = 50$ uM.

Figures 3, 4 and 5 show the following important features. For the same dose, lower light intensity achieves a higher steady-state-efficacy (SSE) in type-I; in contrast to type-II, which has an equal SSE. Type-II process is also affected by the available oxygen. Higher light intensity produces more efficient singlet oxygen, resulting in a higher transient efficacy, in which all intensities reach the same SSE when oxygen is completely depleted. With external oxygen, type-II efficacy increases with time, otherwise, it is governed only by the light dose, i.e., same dose achieves same efficacy. Moreover, type-II has an efficacy following Bunsen Roscoe law (BRL), whereas type-I follows non-BRL. The photopolymerization dynamics may be defined by the availability of oxygen, where both type-I and –II coexist until the oxygen is depleted. For the case that both type-I and type-II exit, the combined effects lead to a higher efficacy than the case of type-I or type-II only. Oxygen may also play critical role in two competing type-I and type-II processes, in which oxygen inhibits free-radical polymerization thereby reducing type-I crosslink efficiency.

3.2   Experimental Data

We shall now present our measured data which will be compared and analyzed by our theoretically predicted features discussed earlier. Figure 6 shows the measured temporal profiles for cell viability for a fixed light intensity of $I_0 = 50$ mW/cm^2, and Ce6 concentration $C_0 = 0.0031$ and 0.0062 uM.

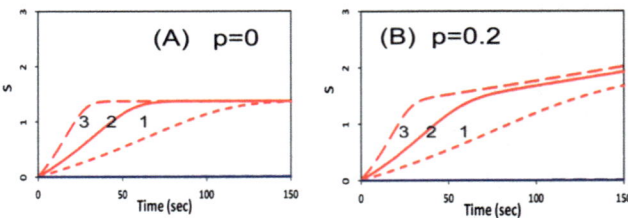

Fig. 4. Same as Fig. 3, but for the type-II S-function, for the case of without (A), and with (B) external oxygen source, with $p = 0$ and $p = 0.2$ (1/s), respectively.

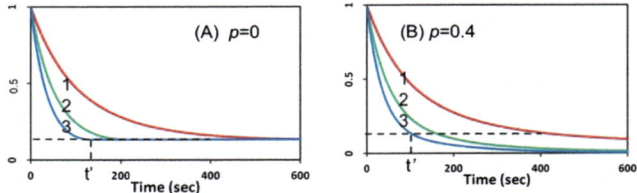

Fig. 5. The calculated temporal profiles for cell viability (CV), without (A), and with (B) external oxygen source, for various PS concentration of 5,10,15 $u$ms (for curve 1, 2, 3), and light intensity of 20 mW/cm^2; also shown is the threshold exposure time (t').

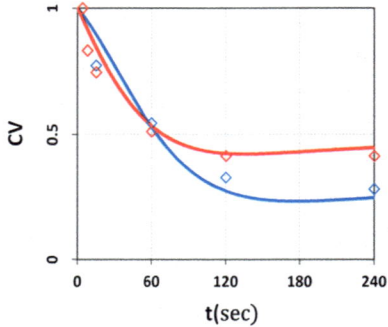

Fig. 6. Measured temporal profiles for cell viability for a fixed light intensity of $I_0 = 50$ mW/cm^2, and Ce6 concentration $C_0 = 0.0031$ and 0.0062 uM, shown by red and green dots; also shown are the calculated curves in red and green, respectively.

Figure 7 shows the measured and the theoretical results for various light intensity at $I_0 = (25, 50, 100, 200)$ mW/cm^2. We note that the theoretical data are based on type-II S function of Eq. (1.b) which is numerically calculated based on the fit effective absorption factor, $A(z,t)$.

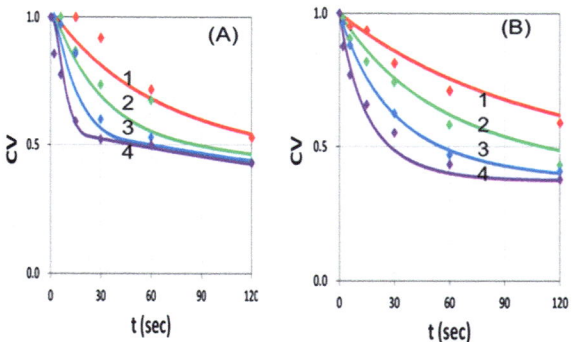

Fig. 7. Same as Fig. 6, but for Ce6 concentration: (A) $C_0 = 0.0031$ uM and (B) 0.0062 uM, for various light intensity at $I_0 = (25, 50, 100, 200)$ mW/cm^2, for curve (1,2,3,4).

3.3   Data Analysis

The measured data shown by Figs. 6 and 7 may be analyzed by our theory as follows. Figure 6 shows that cell viability (CV) is an exponentially deceasing function of the light exposure time (or dose) for a fixed light intensity, and higher PS concentration is more efficient in anti-cancer and has a lower CV. Our theoretical and measured data are comparable to cell viability curves after red-light irradiation of Radachlorin reported in vivo by Klimenko et al. [11], in which their Fig. 5 may be compared with our Fig. 5.

Figure 7 shows that CV, for a fixed Ce6 concentration, is a decreasing function of light intensity, in consistent to our theoretical prediction based on Eq. (1.b), and Figs. 3 and 4, that high intensity kills the cells faster, but has the same steady-state CV as that of low intensity, when the oxygen is completely depleted and Ce6 concentration reaches its steady-state, as shown by Fig. 3(A).

Our empirical modeling demonstrates the following important features:

(i)   Higher light intensity has a faster depletion of oxygen and PS concentration;

(ii)   For the same dose, higher light intensity has a faster rising efficacy, but reach the same steady-state as that of low intensity for type-II PDT (for the case of no external oxygen); in contrast to type-I, in which higher light intensity has lower steady-state efficacy;

(iii) The cell viability (CV) at various conditions are measured and shown in Fig. 3. For a fixed Ce6 concentration, CV is a nonlinear decreasing function of light intensity and exposure time, in consistent to our formula for CV = 1 − Ceff = $\exp(-S2)$.

We should note that the CV and anti-cancer therapy in our in vitro measurements are much less efficient than in vivo having much higher available oxygen from the blood flowing. The anti-cancer efficacy (dominant by type-II mechanism) is limited by the available oxygen and Ce6 in the cell-Ce6-mixed solution. Therefore, it may be enhanced by the resupply of Ce6 and/or external oxygen. The CV reaches its steady-state when oxygen is completely depleted by the light.

4 Conclusions

We have measured the cell viability (CV) in Chlorine e6 (Ce6) solution and under a red LED light exposure at various time and light intensity. The measured data are in consistent with our theoretically predicted features. Anti-cancer efficacy may be enhanced by the resupply of Ce6 and/or external oxygen.

Conflict of Interest. JT Lin is the CEO of New Vision Inc.; KT Chen and HW Liu have no conflict of interest.

References

1. Lin, J.T.: Efficacy S-formula and kinetics of oxygen-mediated (type-II) and non-oxygen-mediated (type-I) corneal cross-linking. Ophthalmol. Res. **8**(1), 1–11 (2018)
2. Lin, J.T., Liu, H.W., Chen, K.T., Cheng, D.C.: Modeling the optimal conditions for improved efficacy and crosslink depth of photo-initiated polymerization. Polymer **11**, 217 (2019). https://doi.org/10.3390/polym11020217
3. Zhu, T.C., Finlay, J.C., Zhou, X., et al.: Macroscopic modeling of the singlet oxygen production during PDT. Proc. SPIE. **6427**, 6427O81–6427O812 (2007)
4. Chen, F.M., Shi, S.: Principles of Tissue Engineering, 4th edn. Elsevier, New York (2014)
5. Pereira, R., Bartolo, P.: Photopolymerizable hydrogels in regenerative medicine and drug delivery. Top. Biomater. 6–28 (2014)
6. Anseth, K.S., Klok, H.A.: Click chemistry in biomaterials, nanomedicine, and drug delivery. Biomacromolecules **17**, 1–3 (2016)
7. Marturano, V., Cerruti, P., Giamberini, M., et al.: Light-responsive polymer micro- and nano-capsules. Polymers **9** (2017). https://doi.org/10.3390/polym9010008
8. Sun, H., Kabb, C.P., Dai, Y., Hill, M.R., Ghiviriga, I., Bapat, A.P., Sumerlin, B.S.: Macromolecular metamorphosis via stimulus-induced transformations of polymer architecture. Nat. Chem. **9**, 817–823 (2018)
9. Qiu, M., Wang, D., Liang, W.Y., Liu, L., Zhang, Y., Chen, X., Sang, D.K., Xing, C., Li, Z., Dong, B., et al.: Novel concept of the smart NIR-light-controlled drug release of black phosphorus nanostructure for cancer therapy. Proc. Natl. Acad. Sci. U.S.A. **115**, 501–506 (2018)
10. Yang, L., Tang, H., Sun, H.: Progress in photo-responsive polypeptide derived nano-assemblies. Micromachines **9**, 296–313 (2018)
11. Klimenko, V.V., Shmakov, S.V., Kaydanov, N.E., et al.: In vitro singlet oxygen threshold dose at PDT with Radachlorin. In: SPIE Proceedings (Optical Society of America, 2017), paper 1041703 (2017)

Investigating the Use of Wearables for Monitoring Circadian Rhythms: A Feasibility Study

Rossana Castaldo[1,2(✉)], Marta Prati[3], Luis Montesinos[1],
Vishwesh Kulkarni[1], Micheal Chappell[1], Helen Byrne[4],
Pasquale Innominato[5], Stephen Hughes[6], and Leandro Pecchia[1]

[1] School of Engineering, University of Warwick, Library Road, Coventry, UK
R.Castaldo.1@warwick.ac.uk
[2] Institute of Advanced Studies, University of Warwick, Coventry, UK
[3] Ingegneria dell'informazione, informatica e statistica,
Università degli Studi di Roma La Sapienza, Rome, Italy
[4] Mathematical Institute, University of Oxford, Oxford, UK
[5] Warwick Medical School, University of Warwick, Coventry, UK
[6] North Wales Clinical Research Centre, Wrexham, UK

Abstract. Circadian rhythms are physiological and behavioural processes that typically recur over 24-h periods.

Researchers show that circadian disruption, a marked break in normal 24-h cycles of circadian rhythms, can cause serious health problems. It could lead to critical illness, cancer, stress, myocardial infarction, diabetes, hypertension and arrhythmias.

Today, circadian rhythms are monitored using blood, salivary and urine hormone tests, such tests are not practical at home and do not provide continuous real-time monitoring. Combining signal processing and artificial intelligence with commercial sensors embedded in smartwatches or clothes that measure physiological and behavioral attributes offers unprecedented and as yet unexplored opportunities to monitor circadian rhythms in real time. This paper presents the initial steps towards the development of a model for real-time monitoring of the circadian rhythms. This model will contribute to transform medicine from primarily intervention-focused to predictive and preventative. Preliminary analysis shows promising results to automatically classify cortisol levels as high or low, based on behavioral and physiological signals monitored by non-invasive wearable sensors.

Keywords: Circadian rhythms · Biomedical signals · Wearable sensors · Machine learning

1 Introduction

"Inner clock adapts our physiology to the dramatically different phases of the day, [...] regulating critical functions such as behavior, hormone levels, sleep, body temperature and metabolism". This phenomenon is known as the biological clock or circadian rhythm [1].

© Springer Nature Switzerland AG 2020
K.-P. Lin et al. (Eds.): ICBHI 2019, IFMBE Proceedings 74, pp. 275–280, 2020.
https://doi.org/10.1007/978-3-030-30636-6_38

Circadian alteration has significant side effects in our life. Among many, it could lead to cardiovascular diseases, cancer and sleep disorders. It can affect lung function, immune function, angiogenesis and many more are significantly influenced by the circadian system, disrupting quality of life [2]. Moreover, recent researches [3] proved that patient with major alterations in circadian cycles are significantly less likely to survive to cancer treatments.

Thus, in order to reduce significant side effects due to circadian alterations also in chronotherapy and chronomedicine, there is the need to develop new methods to determine the state of a person's circadian clock(s) in real-time.

Currently, the methods for circadian measurements are not suitable for continuous and simultaneous monitoring at home. In fact, circadian cycles are measured via laboratory tests (i.e., hormones measured via blood, urine or saliva specimens), which are expensive and not easy to be performed at home. Most recently, actigraphy has been explored for circadian rhythm estimations at home [4]. Nonetheless, benchmark methods are not yet available and non-invasive behavioral (i.e., actigraphy) and physiological monitoring has not been combined yet.

Therefore, the combination of wearable sensors, biomedical signal analysis and machine learning techniques to develop methods and tools to quantify alterations in internal clock could transform medicine from primarily intervention-focused to predictive and preventative.

Several cortisol indices are commonly used in the literature to determine circadian alterations such as amplitude, frequency and phase [5]. In particular, peak-to-trough difference is one of the most used index to assess rhythm alterations [6].

This paper presents a preliminary result from a feasibility study conducted on healthy subjects to identify a model to monitor circadian rhythms (peaks and trough) in real-time using artificial intelligence and unobtrusive wearable behavioral and physiological monitors.

2   Methods and Materials

2.1   Study Participants

8 healthy participants (4 men and 4 women, mean age (SD): 26.2 (3.3) years) in whom no abnormalities were detected by the medical history, were recruited in the study. Baseline characteristics, such as age, height, weight, general health status and use of medications, were collected during a baseline assessment and briefing session. The participants did not report history of heart disease, diabetes, systemic hypertension or hypotension, or sleep-disorders, or consumption of any medication throughout the course of the study, which could alter physiological signals being acquired. They had healthy body mass index (BMI), i.e. between 18.5 and 24.9.

The Biomedical and Scientific Research Ethics Committee of the University of Warwick approved this study (ref. REGO-2018-2205), assuring anonymity and no side effects or possible disadvantages for the participants. All participants were carefully instructed, and informed consent was acquired prior to the experiment. Participants were compensated with a fixed fee.

2.2   Protocol

Participants were asked to wear two different wearable devices for three nights and two consecutive days. The first wearable device, the Zephyr BioPatch, recorded ECG, breathing rate and raw 3-axis accelerations, with a sampling rate of 250 Hz, 18 Hz and 100 Hz respectively. The second one was a wireless data logger, the iButtons, which can be used to obtain a valid measurement of human skin temperature. One iButton was attached to each ankle, and another iButton was attached on each side of the chest, one or two inches below the clavicle in the mid- clavicular line in order to measure distal and proximal body temperature respectively [7]. The temperature sensors took a measurement every 10 min.

In this study, cortisol was used as a marker of circadian rhythm. Participants were instructed on how to take and store saliva samples, so as they could be sent to a specialized laboratory and analyzed for levels of salivary cortisol. Participants were instructed to take a sample immediately upon waking, and then to take further samples every two hours for the rest of the day until they went to bed. Saliva samples were acquired for two consecutive days via Salimetrics® Cortisol Enzyme Immunoassay Kit, which is an immunoassay specifically designed and validated for the quantitative measurement of salivary cortisol. The saliva was collected by the passive drool technique.

For each subject, behavioral and physiological signals were acquired for three nights and two days by wearable devices, and two days' worth of salivary samples were taken.

Participants were asked to report physical activity and food intake [8]. Participants were also asked to complete the Pittsburgh Sleep Quality Index (PSQI) instrument [9] and a consensus sleep diary [10]. The PSQI and sleep diary results were used to compare reported sleep disturbances with alteration in circadian cycles.

All of the participants were asked to maintained ordinary daily schedules during the experiments.

2.3   Data Analysis

The maximum and minimum cortisol levels were obtained for each subject for the two days, and these were labelled respectively as "peak" and "trough". In the cases where the minimum or maximum cortisol level for a period appeared in more than one measurement, then each measurement was also labelled.

Since physical exercise can greatly affect cortisol levels [11], only periods of time during which there were similar levels of activity were considered. For each peak and trough, a window of two hours around the time of the saliva measurement was taken. Within each window of time, activity level and posture were evaluated. The activity as reported from the Zephyr BioPatch represents a measure of second- to-second activity and is sensitive to small movements. In order to reduce this sensitivity, the signal was smoothed using a moving average, with a sample window of 60 s. This smoothed activity, in essence, represents minute-to-minute activity.

In order to control for activity and posture in the two hours window around each peak or trough, only times when activity was less than 0.2 (which corresponds to a level of activity less intense than walking) and the posture was between $-20°$ and $20°$ (which corresponds to times when the chest was roughly upright) were considered.

For each selected window of time, distal and proximal body temperature were also considered. Distal body temperature was calculated as the mean of all measurements from ankle temperature sensors during the selected window of time. Proximal body temperature was calculated as the mean of all measurements from the clavicle temperature sensors during the selected window of time.

For each selected window of time, the RR interval time-series was extracted from ECG records using an automatic QRS detector, WQRS, available in the PhysioNet's toolkit [12]. QRS review and correction was performed using PhysioNet's WAVE. The fraction of total RR intervals labelled as normal-to-normal (NN) intervals was computed as NN/RR ratio. NN/RR ratio was then used to measure the reliability of the data. Records with NN/RR ratio less than 90% threshold were excluded from the analysis. Heart Rate Variability (HRV) analysis was performed on 5 min excerpts using Kubios (version premium) [13]. Time and frequency-domain features were analyzed according to international guidelines [14], while non-linear measures were analyzed as described in [15]. Frequency domain features were extracted from power spectrum estimated with autoregressive (AR) model methods [13]. Finally, 20 HRV features were extracted and examined.

2.4   Statistical Analysis and Classification

Given that HRV features were found non-normally distributed, Median (MD), Median Absolute Deviation (MAD) and interquartile range (IQR) (i.e., non-parametric descriptors) were computed for each repetition. The non-parametric Wilcoxon Signed-Rank Test was used to appraise statistical differences of HRV features and temperature variation between the "peak" and "trough" of cortisol measures.

In order to optimize the performance of the machine learning models, the number of features should be limited by the number of instances of the event to detect (in this instance, a peak or trough in cortisol levels). Furthermore, a reduction in the number of features greatly simplifies the medical interpretation of any results achieved. Therefore, the features selection was performed using relevance and redundancy analysis as described in [16]. Training of the machine-learning models (including the algorithm parameter tuning) was performed using a leave-one-outcross-validation approach on 6 participants. Binary classification performance measures were adopted according to the standards reported in [15]. Five different machine-learning methods were used to train, validate and test the classifiers (SVM, MLP, IBK, RF and LDA); the model was chosen as the classifier achieving the highest Area under the Curve (AUC), which is a reliable estimator of both sensitivity and specificity rates. The model was then tested on the remaining 2 participants.

3   Results and Conclusion

Preliminary analysis shows promising results to automatically detect cortisol levels as high or low (peaks or troughs), based on HRV and temperature data extracted during periods where activity and posture are controlled for. Some moderately successful classifiers were produced. Random Forest outperformed the other classifiers achieving 78% AUC and 73% overall accuracy. These results provide encouragement that such a protocol may be successful with further refinement, and wearable devices (through the measurement of HRV) may indeed be useful in the real-time monitoring of circadian rhythm.

Acknowledgment. We acknowledge the EPSRC-funded grant under the Cyclops Healthcare Network. RC thanks the Institute of Advanced studies at the University of Warwick.

Conflict of Interest. The authors declare that they have no conflict of interest.

References

1. Van Laake, L.W., Lüscher, T.F., Young, M.E.: The circadian clock in cardiovascular regulation and disease: lessons from the nobel prize in physiology or medicine 2017. Eur. Heart J. **39**, 2326–2329 (2017)
2. Eckle, T.: Health impact and management of a disrupted circadian rhythm and sleep in critical illnesses. Curr. Pharm. Des. **21**(24), 3428 (2015)
3. Lévi, F., Okyar, A., Dulong, S., Innominato, P.F., Clairambault, J.: Circadian timing in cancer treatments. Ann. Rev. Pharm. Toxicol. **50**, 377–421 (2010)
4. Smith, M.T., et al.: Use of actigraphy for the evaluation of sleep disorders and circadian rhythm sleep-wake disorders: an American Academy of Sleep Medicine clinical practice guideline. J. Clin. Sleep Med. **14**(07), 1231–1237 (2018)
5. Dorn, L.D., Lucke, J.F., Loucks, T.L., Berga, S.L.: Salivary cortisol reflects serum cortisol: analysis of circadian profiles. Ann. Clin. Biochem. **44**(3), 281–284 (2007)
6. Mormont, M., Levi, F.: Circadian-system alterations during cancer processes: a review. Int. J. Cancer **70**(2), 241–247 (1997)
7. Hasselberg, M.J., McMahon, J., Parker, K.: The validity, reliability, and utility of the iButton® for measurement of body temperature circadian rhythms in sleep/wake research. Sleep Med. **14**(1), 5–11 (2013)
8. de Assis, M.A.A., Kupek, E., Nahas, M.V., Bellisle, F.: Food intake and circadian rhythms in shift workers with a high workload. Appetite **40**(2), 175–183 (2003)
9. Buysse, D.J., Reynolds III, C.F., Monk, T.H., Hoch, C.C., Yeager, A.L., Kupfer, D.J.: Quantification of subjective sleep quality in healthy elderly men and women using the Pittsburgh Sleep Quality Index (PSQI). Sleep **14**(4), 331–338 (1991)
10. Carney, C.E., et al.: The consensus sleep diary: standardizing prospective sleep self-monitoring. Sleep **35**(2), 287–302 (2012)
11. Budde, H., Machado, S., Ribeiro, P., Wegner, M.: The cortisol response to exercise in young adults. Front. Behav. Neurosci. **9**, 13 (2015)

12. Goldberger, A.L., et al.: Physiobank, physiotoolkit, and physionet components of a new research resource for complex physiologic signals. Circulation **101**(23), e215–e220 (2000)
13. Tarvainen, M.P., Niskanen, J.-P.: Kubios HRV user's guide. In: Biosignal Analysis and Medical Imaging Group (BSAMIG), Department of Physics University of Kuopio (2013)
14. Force, T.: Heart rate variability guidelines: Standards of measurement, physiological interpretation, and clinical use. Eur. Heart J. **17**, 354–381 (1996)
15. Melillo, P., Bracale, M., Pecchia, L.: Nonlinear heart rate variability features for real-life stress detection. Case study: students under stress due to university examination (in English). BioMed. Eng. OnLine **10**(1), 1–13 (2011). Article no. 96
16. Castaldo, R., Melillo, P., Izzo, R., Luca, N.D., Pecchia, L.: Fall prediction in hypertensive patients via short-term HRV analysis. IEEE J. Biomed. Health Inf. **21**(2), 399–406 (2017)

Quantitative Reduction in the Dynamic Endothelial Function on Foot Microcirculation in Patients with Diabetes Mellitus

Jia-Jung Wang[1]([✉]), Xuan-Hao Su[1], G. Hung[1], Hsin-Yen He[1], and Wei-Kung Tseng[2]

[1] Department of Biomedical Engineering, I-Shou University, Yida Road, Kaohsiung, Taiwan
wangjj@isu.edu.tw
[2] Department of Cardiology, E-Da Hospital, Kaohsiung, Taiwan

Abstract. Microvascular perfusion on the foot bottom in 39 subjects (Control group: 23 healthy participants; Patient group: 16 patients with diabetes mellitus) was measured with the laser Doppler flowmetry (LDF). Each subject was requested to perform a non-invasive provocation of 37 min, including 8-min baseline, 3-min ankle occlusion, 6-min post-occlusive reactive hyperemia (PORH), and 20-min heating (42 °C) period. By using the wavelet transform, we calculated the power spectral densities (PSD), on one-minute basis, of the 37-min LDF signal. The results indicated that the PSD corresponding to the endothelial NO-independent (PSD_{ENDO1}) and NO-dependent (PSD_{ENDO2}) metabolic activities varied with time in both Control and Patient groups. Patient group showed less PSD_{ENDO1} and PSD_{ENDO2} than those in Control group. In summary, endothelial dysfunction in peripheral microcirculation exists in diabetes patients, apparently as compared with healthy participants.

Keywords: Endothelial function · Microcirculation · Diabetes mellitus · Laser Doppler flowmetry

1 Introduction

Microcirculation is the fundamental part of the human cardiovascular system, mainly responsible for transporting oxygen, carbon dioxide and nutrition to all tissues. Long-term insufficient perfusion in peripheral microcirculation will lead to ischemia or necrosis in tissues or organs. It is obvious that abnormality in peripheral microvascular blood flow may show up earlier than the occurrence of cardiovascular disease [1, 2]. Thus, it is necessary and crucial to uncover some useful parameters to help physicians to initially diagnose the microcirculatory dysfunction, particularly for the microvascular endothelial vasodilatation.

It is known that peripheral microvascular blood perfusion is regulated by several possible mechanisms, including the endothelial nitric oxide (NO) -independent metabolic, endothelial NO-dependent metabolic, neurogenic, myogenic, respiratory, and cardiac activities [3–5]. Among them, endothelial NO-independent and –dependent metabolic activities are directly related to the microvascular endothelium. And, it is

© Springer Nature Switzerland AG 2020
K.-P. Lin et al. (Eds.): ICBHI 2019, IFMBE Proceedings 74, pp. 281–287, 2020.
https://doi.org/10.1007/978-3-030-30636-6_39

believed that the endothelium may regulate microcirculatory blood flow in a dynamic manner [6, 7].

Therefore, the aim of the work was to investigate the dynamic endothelial activities in the foot bottom microcirculation during a non-invasive provocation, and to study whether the endothelial NO-independent or NO-dependent metabolic activity makes more contribution to the microvascular blood perfusion in diabetes patients and healthy subjects.

2   Methods

2.1   Subjects

Twenty-three healthy participants (Control group) and sixteen patients with diabetes mellitus (Patient group) were included in the study. The subjects in Control group had no cardiovascular disease, diabetes mellitus, or renal dysfunction. In Patient group, the subjects with diabetes mellitus had neither peripheral arterial occlusion disease nor renal failure.

2.2   Experimental Protocol

The clinical trial was approved by the Institutional Review Board of the E-DA Hospital, Kaohsiung, Taiwan (no. EMRT04105N), and informed consent was obtained from each participant prior to initiation of the study. Every participant in supine position was asked to carry out a non-invasive provocation of 37-min, including 8-min baseline, 3-min ankle occlusion (by an air cuff inflated up to systolic pressure plus 50 mmHg), 6-min post-occlusive reactive hyperemia (PORH), and 20-min heating (42 °C) period [8]. Microcirculatory perfusion on the foot bottom close to the foot thumb was measured with the laser Doppler flowmetry (LDF) (moorVMS-LDF1, Moor Instrument, USA) and the measuring spot was heated using a heater device (moorVMS-HEAT, Moor Instrument, USA). The ambient temperature of the measuring room was controlled at 27 ± 1 °C in the testing procedure.

2.3   Data Analysis

Every one-minute segment of the LDF signals was analyzed by the wavelet transform algorithm, and its mean power spectral density (PSD) during the one minute was calculated. In the study, the mean powder spectral density of frequency bands of 0.005–0.0095 Hz and 0.0095–0.021 in the skin microvascular LDF signals were selected to correspond to the endothelial NO-independent and NO-dependent metabolic activities (PSD_{ENDO1} & PSD_{ENDO2}), respectively [3].

2.4   Statistics

The quantitative PSD are expressed as mean ± SD. To compare the mean PDS between the control and patient groups, 2-tailed paired t-test was used. A p-value of 0.05 or less was considered statistically significant.

3   Results

The basic information of the healthy participants and the diabetes patients was showed in Table 1. Both age and height appeared significant difference between the patient and the control groups. However, other parameters including the body mass index, weight, systolic pressure, diastolic pressure, and heart rate showed no significant difference in the two groups.

Table 1. Basic data of the subjects

Parameter	Control group (N = 23)	Patient group (N = 10)	p value
Age (year)	28 ± 13	66 ± 13	<0.001
Gender	19M/4F	12M/4F	
Height (cm)	171 ± 7	160 ± 7	<0.001
Weight (kg)	68.8 ± 14.4	68.2 ± 10.0	0.907
Body mass index	24.0 ± 5.2	25.9 ± 2.3	0.290
Systolic pressure (mmHg)	115.5 ± 13.5	125.7 ± 15.1	0.055
Diastolic pressure (mmHg)	78.5 ± 8.9	77.3 ± 7.3	0.726
Heart rate (beats/min)	74.6 ± 10.4	6.5 ± 12.7	0.612

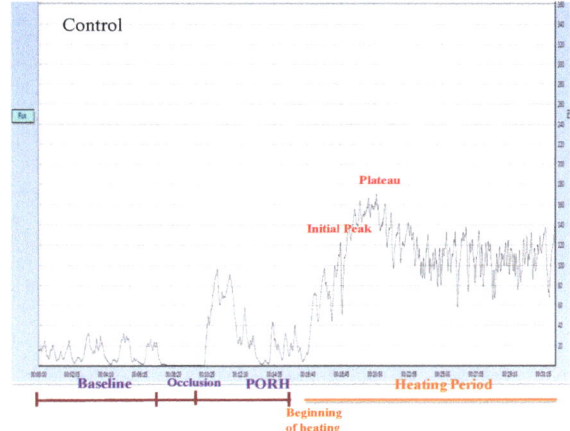

Fig. 1. Typical time course of perfusion signal record measured from a healthy participant

One typical LDF signal from a normal participant and a typical LDF signal from a diabetes patient are displayed in Figs. 1 and 2, respectively. Clearly, the amplitude of the two LDF signals become large immediately after the 3-min occlusion. In the heating period, the LDF signals first approach an initial peak and later a plateau. Also, there are noticeable fluctuations in both microvascular perfusion signals.

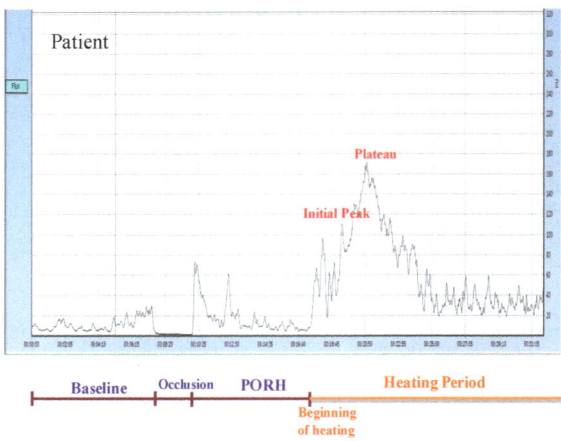

Fig. 2. Typical time course of perfusion signal record measured from a patient with diabetes mellitus

Figures 3 shows the dynamic PSD_{ENDO1} during the baseline, PORH and heating period in Control and Patient groups. The one-minute based PSD_{ENDO1} of the patient group was smaller than that of the control group, although no significant difference existed. Similarly, as compared with Patient group, Control group has greater dynamic PSD_{ENDO2}, as shown in Fig. 4.

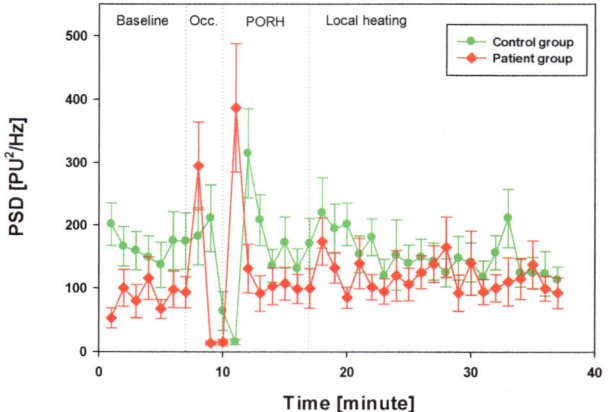

Fig. 3. Dynamic Endothelial NO-independent metabolic activities (PSDENDO1) in the control (N = 23) and patient (N = 16) groups

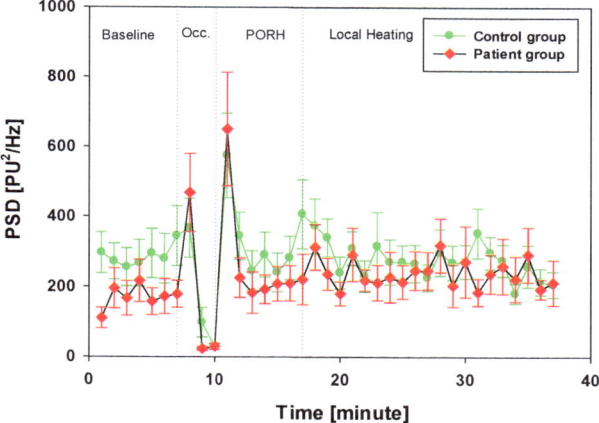

Fig. 4. Dynamic Endothelial NO-dependent metabolic activities (PSDENDO2) in the control (N = 23) and patient (N = 16) groups

For both groups, the one-minute based PSD_{ENDO2} is always significantly greater than PSD_{ENDO1} during the 37-min non-invasive provocation, as shown in Figs. 5 and 6.

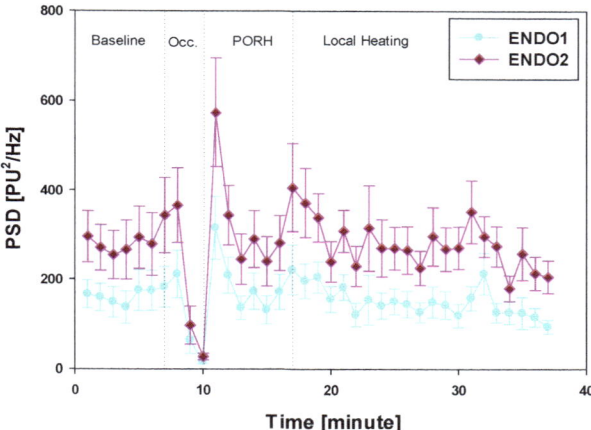

Fig. 5. Comparison between the endothelial NO-independent (PSDENDO1) and the NO-dependent (PSDENDO2) activities in Control group (N = 23)

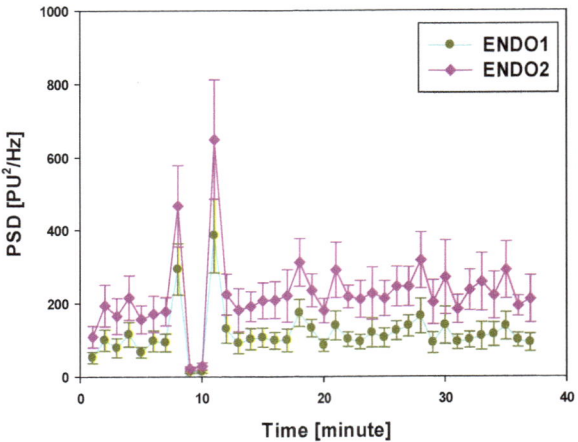

Fig. 6. Comparison between the endothelial NO-independent (PSDENDO1) and the NO-dependent (PSDENDO2) activities in Patient group (N = 16)

4   Discussion

Through the frequency-domain analysis of LDF signals, the PSD of the specific frequency bands that relate closely to microvascular endothelial function is found to vary with time in both healthy diabetes subjects. This indicates that the endothelium may dynamically modulate the microcirculatory blood flow.

Since PSD_{ENDO2} is always greater than PSD_{ENDO1} in the skin microcirculation, it means that the endothelial NO-dependent activity plays a more important role in regulating microcirculatory perfusion than the endothelial NO-independent activity.

In the study, we find that the patient group shows lower PSD_{ENDO2} and PSD_{ENDO1}. As a result, patients with diabetes mellitus have impaired endothelial function in peripheral microcirculation. This is consistent with previous investigations [9, 10]. Furthermore, both PSD_{ENDO2} and PSD_{ENDO1} may become helpful indicators for examining the degree of severity in peripheral microcirculation in diabetes patients.

5   Conclusions

Separate contribution of the endothelial NO-independent and NO-dependent metabolic activities to the microvascular perfusion is explored in healthy participants and diabetes patients. The endothelial NO-dependent activity appears more significant than the endothelial NO-independent activity in both the control and diabetes groups. Also, the patients with diabetes mellitus have decreased endothelial function in modulating peripheral microvascular blood perfusion, as compared with healthy subjects.

Acknowledgment. The authors would like to express thanks to the staffs in the Department of Cardiology, I-Da Hospital, Taiwan, for their help and support in performing clinical trials. Also, thanks go to the Ministry of Science and Technology, Taiwan, for its funding support (MOST 105-2221-E-214 -012 -MY3).

Conflict of Interest. The authors declare that they have no conflict of interest in the paper.

References

1. Rousit, M., Cracowski, J.L.: Non-invasive assessment of skin microvascular function in humans: an insight into methods. Microcirculation **19**, 47–64 (2012)
2. Rossi, M., Carpi, A., Di Maria, C., et al.: Spectral analysis of laser Doppler skin blood flow oscillations in human essential arterial hypertension. Microvasc. Res. **72**, 34–41 (2006)
3. Mizeva, I., Frick, P., Podtaev, S.: Relationship of oscillating and average components of laser Doppler flowmetry signal. J. Biomed. Opt. **21**, 85002 (2016). https://doi.org/10.1117/1. JBO.21.8.085002
4. Cracowski, J.L., Minson, C.T., Salvat-Melis, M., et al.: Methodological issues in the assessment of skin microvascular endothelial function in humans. Trends Pharmacol. Sci. **27**, 503–508 (2006)
5. Roustit, M., Cracowski, J.L.: Assessment of endothelial and neurovascular function in human skin microcirculation. Trends Pharmacol. Sci. **34**, 373–384 (2013). https://doi.org/10. 1016/j.tips.2013.05.007
6. Hodges, G.J., Mallette, M.M., Martin, Z.T., et al.: Effect of sympathetic nerve blockade on low-frequency oscillations of forearm and leg skin blood flow in healthy humans. Microcirculation **24**(7) (2017). https://doi.org/10.1111/micc.12388
7. Mizeva, I., Makovik, I., Dunaev, A., et al.: Analysis of skin blood microflow oscillations in patients with rheumatic diseases. J. Biomed. Opt. **22**, 70501 (2017). https://doi.org/10.1117/ 1.JBO.22.7.070501
8. Iredahl, F., Löfberg, A., Sjöberg, F., et al.: Non-Invasive measurement of skin microvascular response during pharmacological and physiological provocations. PLoS ONE **10**(8), e0133760 (2015). https://doi.org/10.1371/journal.pone.0133760
9. Jonasson, H., Bergstrand, S., Nystrom, F.H., et al.: Skin microvascular endothelial dysfunction is associated with type 2 diabetes independently of microalbuminuria and arterial stiffness. Diab. Vasc. Dis. Res. **14**, 363–371 (2017)
10. Clough, G.F., Kuliga, K.Z., Chipperfield, A.J.: Flow motion dynamics of microvascular blood flow and oxygenation: evidence of adaptive changes in obesity and type 2 diabetes mellitus/insulin resistance. Microcirculation **24**(2) (2017). https://doi.org/10.1111/micc. 12331

Promises and Challenges in the Use of Wearable Sensors and Nonlinear Signal Analysis for Balance and Fall Risk Assessment in Older Adults

Luis Montesinos[1,2]([✉]), Rossana Castaldo[1,3], and Leandro Pecchia[1]

[1] School of Engineering, University of Warwick, Library Road, Coventry, UK
`l.montesinos-silva@warwick.ac.uk`
[2] Escuela de Ingenieria y Ciencias, Tecnologico de Monterrey,
Mexico City, Mexico
[3] Institute of Advanced Study, University of Warwick, Coventry, UK

Abstract. The rise of wearable technologies is enabling novel ways of assessing balance and risk of falling in later life. Wearable inertial sensors are a promising addition to clinical balance assessment tools since they provide an objective and accurate fall risk assessment. Moreover, wearable devices also enable the ambulatory monitoring of physiological and behavioural variables, which can be used to infer health status and health-related behaviours linked to impaired balance and fall risk (e.g. sleep disturbances and poor sleep quality). This situation could potentially expand the prevailing paradigm in fall prevention, from the current one mainly involving the occasional assessment of risk factors to a new paradigm also including the continuous monitoring and detection of short-lived factors that might result in an imminent fall. Additionally, the diffusion of the dynamical systems theory and methods within the medical research community is inspiring a new approach to the study of ageing and balance in older adults. In particular, nonlinear signal analysis methods could potentially provide with further information on the underlying control mechanisms in ageing and produce more sensitive measures of fall risk. However, there are several challenges in the adoption of these devices and methods, which still preclude a firm conclusion on their clinical value. This paper summarises three studies performed to address some of these challenges and distils the lessons learnt from them. Collectively, the findings of this research confirm that these sensors and methods could improve currents tools and practices for balance and fall risk assessment, and provides some insights concerning their optimal use.

Keywords: Wearable sensors · Nonlinear signal analysis · Balance · Fall risk · Fall prevention

© Springer Nature Switzerland AG 2020
K.-P. Lin et al. (Eds.): ICBHI 2019, IFMBE Proceedings 74, pp. 288–295, 2020.
https://doi.org/10.1007/978-3-030-30636-6_40

1   Introduction

Balance is a crucial ability for successfully performing the activities of daily life. This ability emerges from the complex integration of sensory, motor and control systems. Namely, the visual, vestibular, somatosensory, musculoskeletal and central nervous systems [1]. Impairment in any of these systems can result in a balance control deficit. Specific medical conditions, the progressive decline of function in the course of healthy ageing or some behavioural factors (e.g. use of multiple medications) may cause such impairment [2]. Falls are the most severe consequence of impaired balance, given their high prevalence and impact on morbidity and mortality, as well as in socioeconomic terms [3]. Consequently, a score of researchers and clinicians have made great efforts in trying to gain an understanding of balance control and in developing tools to assess its status at any point in time [1].

The rise of wearable technologies is enabling novel ways of assessing balance and the risk of falling in older adults. In particular, wearable inertial sensors represent a promising complement to clinical balance assessment tools. By providing detailed information on the timing and kinematics of functional tasks (e.g. walking), they have the potential to provide an objective and accurate fall risk assessment.

Moreover, wearable technologies are also enabling the continuous monitoring of physiological and behavioural variables (e.g. heart rate and physical activity), which can be used to infer health status and health-related behaviours linked to impaired balance and increased risk of falling [4]. This situation can potentially expand the prevailing paradigm in fall prevention, from the current one focusing on the occasional assessment of risk factors and changes in the balance control system to a new paradigm including also the continuous monitoring and detection of short-lived factors that might result in an imminent fall (e.g. sleep quantity and quality).

Furthermore, the diffusion of the dynamical systems theory and methods within the medical research community has inspired a new approach to the study of ageing and balance in older adults [5]. Various quantitative descriptors of nonlinear dynamics have been put forward for the analysis of balance data (e.g. entropy measures). These descriptors can potentially provide with further information on the underlying control mechanisms in ageing and represent more sensitive indicators of fall risk.

However, there are several challenges in the adoption of wearable sensors and nonlinear signal analysis methods for the assessment of balance and fall risk. These challenges need to be tackled in order to prove the clinical value of these devices and methods. This paper summarises three studies performed to address some of these challenges and distils the lessons learnt from them.

1.1   Wearable Inertial Sensors for Fall Risk Assessment and Prediction in Older Adults

Wearable inertial sensors are microelectronic devices integrating accelerometers and gyroscopes. Some studies have used these sensors to produce instrumented versions of clinical balance assessment tools, in order to provide objective and accurate indicators of balance problems and fall risk [6]. However, the variety in sensor placements, movement tasks and measured variables has precluded a consensus on their clinical relevance [7].

This study aimed to synthesise and analyse the empirical evidence regarding the use of wearable inertial sensors for fall risk assessment and prediction in older adults (over 60 years), in order to identify the optimal sensor-based testing protocol (i.e. sensor placement, movement task and measured variables).

1.2   Approximate Entropy and Sample Entropy in Force Plate-Based Human Balance Evaluation

Balance control in standing is achieved by continually reconfiguring ground reaction forces under the feet to counteract the movements of the body's centre of mass. The central point of application of those reaction forces is called the centre of pressure (CoP). CoP displacement is one of the most popular techniques for measuring balance in standing [1].

CoP excursions are usually characterised using some time- and frequency-domain measures (e.g. amplitude and median frequency of the CoP oscillations). However, these measures are not sensitive to structural variations in CoP excursions produced by the nonlinearities of the balance control system.

Approximate entropy (ApEn) and sample entropy (SampEn) have been put forward as a way to quantify the level of regularity in CoP time-series, a descriptor of the nonlinear dynamics of balance control. This study aimed: (1) to determine the ability of ApEn and SampEn to discriminate between non-fallers and fallers; and, (2) to determine the optimal input parameters needed for the calculation of ApEn and SampEn in order to reveal the differences between non-fallers and fallers.

1.3   Day-to-Day Variations in Sleep Quality and Balance

Since sleep disturbances and poor sleep quality have been linked with future risk of falling [8, 9], continuous sleep monitoring could be relevant for fall prevention. This study investigated the associations between day-to-day variations in sleep quality measured via wearable devices and balance in standing. Namely, this study investigated: (1) the potential use of wearable devices for monitoring day-to-day variations in sleep quantity and quality; and, (2) the sensitivity of the balance control system to day-to-day variations in sleep quality.

2   Methods and Materials

2.1   Wearable Inertial Sensors for Fall Risk Assessment and Prediction in Older Adults

A systematic review and meta-analysis of relevant studies were performed. Namely, studies that used wearable inertial sensors for discriminating fallers from non-fallers were systematically reviewed. Standard methods for the analysis of categorical data were used to identify optimal combinations of sensor placement, movement task and measured variables. Additionally, standard methods for the meta-analysis of continuous variables were used to identify significant features for the discrimination between fallers and non-fallers. A detailed description of the methods used in this study can be found elsewhere [10].

2.2 Approximate Entropy and Sample Entropy in Force Plate-Based Human Balance Evaluation

A public dataset of CoP time-series was used [11]. ApEn (m, r, N) and SampEn (m, r, N) were calculated for 72 different input parameter combinations (m: subseries length, r: tolerance and N: data length). Subjects were grouped in young adults (age < 60, n = 85), and older adults (age $\geq$ 60) with (n = 18) and without (n = 56) falls in the last year. The ability of ApEn and SampEn to discriminate between groups was investigated with a mixed ANOVA. The sensitivity of ApEn and SampEn to input parameters was investigated with a three-way ANOVA.

Additionally, five linear measures of CoP displacement were also computed as described elsewhere [6]: total length, amplitude, standard deviation, mean velocity, total mean velocity and area. These measures were computed in order to compare their ability to discriminate between groups to that of ApEn and SampEn.

A detailed description of the methods used in this study can be found elsewhere [12].

2.3 Day-to-Day Variations in Sleep Quality and Balance

Study participants underwent in-home sleep and lab-based balance assessment for two consecutive nights and days, respectively. Sleep assessment was performed using: (1) a wearable device to collect electrocardiography (ECG) and chest actigraphy (3D accelerations) data during sleep, and; (2) a sleep diary. Balance testing was performed via foot CoP displacement using a pair of instrumented insoles. Sleep quantity and quality were characterised by: (1) sleep parameters extracted from the sleep diary; (2) activity level measures computed from 3D body accelerations; and, (3) heart rate variability measures computed from the ECG recordings. Three CoP displacement measures characterised balance: area, amplitude and standard deviation. Inter-session differences for all these measures were investigated using suitable paired statistical tests [13].

3 Results and Discussion

3.1 Wearable Inertial Sensors for Fall Risk Assessment and Prediction in Older Adults

Thirteen studies out of 481 database records were included in the review and meta-analysis. The most common sensor placements were the lower back, shins and feet. The more frequent movement tasks were unperturbed standing, walking, and getting up from a chair and sitting down (i.e. sit-to-stand/stand-to-sit transitions). Ninety-three distinct measured variables were identified in the selected studies, which were categorised in linear acceleration, angular velocity, spatial, temporal, frequency and non-linear measures.

Altogether, the results of the data analysis suggest the instrumented Timed Up and Go test [14] is a suitable tool for discriminating non-fallers and fallers, provided that the inertial sensors are placed on the shins and angular velocity, temporal (e.g. total time and step time) and spatial (e.g. number of steps) measures are computed.

Additionally, some studies stood out for their novel approach to the problem. In particular, the studies by Toebes *et al.* [15] and Riva *et al.* [16] found significant associations between fall risk and nonlinear descriptors of gait dynamics (e.g. the maximum Lyapunov exponent, multiscale entropy and recurrence quantification analysis). Moreover, Rispens *et al.* [17] and van Schooten *et al.* [18, 19] found significant associations between fall risk and ambulatory gait measures.

3.2   Approximate Entropy and Sample Entropy in Force Plate-Based Human Balance Evaluation

A significant three-way interaction between m, r and N confirmed the sensitivity of ApEn and SampEn to the input parameters. However, SampEn showed more consistent behaviour over different parameter combinations.

Moreover, ApEn and SampEn exhibited a higher sensitivity to differences between groups than linear measures. Indeed, ApEn and SampEn were able to discriminate between older adults with and without falls in the last 12 months, whereas linear measures were not. In other words, while non-fallers and fallers exhibited commensurable CoP displacements regarding magnitude (i.e. total length, amplitude and area), variability (i.e. standard deviation) and velocity, they manifested differences in CoP time-series structure (more specifically, in regularity). It suggests that fallers suffer from balance impairments of a different nature to those produced by normal ageing.

Additionally, SampEn exhibited a higher sensitivity to differences between groups than ApEn. These differences were mostly observed for CoP time-series in the anterior-posterior direction with a duration of 60-s ($N = 1200$ data points). Importantly, those differences were observed for specific combinations of m and r, highlighting the importance of an adequate selection of input parameters.

Altogether, these results suggest that future studies should favour SampEn over ApEn and longer time-series (≥ 60 s) over shorter ones (e.g. 30 s). The use of parameter combinations such as SampEn ($m = \{4, 5\}$, $r = \{0.25, 0.3, 0.35\}$) is recommended.

3.3   Day-to-Day Variations in Sleep Quality and Balance

Twenty volunteers (12 females and 8 males; age: 28.8 ± 5.7 years, body mass index: 23.4 ± 3.4 kg/m^2, resting heart rate: 63.1 ± 8.7 bpm) with no history of sleep disorders or balance impairments participated in the study. Six participants showed no variation in sleep quality over two consecutive nights, whereas 14 participants showed a variation in sleep quality over two consecutive nights. Participants with a day-to-day deterioration in sleep quantity and quality (i.e. decreased duration and increased fragmentation, increased nocturnal activity and decreased heart rate variability) also exhibited significant changes in balance (i.e. larger CoP area, amplitude and standard deviation). Conversely, subjects with no significant alterations in sleep quantity and quality showed no significant changes in CoP displacements.

Altogether, the results of this study suggest that wearable devices can be used for monitoring day-to-day variations in sleep quantity and quality. Moreover, these results also suggest that the balance control system is sensitive to day-to-day variations in sleep quantity and quality.

4   Conclusions

Wearable sensors and nonlinear signal analysis methods are enabling novel ways of assessing balance and fall risk in older adults. However, their adoption for research and clinical practice poses some challenges. The studies summarised in this paper addressed some of those challenges and provided some insights concerning their optimal use. Collectively, the findings of this research confirm that these sensors and methods can improve currents tools and practices in balance and fall risk assessment.

Wearable inertial sensors offer the means for developing instrumented versions of clinical balance assessment tools. However, selecting a suitable combination of sensor placement, movement task and measured variable is crucial for discriminating between subjects at high and low risk of falling. Moreover, there is evidence suggesting that these sensors can be used for the ambulatory assessment of fall risk.

Moreover, wearable devices offers the means for continuously monitoring physiological and behavioural variables, which can be used to infer outcomes linked to impaired balance and increased risk of falling. This research proved that these devices could be used to detect day-to-day variations in sleep quantity and quality, which in turn shown associations with variations in balance. This situation can potentially expand the prevailing paradigm in fall prevention, from the current one focusing on the occasional assessment of risk factors and changes in the balance control system to a new paradigm including also the continuous monitoring and detection of short-lived factors that might result in an imminent fall.

Finally, nonlinear methods proved to be more sensitive to group differences in balance (non-fallers versus fallers) than linear measures. However, the suitable selection of the input parameters required for their computation proved to be of paramount importance to achieve favourable results.

Acknowledgement. The work of L. Montesinos was supported by a scholarship awarded by CONACyT, the Mexican National Council for Science and Technology (409248). The work of R. Castaldo was supported by the University of Warwick through the Institute of Advanced Study's Early Career Fellowship and an EPSRC IAA grant (EP/R511808/1).

Conflict of Interest. The authors declare that they have no conflict of interest.

References

1. van Dieën, J.H., Pijnappels, M.: Balance control in older adults. In: Barbieri, F.A., Vitório, R. (eds.) Locomotion and Posture in Older Adults, pp. 237–262. Springer, Cham (2017)
2. Ambrose, A.F., Paul, G., Hausdorff, J.M.: Risk factors for falls among older adults: a review of the literature. Maturitas **75**, 51–61 (2013)
3. Peel, N.M.: Epidemiology of falls in older age. Can. J. Aging Rev. Can. Vieil. **30**, 7–19 (2011)
4. Melillo, P., Castaldo, R., Sannino, G., Orrico, A., De Pietro, G., Pecchia, L.: Wearable technology and ECG processing for fall risk assessment, prevention and detection. In: 2015 37th Annual International Conference of the IEEE, Engineering in Medicine and Biology Society (EMBC), pp. 7740–7743. IEEE (2015)
5. Moraes, R., Mauerberg-de Castro, E.: Complex systems approach to the study of posture and locomotion in older people. In: Barbieri, F.A., Vitório, R. (eds.) Locomotion and Posture in Older Adults, pp. 3–20. Springer, Cham (2017)
6. Howcroft, J., Kofman, J., Lemaire, E.D.: Review of fall risk assessment in geriatric populations using inertial sensors. J. NeuroEng. Rehabil. **10**, 91 (2013)
7. Sun, R., Sosnoff, J.J.: Novel sensing technology in fall risk assessment in older adults: a systematic review. BMC Geriatr **18**, 14 (2018)
8. Stone, K.L., Blackwell, T.L., Ancoli-Israel, S., Cauley, J.A., Redline, S., Marshall, L.M., Ensrud, K.E.: Sleep disturbances and risk of falls in older community-dwelling men: the outcomes of sleep disorders in older men (MrOS Sleep) Study. J. Am. Geriatr. Soc. **62**, 299–305 (2014). For the Osteoporotic Fractures in Men Study Group
9. Takada, S., Yamamoto, Y., Shimizu, S., Kimachi, M., Ikenoue, T., Fukuma, S., Onishi, Y., Takegami, M., Yamazaki, S., Ono, R., Sekiguchi, M., Otani, K., Kikuchi, S., Konno, S., Fukuhara, S.: Association between subjective sleep quality and future risk of falls in older people: results from LOHAS. J. Gerontol. Ser. A **73**, 1205–1211 (2018)
10. Montesinos, L., Castaldo, R., Pecchia, L.: Wearable inertial sensors for fall risk assessment and prediction in older adults: a systematic review and meta-analysis. IEEE Trans. Neural Syst. Rehabil. Eng. **26**, 573–582 (2018)
11. Santos, D.A.D., Duarte, M.: A public data set of human balance evaluations (2016)
12. Montesinos, L., Castaldo, R., Pecchia, L.: On the use of approximate entropy and sample entropy with centre of pressure time-series. J. NeuroEng. Rehabil. **15**, 116 (2018)
13. Montesinos, L., Castaldo, R., Cappuccio, F.P., Pecchia, L.: Day-to-day variations in sleep quality affect standing balance in healthy adults. Sci. Rep. **8**, 17504 (2018)
14. Podsiadlo, D., Richardson, S.: The timed "Up & Go": a test of basic functional mobility for frail elderly persons. J. Am. Geriatr. Soc. **39**, 142–148 (1991)
15. Toebes, M.J.P., Hoozemans, M.J.M., Furrer, R., Dekker, J., van Dieën, J.H.: Local dynamic stability and variability of gait are associated with fall history in elderly subjects. Gait Posture **36**, 527–531 (2012)
16. Riva, F., Toebes, M.J.P., Pijnappels, M., Stagni, R., van Dieën, J.H.: Estimating fall risk with inertial sensors using gait stability measures that do not require step detection. Gait Posture **38**, 170–174 (2013)
17. Rispens, S.M., van Schooten, K.S., Pijnappels, M., Daffertshofer, A., Beek, P.J., van Dieën, J.H.: Identification of fall risk predictors in daily life measurements: gait characteristics' reliability and association with self-reported fall history. Neurorehabil. Neural Repair **29**, 54–61 (2015)

18. van Schooten, K.S., Pijnappels, M., Rispens, S.M., Elders, P.J.M., Lips, P., van Dieën, J.H.: Ambulatory fall-risk assessment: amount and quality of daily-life gait predict falls in older adults. J. Gerontol. A Biol. Sci. Med. Sci. **70**, 608–615 (2015)
19. van Schooten, K.S., Pijnappels, M., Rispens, S.M., Elders, P.J., Lips, P., Daffertshofer, A., Beek, P.J., van Dieen, J.H.: Daily-life gait quality as predictor of falls in older people: a 1-year prospective cohort study. PLoS ONE **11**, e0158623 (2016)

Arrhythmia Detection Using Curve Fitting and Machine Learning

Po-Chuan Chiu$^{(\boxtimes)}$, Han-Chien Cheng, and Shu-Nung Yao

Department of Electrical Engineering,
National Taipei University, Taipei, Taiwan (ROC)
ntpu410187026@gmail.com, snyao@gm.ntpu.edu.tw

Abstract. Electrocardiogram (ECG) is a graph that depicts blood circulation through the heart. ECG is also used for depicting the state of health of an individual and is helpful in disease diagnosis. The target of this work is to check the application of curve fitting on ECG signals based on the Fourier series analysis method. When ECG signals are approximated by the Fourier series model, the fitting for the cardiac cycle is used for judging arrhythmias. The data used here was sourced from the MIT-BIH arrhythmia database, and only ECG recordings were utilized for the purpose of this study. The study has presented efficient methods for signal identification with the help of fitting parameters and ECG classification.

Keywords: ECG · Fourier series · Noise removal · Curve fitting

1 Introduction

Physicians have to face a large number of patients daily with very limited time at their disposal to attend these patients. Hence, the methods with fast and accurate judgment cardiac status play a vital role in diagnosis for arrhythmia in the early stages. Arrhythmia is a general term for heartbeat abnormalities which contains a variety of abnormal patterns. These patterns can be classified into three categories: heart rhythm, chronic heart rhythm, and irregular contraction. In general, heartbeat above 100 times per minute in adults represents an over high heart rate and below 60 times per minute refers to an over slow heart rate. The rate at which heartbeat accelerates is slightly faster than that of exhaling. In [1], it has been observed that the use of the Fourier series can construct the original status precisely since the result of an electrocardiogram (ECG) signal is periodic. Recent researches tend to compare the ECG signals with a normal sinus rhythm in order to identify the morphology differences between each heartbeat, time interval, and waveform. QRS waves of the ECG signal characterize the activity of the heart. Hence, it is the most obvious section for tracing disease visually. Various methods of preprocessing ECG signals and features extracting in QRS waves have been addressed in [2–5] which can be used to achieve high accuracy classification in arrhythmia.

© Springer Nature Switzerland AG 2020
K.-P. Lin et al. (Eds.): ICBHI 2019, IFMBE Proceedings 74, pp. 296–303, 2020.
https://doi.org/10.1007/978-3-030-30636-6_41

2   Methodology

Most of the ECG signals used for this paper are from MIT-BIH arrhythmia database. Different methods are used for judging ECG signals and to identify the existence of arrhythmia. These methods are preprocessing ECG data, and extracting features.

The flow chart as shown in Fig. 1 interprets how to perform data preprocessing of ECG, features extraction, and arrhythmia detection [4]. The proposed method is to scrapbook the raw ECG data as well as contrast the differences. With the help of this approach, we are able to conclude if the patient is suffering from arrhythmia or not.

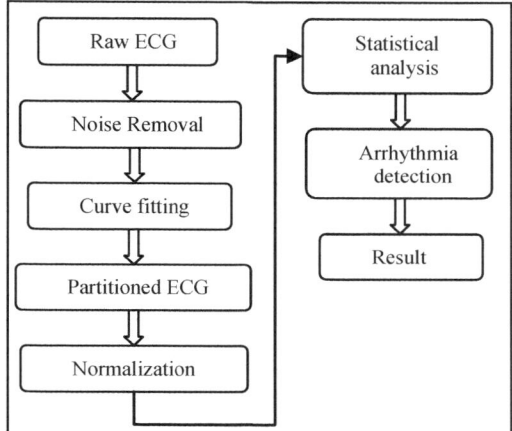

Fig. 1. Diagram of ECG signal processing and arrhythmia interpretation

2.1   Preprocessing

The mathematicians found that periodic functions can be represented as the sum of sinusoidal functions and cosine functions. In this research, we have calculated the coefficients and frequency of Fourier series which were based on the fitting algorithm [6]:

$$f(t) = A_0 + \sum_{n=1}^{N} A_n \cdot cos\left(\frac{2\pi nt}{T}\right) + B_n \cdot sin\left(\frac{2\pi nt}{T}\right), \tag{1}$$

where $t = t_1, t_2, \ldots, t_K$ is the time index. A_0, A_n and B_n are the Fourier coefficients, n means the order of Fourier series, T is the period.

In software build-in fitting function, Fourier series can only be expanded into the eighth order. Accordingly, a normal equation is adopted which can extend the orders easily. Figure 2 shows the original ECG signal and simulated curve, the former one presents an individual's heartbeats and physiological activities, such as slightly respiratory noise, the latter appears ideal trend of the former ECG. Because common electrodes introduce noises caused by loose contact, motion artifact and baseline drift, moving average (MA) was used to recover the original appearance of ECG [7].

$$
\begin{bmatrix}
1 & \cos\left(\frac{2\pi t_1}{T}\right) & \sin\left(\frac{2\pi t_1}{T}\right) & \cdots & \sin\left(\frac{2\pi N t_1}{T}\right) \\
1 & \cos\left(\frac{2\pi t_2}{T}\right) & \sin\left(\frac{2\pi t_2}{T}\right) & \cdots & \sin\left(\frac{2\pi N t_2}{T}\right) \\
\vdots & \vdots & \vdots & \vdots & \vdots \\
1 & \cos\left(\frac{2\pi t_K}{T}\right) & \sin\left(\frac{2\pi t_K}{T}\right) & \cdots & \sin\left(\frac{2\pi N t_K}{T}\right)
\end{bmatrix}
\begin{bmatrix}
A_0 \\ A_1 \\ B_1 \\ \vdots \\ B_N
\end{bmatrix}
=
\begin{bmatrix}
y(t_1) \\ y(t_2) \\ \vdots \\ \vdots \\ y(t_K)
\end{bmatrix}
\tag{2}
$$

$$
\begin{bmatrix}
A_0 \\ A_1 \\ B_1 \\ \vdots \\ B_N
\end{bmatrix}
=
\begin{bmatrix}
1 & \cos\left(\frac{2\pi t_1}{T}\right) & \sin\left(\frac{2\pi t_1}{T}\right) & \cdots & \sin\left(\frac{2\pi N t_1}{T}\right) \\
1 & \cos\left(\frac{2\pi t_2}{T}\right) & \sin\left(\frac{2\pi t_2}{T}\right) & \cdots & \sin\left(\frac{2\pi N t_2}{T}\right) \\
\vdots & \vdots & \vdots & \vdots & \vdots \\
1 & \cos\left(\frac{2\pi t_K}{T}\right) & \cos\left(\frac{2\pi t_K}{T}\right) & \cdots & \sin\left(\frac{2\pi N t_K}{T}\right)
\end{bmatrix}^{-1}
\begin{bmatrix}
y(t_1) \\ y(t_2) \\ \vdots \\ \vdots \\ y(t_K)
\end{bmatrix}
\tag{3}
$$

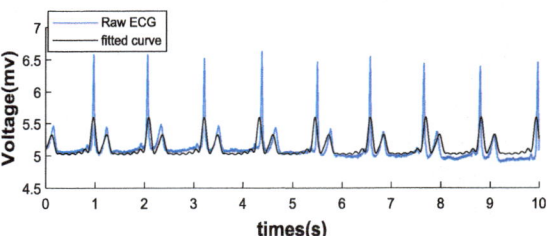

Fig. 2. ECG raw data and fitting curve

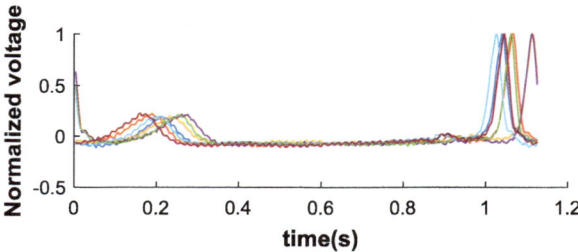

Fig. 3. Overlay of the segment data of normal sinus rhythm

In (2) and (3), $A_{0...N}, B_{1...N}$ are Fourier series' coefficients, $y(t)$ is the original ECG signal. $\mathbf{H}^{-1}$ denotes the inverse matrix of $\mathbf{H}$.

$$\hat{y}(t) = A_0 + \sum_{n=1}^{N} A_n \cdot \cos\left(\frac{2\pi nt}{T}\right) + B_n \cdot \sin\left(\frac{2\pi nt}{T}\right) \tag{4}$$

After rebuilding Fourier series, we obtain the simulative fitting data $\hat{y}(t)$ as shown in (4). The least squares approximation then computes the minimum error of the reconstructed ECG signal by (5), looking for suitable T in (1).

$$D = \min \sum_{t=0}^{T} (y(t) - \hat{y}(t))^2 \tag{5}$$

2.2   Features Extraction

Least squares approximation (5) aids in finding optimal heartbeat cycle by Fourier series' curve fitting that provides a standard for signal segmentation. Overlay and normalization of the segment ECG data which was cut after each cycle passed through. Normal sinus rhythm was expected to exhibit almost coincident figures as shown in Fig. 3, whilst the others abnormal symptoms are in contrast.

In order to calculate the degree of data dispersion, standard deviation (SD) as shown in (6) was applied to find the diversities between segments.

$$SD(t) = \sqrt{\frac{1}{M} \sum_{j=1}^{M} \left(x_j(t) - \mu(t)\right)^2}, \tag{6}$$

where M is the number of segments, μ is the average and x_j is the data point.

Figures 4 and 5 depict the distribution of SD in the black dashed line. The differences of heartbeats were separated from the whole original ECG signal. Based on the standard deviation at the same time point on overlay ECG graph, integration was operated to sum the area trapped from SD and time axis.

$$C_g = \left(\int_0^T SD(t)dt\right)/T \tag{7}$$

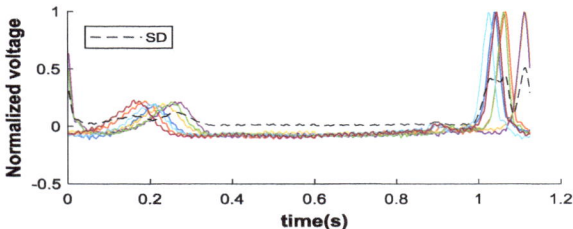

Fig. 4. Standard deviation of normal sinus rhythm

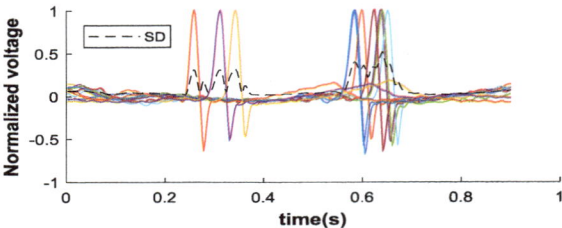

Fig. 5. Standard deviation of abnormal sinus rhythm

In (7), T is a period of a heartbeat, and was decided by the minimum error of the fitting function. C_g represents the average area of the gth subject in a second and was organized in Table 1, which shows the categories of arrhythmia, and average SD area.

Table 1. Extraction values of ECG signal features from ECG data

ECG data	Period	Average SD area
AFIB_1	0.91	0.149
AFIB_3	1.21	0.140
AFIB_6	1.35	0.154
AFIB_8	0.83	0.112
AFL_2	0.44	0.234
AFL_5	1.04	0.203
AFL_6	1.21	0.149
AFL_8	1.35	0.214
APB_1	0.83	0.159
APB_4	0.69	0.232
APB_5	0.84	0.139
APB_7	0.56	0.257
NSR_1	0.77	0.072
NSR_3	0.71	0.089
NSR_6	0.86	0.077
NSR_8	0.85	0.066
NSR_10	0.71	0.100
NSR_13	0.7	0.054
NSR_14	1.13	0.057
NSR_16	1.01	0.065
NSR_17	0.75	0.054
NSR_20	0.69	0.051
NSR_21	1.21	0.055
NSR_23	1.12	0.067

2.3 Arrhythmia Detection

There are 48 samples containing normal sinus rhythm (NSR), atrial flutter (AFL), atrial fibrillation (AFIB), atrial premature beats (APB), and taking up 24, 8, 8, and 8 in total, respectively. To achieve features extraction from ECG data, we proposed to use k-means clustering to divide them into two groups, normal and abnormal.

Research selects K data in the dataset as the initial group center, randomly. Then, the shortest distance is calculated from each group data to the group center. After that, the group center is recomputed by using the classification which was arrived earlier. Finally, the last two steps are repeated until the distances converge.

$$J = \sum_{r=1}^{K} \sum_{C_j \in V_r} \left(C_j - C_r \right)^2 \tag{8}$$

In (8), the variable K is used to cluster a certain quantity, C_r means the optimal group center which is obtained by calculating the summation of minimum distance from all data C_j to the group V_r center. In our case, K is equal to 2, representing abnormal and normal ECG signals and C_j is the average SD area of the jth subject as shown in (7).

Table 2. Arrhythmia cluster by using average SD area

ECG data	Arrhythmia cluster	ECG data	Arrhythmia cluster
AFIB_1	2	NSR_1	2
AFIB_2	1	NSR_2	2
AFIB_3	1	NSR_3	2
AFIB_4	1	NSR_4	2
AFIB_5	2	NSR_5	2
AFIB_6	1	NSR_6	2
AFIB_7	2	NSR_7	2
AFIB_8	1	NSR_8	2
AFL_1	1	NSR_9	2
AFL_2	1	NSR_10	2
AFL_3	1	NSR_11	2
AFL_4	1	NSR_12	2
AFL_5	1	NSR_13	2
AFL_6	1	NSR_14	2
AFL_7	2	NSR_15	2
AFL_8	1	NSR_16	2
APB_1	1	NSR_17	2
APB_2	1	NSR_18	2
APB_3	1	NSR_19	2
APB_4	1	NSR_20	2
APB_5	1	NSR_21	2
APB_6	1	NSR_22	2
APB_7	1	NSR_23	2
APB_8	1	NSR_24	2

3   Results and Discussion

48 samples of ECG data were tested for the algorithm. Extracted values of features from ECG signals are presented in Table 1. The classified result as shown in Table 2 of arrhythmia was based on features extraction values with k-means clustering. Table 3 [5, 8, 9] presents the arrhythmia classification of all data by using the proposed algorithm, then compares it with the medical diagnosis and the performance between the different algorithms.

The results show that the proposed algorithm is able to determine whether people are suffering from arrhythmia. Any additional condition in the heartbeats which causes abnormal heart rate will classify into arrhythmia, such us AFL, AFIB, APB, LBBB, RBBB, and so on. The results are comparably accurate.

Table 3. Comparison of arrhythmia detection algorithms [5, 8, 9]

Item	Accuracy (%)
LINEAR & CHOATIC features In GDA+SOM+MLP	95%–98%
Neuron fuzzy network	97%
Wavelet transform & RBF networks	92%–99%
NN layer 300 with Daubechies 6 Wavelet	87%
Mentioned three features & DFA	89%–98%
TreeBoost hierarchical	91%–93%
Proposed	91%–93%

4   Conclusion

The aim of this work was to create a dichotomy algorithm to detect and test for indications of heart disease and to propose a feature extraction method that uses Fourier series principles to capture the original data information in each period of the acquired signal to integrate the deviations that may be indicative of disease. Compared to other studies, the research architecture here is absorbed in once complete heartbeat rather than concentrating on specific intervals, such as QRS complex. The method can not only measure the heart rate and arrhythmia but also figure out which cycle and heart position occur variation. The results indicate that the algorithm can support physicians in the process of diagnosis. In addition, using this configuration in conjunction with a wearable device helps the construction of long-term care (LTC).

Acknowledgment. This work was supported in part by the Ministry of Science and Technology in Taiwan under Grant MOST 107-2221-E-305-010-MY2.

Conflict of Interest. The authors declare that they have no conflict of interest.

References

1. Kubicek, J., Penhaker, M., Kahankova, R.: Design of a synthetic ECG signal based on the fourier series. In: Proceedings of IEEE 2014 International Conference on Advances in Computing, Communications and Informatics, New Delhi, India, pp. 1881–1885 (2014)
2. He, C., Li, W., Chik, D.: Waveform compensation of ECG data using segment fitting functions for individual identification. In: 2017 13th International Conference on Computational Intelligence and Security (CIS), Hong Kong, pp. 475–479 (2017)
3. Tavakoli, V., Sahba, N., Hajebi, N.: A fast and accurate method for arrhythmia detection. In: Proceedings of IEEE 2009 Annual International Conference of the IEEE Engineering in Medicine and Biology Society, Minneapolis, MN, pp. 1897–1900 (2009)
4. Rahman, M., Nasor, M.: An algorithm for detection of arrhythmia. In: Proceedings IEEE 2011 1st Middle East Conference on Biomedical Engineering, Sharjah, United Arab Emirates, pp. 243–246 (2011)
5. Ahmed, R., Arafat, S.: Cardiac arrhythmia classification using hierarchical classification model. In: Proceedings of IEEE 2014 6th International Conference on Computer Science and Information Technology, Amman, pp. 203–207 (2014)
6. Chen, H., Wang, C., Chen, T., Zhao, X.: Feature selecting based on fourier series fitting. In: Proceedings of IEEE 2017 8th IEEE International Conference on Software Engineering and Service Science, Beijing, pp. 241–244 (2017)
7. Chen, H.C., Chen, S.W.: A moving average based filtering system with its application to real-time QRS detection. In: Proceedings of IEEE 2003 Computers in Cardiology, Thessaloniki Chalkidiki, Greece, pp. 585–588 (2003)
8. Rouhani, M., Soleymani, R.: Neural networks based diagnosis of heart arrhythmias using chaotic and nonlinear features of HRV signals. In: Proceedings of IEEE 2009 International Association of Computer Science and Information Technology - Spring Conference, Singapore, pp. 545–549 (2009)
9. Dewangan, N.K., Shukla, S.P.: ECG arrhythmia classification using discrete wavelet transform and artificial neural network. In: Proceedings of IEEE 2016 International Conference on Recent Trends in Electronics, Information & Communication Technology (RTEICT), Bangalore, pp. 1892–1896 (2016)

Combining Multi-classifier with CNN in Detection and Classification of Breast Calcification

Kuan-Chun Chen[(✉)], Chiun-Li Chin, Ni-Chuan Chung, and Chin-Luen Hsu

Department of Medical Informatics, Chung Shan Medical University, No. 110, Section 1 Jianguo North Road, Taichung, Taiwan
cgc2367014@gmail.com

Abstract. Breast calcification or microtumors screening can early detect breast cancer that can make the disease easier to treat. At present, the segmentation of breast calcifications relies on the delineate by doctors. The process is time-consuming, and the benefits are not readily apparent. None of the paper has been discussed on combining automatically delineate and classify the breast calcifications to benign or malignant in previous research. According to the above reasons, we proposed an approach on combining Cascade Adaboost with CNN to delineate breast calcifications in mammogram and classify breast calcifications to benign or malignant by the CNN we trained. The ability of classification in Cascade Adaboost algorithm is better than Adaboost algorithm, it can significantly reduce the time cost by classification in CNN and speed up the process time. In this paper, we compare our method with the architecture of R-CNN combining CNN, and the experimental results show that by using Cascade Adaboost combined with CNN can detect calcification more accurately and classify it into benign or malignant. We hope that by using the approach in this work can help doctors to detect and diagnose breast calcifications in less time.

Keywords: Breast calcification · Cascade Adaboost · Deep learning · CNN · Benign or malignant

1 Introduction

In previous research, none of the paper has been discussed on combining automatically delineate and classify the breast calcifications to benign or malignant [1, 2]. The diagnosis of breast cancer nowadays relies on doctors to interpret mammogram images and classify the calcification to benign or malignant through professional knowledge or accumulation of experience, hence automatically classifying calcification plays an important role in diagnosing breast cancer [3]. The classification in breast calcification in recent uses Breast Image Reporting and Data Analysis System (BI-RADS) to evaluate and label [4]. However, this process cost a lot of time, exhaustion and pressure to affect the judgment of results by the physician. Based on the above questions, we developed a system that can automatically detect the breast calcification and classify it to benign or malignant. Gao et al. [5] use Cascade Adaboost algorithm to detect

© Springer Nature Switzerland AG 2020
K.-P. Lin et al. (Eds.): ICBHI 2019, IFMBE Proceedings 74, pp. 304–311, 2020.
https://doi.org/10.1007/978-3-030-30636-6_42

human's head images from the surveillance camera and use the convolutional neural network (CNN) to classify whether it is a head image. Rouhi et al. [6] proposed the classification of benign and malignant breast tumors and found that CNN is better used in region growing method for tumor classification. In the CNN model, using less layers of AlexNet as a model can increase the overall processing speed [7].

Based on the literature review, we can find that there are few studies in the detection and classification of breast calcification, especially some micro calcifications cannot be clearly detected as benign or malignant. Most reviews are aiming to identify whether there is a tumor caused by a wide range of calcification in mammogram images. Therefore, we propose a method combining the Cascade Adaboost algorithm with CNN to automatically detect the calcification and analyze whether it is benign or malignant. To prevent the overfitting situation happens, Srivastava et al. [8] shows that using dropout can effectively improve the classification of the neural network, thus we add dropout to the deep learning network and adjust it. Last, we compare our method with R-CNN combining CNN to evaluate the method. This paper presents the following contributions:

1. Improved the time-consuming process of delineate calcification and analyze whether it is benign or malignant, assisting physicians in interpreting the medical images.
2. After the automatic detection of the calcification, we use the CNN model to confirm the action of feature extraction in order to increase the accuracy of delineating the correct calcification.

This paper is divided into four sections. The rest of the paper is organized as follows: In Sect. 2, we introduce the method we proposed and describe the framework of CNN. Section 3 is the experimental results of this paper and the conclusions of this paper will be mentioned in Sect. 4.

2   Materials and Method

The proposed method used in this paper is to develop a breast calcification classification system using the combination of cascade Adaboost algorithm and CNN deep learning algorithm. The system will first do the image preprocessing, and the calcification will be aligned to the center by normalizing. Then, the preprocessed images will input to the training and testing network.

2.1   Mammogram Image Preprocessing

In order to improve the accuracy of identification, pre-processing is a necessary step to form the dataset. All images in the dataset will perform pre-processing first, so we try to normalize the location of calcification and increase the image contrast enhancement, the description will be introduced as follows.

(a) *Normalized location of breast calcifications*

The breast calcification dataset used in this paper is delineated by the physician, but the calcification delineated will not completely align in the center of the image. Therefore, we use the algorithm to normalize the location of delineated calcification image [9]. We move the location of the calcification to the middle of the image to improve the identification and analysis of the system. Figure 1 shows the result of normalizing the location of breast calcifications.

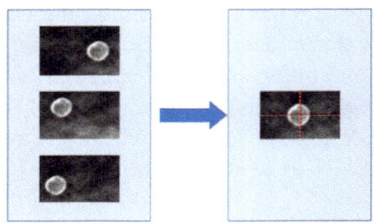

Fig. 1. Location normalization result image

(b) *Contrast normalization*

Contrast normalization is often used in the classification of medical images. Some mammogram images we collected meet poor contrast problems during training, which may cause it hard to classify to labels. As a consequence, we solve this problem by increasing the contrast of mammogram images, reducing the pixel values from the noise due to external factors. To make the features in the image more prominent, we calculate the average brightness of each mammogram image and subtract the average value of each pixel in the image. As shown in the Eq. (1), where $X_{i,j}$ represents the vector of each image ($X \in \mathbb{R}^{r \times r}$), $\bar{X}$ represents the average of the image brightness $X_{i,j}$, and $x'_{i,j}$ shown in the Eq. (2) is the vector for contrast normalizing. Figure 2(a) and (b) is respectively the original image and the normalized image.

$$\bar{X} = \frac{1}{r^2} \sum_{i,j} x_{i,j} \tag{1}$$

$$x'_{i,j} = x_{i,j} - \bar{X} \tag{2}$$

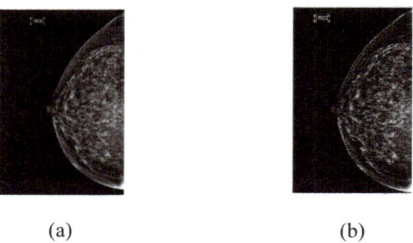

(a)   (b)

Fig. 2. (a) is Original image and (b) is normalized image

2.2   Cascade Adaboost Algorithm

The Adaboost algorithm combines multiple weak classifiers into a strong classifier. During the training process, the weak classifier with high accuracy will be given a larger weight and combine to a strong classifier which leads to a better training result, and the most important thing is that it does not cause overfitting problems by using this algorithm [10]. The Cascade Adaboost used in this paper inherits the advantages of Adaboost and connected multiple Adaboost to learn specific features to achieve better training efficiency and effectiveness. The Cascade classifier is shown in Fig. 3.

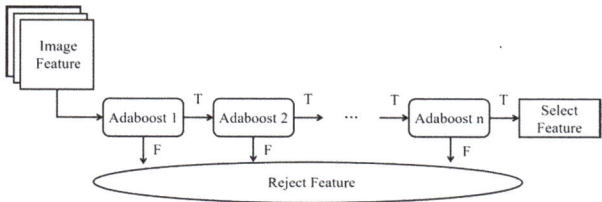

Fig. 3. Cascade Adaboost classifier

2.3   Combining Cascade Adaboost with CNN Method

The main architecture of this paper is combining CNN with Cascade Adaboost. Cascade Adaboost algorithm consists of multiple strong classifiers, which can select the classifier type and determine the number of classifiers according to the training samples and results. After pre-training these data, the Cascade Adaboost algorithm can quickly find multiple features in a new image and input these features into the next step. The CNN classification will review the process, filter the incorrect features, delineate the calcification and analysis whether it is benign or malignant in a mammogram. As shown in Fig. 4, after the image is input to the system, it can label and delineate the calcification in the mammogram, combining CNN to automatically select the breast calcification in the image for classifying it into benign and malignant. We also compare the method of combining R-CNN and CNN with the method proposed in this paper to see whether the calcification is benign or malignant, presenting it in the experimental results.

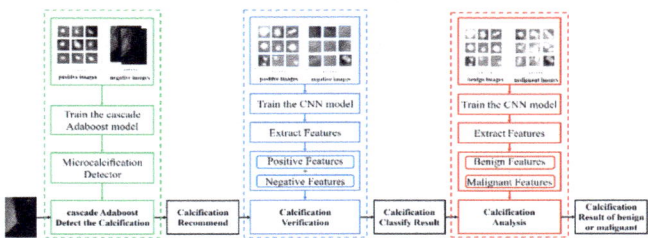

Fig. 4. System architecture

2.4   CNN Model Based on AlexNet

In this paper, we use AlexNet as the baseline of our CNN model with ReLU and dropout simultaneously to make great breakthroughs in image recognition and classification. We want to achieve high accuracy and high processing rate with a simple architecture, hence we choose this model as the architecture of this paper. The CNN architecture is shown in Fig. 5.

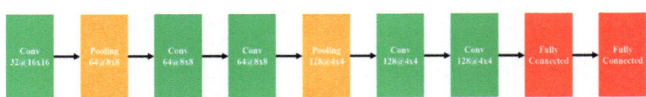

Fig. 5. Our proposed CNN models

In training model, we input the size of 16×16 calcification image to our proposed CNN model. Our CNN architecture generally has 5 convolutional layers, 2 pooling layers, and 2 fully-connected layers. In comparison to original AlexNet, it reduces a pooling layer to avoid image being too small to train. In addition, we use dropout to avoid the problem that training accuracy is higher than the testing result and adjust the learning rate.

3   Results

In this section, we introduce our dataset and development environment first. Then we evaluate the method we proposed and compared it with the others. Last, we show results for automatically delineate and classify the breast calcification to benign or malignant.

3.1   Dataset

The datasets used in this paper is provided by the department of medical imaging in Chung Shan Medical University Hospital, and all mammogram images were taken in craniocaudal (CC) and mediolateral oblique (MLO) views. We select two datasets to perform training and testing: dataset1 and dataset2. In dataset1, there are 2200 images, which included 1100 calcifications and 1100 non-calcifications images. In dataset2, there are 1940 images that are respectively 970 benign calcifications and 970 malignant calcifications. Both of the datasets use 80% of the data for training and 20% of the data for testing. Dataset1 is for classifying whether it is breast calcification, and the other is analyzing whether the breast calcification is benign or malignant. Figure 6(a) and (b) shows the delineation image of benign and malignant calcification.

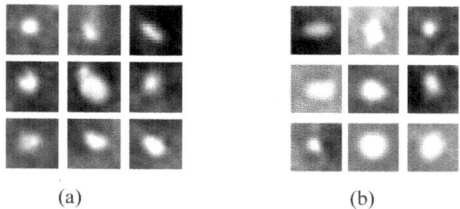

Fig. 6. (a) and (b) is respectively Benign and malignant calcification images

3.2 Development Environment

The experiments run on an operating system of Windows with 8 GB RAM, i7-8750HQ 2.2 GHz CPU and NVIDIA GTX 1060 GPU. We use Anaconda 3 to construct the Tensorflow learning framework and run the CNN model with Python. We also use CUDA 9.0 introduced by NVIDIA integration technology, which enabled parallel computing on NVIDIA graphics processors to speed up training time. In addition, we used Python's GUI library Tkinter to create an identification system for breast calcification detection, which increases the fluency in using the system.

3.3 Identification of Breast Calcification

We compared two methods: Cascade Adaboost combining with CNN and R-CNN combining with CNN, studying the relationship between network parameter and overall accuracy. Additionally, we compared the accuracy between handcraft and CNN, and the handcraft method is the result of delineating calcification in mammogram images by physicians. Finally, we select the best result as our proposed architecture on automatic detection and classification of breast calcification in this work.

We use AlexNet as our basic CNN model and test whether adjusting the parameters in a neural network can get better results. Due to the cropped image size is 16×16 after the images input to the Cascade Adaboost, we reduce one pooling layer in AlexNet to avoid the images size being too small to train. By using four different kinds of dropout in the fully-connected layer and three different values of learning rate, we compare the accuracy of these testing parameters and the results are shown in Table 1.

Table 1. Fine tune dropout and learning rate

Item	Dropout	Learning rate	Accuracy (%)
Dropout	–	0.0001	71.0%
	0.3	0.0001	72.6%
	0.5	0.0001	71.2%
	0.8	0.0001	68.1%
Learning rate	–	0.001	74.2%
	–	0.0001	71.1%
	–	0.00001	66.9%

3.4　The Result of Classifying Delineated Breast Calcification

According to the results of Table 1, we compare three methods: handcraft with CNN, R-CNN with CNN and Cascade Adaboost with CNN. The accuracy result is shown in Table 2.

Table 2. Methods comparing

Method	Accuracy (%)
Handcraft + CNN	90.2%
R-CNN + CNN	81.5%
Cascade Adaboost + CNN	83.4%

According to the results of Table 2, we can know that by using the method handcraft with CNN under the condition of dropout set as 0.3 and learning rate set as 0.001 has the best performance, which accuracy is 90.2%. However, delineating the breast calcification by doctors is cost a lot of time and it is easy to affect the result caused by exhaustion and other mental condition. In addition, the other two results in table show that the method proposed in this paper has better performance. It not only reduces the classification time of CNN but leads great results to accuracy and speed of processing.

4　Conclusions

In this paper, we proposed a method to detect the breast calcification and classify it to benign or malignant which combined with Cascade Adaboost algorithm and CNN. The Cascade Adaboost will delineate the calcification after we input the mammogram images and CNN will automatically classify it to benign or malignant, which can assist doctors to diagnose breast calcification. Furthermore, we compare our method with R-CNN combining CNN. The result shows that the method that we proposed have better performance.

According to the experimental results, we found some cases show error results and the reasons are the color of calcification is too close to the breast tissue, the shape of calcification is too similar to the mammary gland, etc. To avoid these situations, we will train more mammogram to detect variable and difficult shape of calcification. In the future, we can train some computed tomography (CT) images that included organ may have calcification, such as liver or kidney, to provide physicians with a more comprehensive function on diagnosis. We expected to build a system that can effectively assist doctors in improving the accuracy of diagnosis on breast calcification, make early detection of breast cancer and increase the survival rate of patients.

Conflict of Interest. The authors declare that they have no conflict of interest.

References

1. Yousefi, M., Krzyżak, A., Suen, C.Y.: Mass detection in digital breast tomosynthesis data using convolutional neural networks and multiple instance learning. Comput. Biol. Med. **96**, 283–293 (2018)
2. Chougrad, H., Zouaki, H., Alheyane, O.: Deep convolutional neural networks for breast cancer screening. Comput. Methods Programs Biomed. **157**, 19–30 (2018)
3. Sawaguchi, S., Nishi, H.: Slightly-slacked dropout for improving neural network learning on FPGA. ICT Express **4**, 75–80 (2018)
4. Jung, H.K., Kuzmiak, C.M., Kim, K.W., et al.: Potential use of American college of radiology BI-RADS mammography atlas for reporting and assessing lesions detected on dedicated breast CT imaging: preliminary study. Acad Radio **24**, 1395–1401 (2017)
5. Gao, C., Li, P., Zhang, Y., et al.: People counting based on head detection combining Adaboost and CNN in crowded surveillance environment. Neurocomputing **208**, 108–116 (2016)
6. Rouhi, R., Jafari, M., Kasaei, S., et al.: Benign and malignant breast tumors classification based on region growing and CNN segmentation. Expert Syst. Appl. **42**, 990–1002 (2015)
7. Wang, R., Xu, J., Han, T.X.: Object instance detection with pruned AlexNet and extended training data. Signal Process-Image **70**, 145–156 (2018)
8. Srivastava, N., Hinton, G., Krizhevsky, A., et al.: Dropout: a simple way to prevent neural networks from overfitting. Mach. Learn. Res. **15**, 1929–1958 (2014)
9. Khan, M.F., Khan, E., Abbasi, Z.A.: Image contrast enhancement using normalized histogram equalization. OPTIK **24**, 4868–4875 (2015)
10. Cao, Y., Miao, Q.G., Liu, J.C., et al.: Advance and prospects of AdaBoost algorithm. Acta Automatica Sinica **39**, 745–758 (2013)

Evaluation of Left Ventricular Ejection Fraction Obtained from ^{201}Tl Myocardial Perfusion Scan by CZT Cardiac Camera

Hsiao-Ling Chiang[1,2], Chien-Hsin Ting[1], Cheng-Pe Chang[1],
Bang-Hung Yang[1,2], Jyh-Shyan Leu[3], Chi-Long Juang[4(✉)],
and Wen-Sheng Huang[1,5(✉)]

[1] Department of Nuclear Medicine, Taipei Veterans General Hospital,
No. 201, Sec. 2, Shipai Rd, Beitou District, Taipei 11217, Taiwan (R.O.C.)
jolin0829@gmail.com, wshuang01@gmail.com
[2] Taipei Association of Radiological Technologists, TAMRT, Taipei, Taiwan
[3] Department of I & D, TV BU, TPV Technology Group, Taipei, Taiwan
[4] Department of Radiological Technology,
Yuanpei University, Hsinchu, Taiwan
cljuang@mail.ypu.edu.tw
[5] Department of Nuclear Medicine, Tri-Service General Hospital,
Taipei, Taiwan

Abstract. Taking advantage of high energy and spatial resolution and high count sensitivity, the ultrafast cardiac γ-camera with cadmium-zinc-telluride (CZT)-based detectors has become popular in practice for myocardial perfusion imaging (MPI). The shorter imaging time with better imaging quality using CZT detectors compared to conventional ones makes it feasible to perform the left ventricular ejection fraction (LVEF) in the meantime of doing ^{201}Tl MPI. The aim of this study was to compare LVEF from ^{201}Tl MPI using a CZT with that from first-pass radionuclide angiography (FPRA) using a NaI camera.

A total of 117 patients (aged 81 ± 13 years old) were collected. All underwent ^{201}Tl MPI using a CZT camera (Discovery NM530c) and FPRA using a conventional camera (Symbia E Signal Head System) in 2 wks. Correlations of LVEF obtained from these two examinations were evaluated by SPSS 20.0 statistical software.

Our results showed that the mean LVEF measured from MPI and FPRA were $54 \pm 18\%$ and $51 \pm 16\%$, respectively. A good linear correlation was found between both methods (r: 0.861, $p < 0.0001$). It also showed a good agreement and LVEF prediction rates (k = 0.83) obtained from these two measurements. Tl-201 MPI with CZT camera is thus capable to offer a reliable clinical LVEF references.

Keywords: Cadmium-Zinc-Telluride (CZT) ·
^{201}Tl Myocardial Perfusion Imaging (MPI) ·
First-Pass Radionuclide Angiography (FPRA) ·
Left Ventricular Ejection Fraction (LVEF)

Presenting Author—H.-L. Chiang.
H.-.L. Chiang and C.-H. Ting—Contribute equally.

K.-P. Lin et al. (Eds.): ICBHI 2019, IFMBE Proceedings 74, pp. 312–319, 2020.
https://doi.org/10.1007/978-3-030-30636-6_43

1   Introduction

The γ-camera has been further innovated with the application of the cadmium zinc telluride (CZT) detector. It not only enhanced imaging sensitivity 8-10 times higher than that of conventional detectors [1], but also improved energy resolution and spatial resolution [2]. ^{201}Tl myocardial perfusion Imaging (MPI) has served as a clinically useful means in evaluating disease severity, therapeutic planning and prognosis of coronary artery disease [3]. The CZT cardiac camera has displayed a reliable and high-quality of MPI [4] with a low tracer dose [5, 6], a reduced scan time to 5 min [7], and a potential to estimate left ventricular ejection fraction (LVEF) in the meantime of MPI [8].

Traditionally, the major radioactive tracer used in the first-pass radionuclide angiography (FPRA) to estimate the LVEF is free ^{99m}Tc (Technetium) or its derivatives such as ^{99m}Tc-DTPA. The parent nuclides ^{99}Mo are supplied by medical reactors. However, closed the Chalk River reactor results in concerns of rising price or supplying shortage of ^{99m}Tc. In contrast, ^{201}Tl is generated from the cyclotrons. If ^{201}Tl MPI can provide reliable LVEF information for clinical use, it would be a practical alternative to clinically assess cardiac function pre-operative anesthesia and chemotherapy and target treatment.

2   Materials and Methods

The retrospective study was approved by the Institutional Review Board (No. 2018-05-001-AC) and was performed from Jan. 2015 to Dec. 2016 at Department of Nuclear Medicine, Taipei Veterans General Hospital. Data from 117 patients (81 males and 36 females, aged 81 $\pm$ 13 years) were analyzed. All of them underwent ^{201}Tl MPI using a CZT cardiac camera (Discovery NM530c, GE Healthcare, Haifa, Israel) and ^{99m}Tc FPRA using a conventional camera (Symbia E Signal Head System, SIEMENS Medical Solutions, IL, USA) in 2 wks. Imaging procedures and processing parameters of both methods are described as following.

2.1 ^{201}Tl Myocardial Perfusion Scan

Two mCi of ^{201}Tl were intravenously injected to patients in standard supine position for MPI; the image was collected twice with a stress phase obtained first and a rest phase collected 3 h later [9] using GE Discovery NM530 with the following imaging parameters: energy window is set to -14% and $+23\%$ for energy peak 70 keV and $\pm9\%$ for energy peak 167 keV. Electrocardiography receiving range sets to heart rate ±20, each heart period was divided into 8 images, 300 s per image. Imaging data were processed using the Emory Cardiac Toolbox software and the low-pass butter worth filter (cut-off 0.28, order 15). The images were then reconstructed and the blood flow volume that used to estimate the LVEF could be determined from the left ventricular end diastolic volume and the end systolic volume. All LVEF data were obtained in the rest phase.

2.2   First-Pass Radionuclide Angiography

Twelve mCi of free ^{99m}Tc external jugular vein bolus injection was performed for FPRA using Seimens Symbia E Singal Head System equipped with a low-energy collimator with a peak energy of 140 keV $\pm$ 10% in list mode. The matrix size was 64×64 pixels, each image was set to 0.05 s and the image time was 40 s. The ventricular time activity curve was obtained by dividing the right ventricle, pulmonary artery, left ventricle, and aorta by the region of interesting (ROI) technique, then the LVEF could be obtained from the difference between left ventricular end diastolic counts and end systolic counts.

3   Statistics

Correlations of LVEF values obtained from both methods were evaluated using SPSS 20.0 statistical software. Two-way ANOVA was applied to analyze effects of gender and BMI on FPRA and MPI. The Pearson product-moment correlation was applied to observe the linearity of LVEF between both examinations in different subgroups and plotted as scatter diagrams and the determinant coefficient R^2 of the linear regression equation. Interclass correlation coefficient (ICC) was applied for reproducibility of the two methods. The KAPPA coefficient of the chi-square test was used to predictive consistency of these two tests. Data were expressed as mean $\pm$ SD, $p < 0.05$ was set as statistically significant.

4   Result

There are 117 patient data collected in this study, and the characteristics of the subjects were summarized in Table 1.

Table 1. Subject characteristics (n = 117)

Characteristics	Value
Age (years)	68 $\pm$ 13
Male/Female (n)	81/36
Height (cm)	163 $\pm$ 8
Weight (Kg)	69 $\pm$ 14
BMI (Kg/M2)	26 $\pm$ 5

The averaged LVEFs obtained from MPI were 50.68 $\pm$ 16.02 and FPRA were 53.56 $\pm$ 18.22, their box plots were shown in Fig. 1. Table 2 listed the descriptive statistics of all measurements.

Only BMI had significant effects on FPRA (p = 0.030) compared with gender, (p = 0.471) while both gender (p = 0.013) and BMI (p = 0.015) had significant effects on MPI.

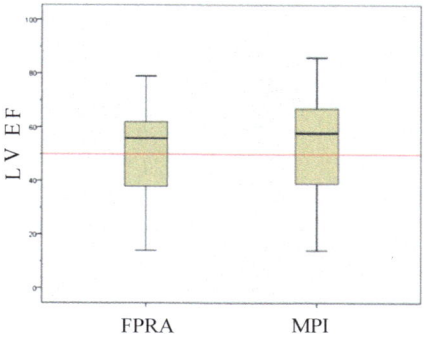

Fig. 1. The box plot of the LVEF obtained from MPI and FPRA

Table 2. Descriptive statistics

	No	EF$_{min}$	EF$_{max}$	EF$_{avg}$
Total subject FP	117	14	79	50.68 ± 16.02
Total subject MP	117	14	86	53.56 ± 18.22
Male FP	81	14	72	49.06 ± 15.67
Male MP	81	14	83	49.58 ± 17.37
Female FP	36	17	79	54.31 ± 16.42
Female MP	36	24	86	62.53 ± 17.07
Normal BMI FP	37	14	74	48.68 ± 18.09
Normal BMI MP	37	14	83	50.08 ± 17.90

High correlations in total subjects ($r = 0.861$, $p < 0.0001$), male ($r = 0.875$, $p < 0.0001$) and female ($r = 0.857$, $p < 0.0001$) subgroups, and in normally ranged BMI (18.5–24.0) subjects ($r = 0.927$, $p < 0.0001$) were also noted between the two methods. Their scatter diagrams and the determinant coefficient R^2 of the linear regression equation were each plotted in Figs. 2, 3, 4 and 5.

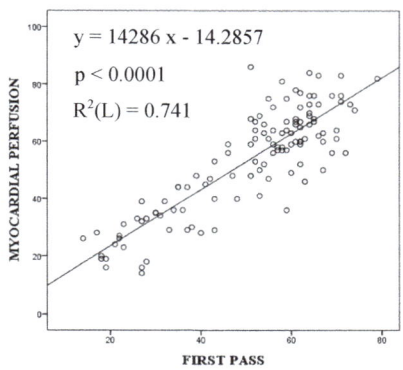

Fig. 2. Scatter diagram of the total subjects

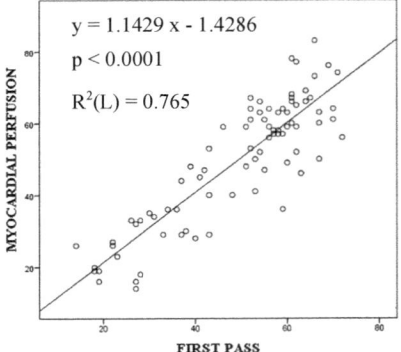

Fig. 3. Scatter diagram of the male subjects

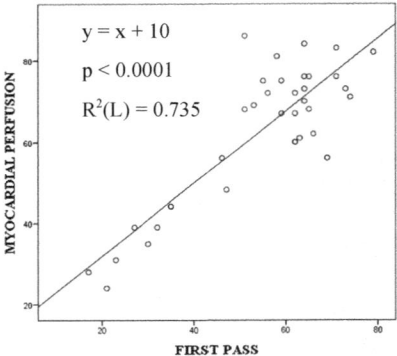

Fig. 4. Scatter diagram of the female subjects

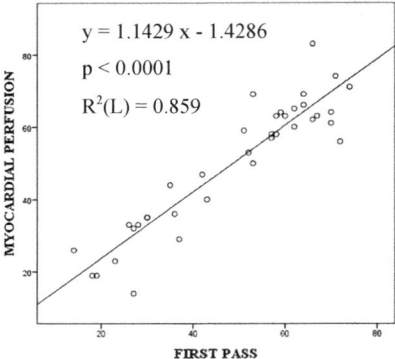

Fig. 5. Scatter diagram of the normal BMI subjects

Figure 6 showed excellent reproducibility of the two methods (ICC = 0.843).

LVEF is an indicator for clinical judgment of cardiac function. The World Health Organization recommending a normal LVEF should be ≥50% at rest [10]. Thus, we further divided LVEF into 2 group, i.e. ≥ or <50% for heart functional prediction. The LVEF ≥50% was 76 cases in MPI group and 74 cases in FPRA group. Observed agreement of both groups were excellent (92.3%), representing probability of both test results was consistent. Chance agreement representing the expected probability of both test results was 53.7%. The KAPPA coefficient κ of the chi-square test was 0.83 (p < 0.0001), indicating that the predictive consistency of both tests was almost perfect.

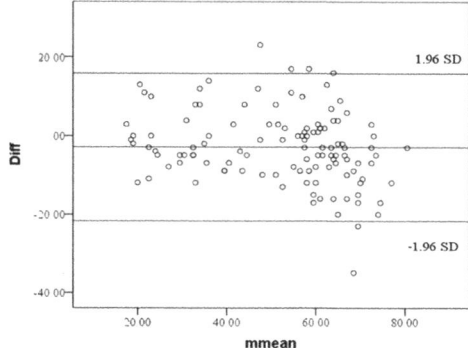

Fig. 6. Consistency of the two LV EFs using Bland - Altman Plot.

5 Discussion

The averaged means of both FPRA and MPI groups as shown in Fig. 1 were quite close; their standard deviations almost overlapped each other indicating a similar power of for LVEF measurements.

The Pearson product-moment correlation coefficient (γ = 0.861, 0.875, 0.857 and 0.927, respectively) and scatter diagram (R^2 = 0.741, 0.765, 0.735 and 0.859, respectively) with $p < 0.0001$ in all subgroups revealed high correlations between these two tests. Our results also showed an excellent reproducibility (ICC = 0.843), indicating great consistency between both tests.

Using the Bland-Altman Plot, it showed that most of the data points were located within the confidence interval, again, indicating high consistency between both tests. Of note, scattering on the high LVEF portions of the figure is slightly dilated, esp. those with LVEF ≥50%. It is shown that the LVEF using MPI method appeared slightly overestimated as it is ≥50%. However, such an overestimation does not impact clinical decision making of the cardiac function evaluation i.e. normal or abnormal.

In our Institute, cardiac function should be assessed for surgical anesthesia, and chemotherapy and/or target treatment for breast cancer. Many target-drugs, such as vascular endothelial growth factor inhibitors or mammalian target of rapamycin (mTOR) inhibitors can cause decreased cardiac function, myocardial infarction or even heart failure. Thus, LVEF should be monitored before, during, and periods after treatment to assess possibly cardiac insult. The treatment should be discontinued in case of left ventricular dysfunction.

The KAPPA coefficient of the chi-square test showed almost perfect in consistency between both tests ($\kappa = 0.83$, $p < 0.0001$), indicating LVEF using MPS method was highly accurate in predicting heart dysfunction.

While LVEFs of MPS in female and obesity subgroups had partial discrepancy from that of FPRA method, good accuracy remained. Accordingly, LVEFs obtained from MPS can overcome clinical false positives caused by attenuation effects in obese patients and female breasts and false negatives caused by myocardial generalized ischemia [13–15].

To achieve a lower irradiation, a better image quality and to offer an accurately clinical information are aims of nuclear cardiology. A half dosed ^{201}Tl MPI using CZT cardiac camera, even in obese patients appeared to be capable to fulfill the above mentioned requirements and achieve a comparable image quality as conventional cameras [11, 12].

The overestimated results with LVEF $\geq 50\%$ using MPI method was observed in the study, however, it might be little influent the clinical decision of whether the heart function is normal or not.

6   Conclusion

The LVEF obtained from MPI using the CZT camera had similar clinical reference values to that obtained from traditional FPRA. Thus, LVEFs using MPS could be an alternative of those using FPRA and serve as a safety guide for patients receiving different surgical anesthesia, certain chemo- or target therapies, especially in the nightmare of ^{99m}Tc shortage.

Acknowledgment. The author wishes to acknowledge Dr. Kang-Ping Lin in commenting on the draft of this chapter. This study was in part supported by Ministry of Science and Technology under grant MOST103-2314-B-371-004-MY3.

Conflict of Interest. The authors declare that they have no conflict of interest.

References

1. Gambhir, S.S., Berman, D.S., Ziffer, J., Nagler, M., et al.: A novel high-sensitivity rapid-acquisition single-photon cardiac imaging camera. J. Nucl. Med. **50**, 635–643 (2009)
2. Ben-Haim, S., Kennedy, J., Keidar, Z.: Novel cadmium zinc telluride devices for myocardial perfusion imaging-technological aspects and clinical applications. Semin. Nucl. Med. **46**, 273–285 (2016)
3. Lugomirski, P., Chow, B., Ruddy, T.: Impact of SPECT myocardial perfusion imaging on cardiac care. Expert Rev. Cardiovasc. Ther. **12**, 1247–1249 (2014)

4. Songy, B., Lussato, D., Guernou, M., Queneau, M., Geronazzo, R.: Comparison of myocardial perfusion imaging using thallium-201 between a new cadmium-zinc-telluride cardiac camera and a conventional SPECT camera. Clin. Nucl. Med. **36**, 776–780 (2011)
5. Mouden, M., Timmer, J.R., Ottervanger, J.P., et al.: Impact of a new ultrafast CZT SPECT camera for myocardial perfusion imaging: fewer equivocal results and lower radiation dose. Eur. J. Nucl. Med. Mol. Imaging **39**, 1048–1055 (2012)
6. Songy, B., Guernou, M., Lussato, D., et al.: Low-dose thallium-201 protocol with a cadmium-zinc-telluride cardiac camera. Nucl. Med. Commun. **33**, 464–469 (2012)
7. Duvall, W., Croft, L., Ginsberg, E., et al.: Reduced isotope dose and imaging time with a high-efficiency CZT SPECT camera. J. Nucl. Cardiol. **18**, 847–857 (2011)
8. Kliner, D., Wang, L., Winger, D., et al.: A prospective evaluation of the repeatability of left ventricular ejection fraction measurement by gated SPECT. J. Nucl. Cardiol. **22**, 1237–1243 (2015)
9. Ishihara, M., Taniguchi, Y., Onoguchi, M., et al.: Optimal thallium-201 dose in cadmium-zinc-telluride SPECT myocardial perfusion imaging. J. Nucl. Cardiol. **25**, 947–954 (2018)
10. Gerard, J., Bryan, D.: Principles of Anatomy and Physiology. Wiley, Hoboken (2011)
11. Kincl, V., Kamínek, M., Vašina, J.D., et al.: Feasibility of ultra low-dose thallium stress-redistribution protocol including prone imaging in obese patients using CZT camera. Int. J. Cardiovasc. Imaging **32**, 1463–1469 (2016)
12. De Lorenzo, A., Peclat, T., Amaral, A.D., et al.: Prognostic evaluation in obese patients using a dedicated multipinhole cadmium-zinc telluride SPECT camera. Int. J. Cardiovasc. Imaging **32**, 355–361 (2016)
13. Mettler Jr., F.A., Guiberteau, M.J.: Essentials of Nuclear Medicine Imaging, 4th edn. Saunders, Philadelphia (1998)
14. Depuey, G., Rozanski, A.: Using gated technetium-99msestamibi SPECT to characterize fixed myocardial defects as infarct or artifact. J. Nucl. Med. **36**, 952–955 (1995)
15. Steven, B., Anita, M.D.: Artifacts and pitfalls in myocardial perfusion imaging. J. Nucl. Med. **34**, 193–211 (2006)

Cardiopulmonary Resuscitation Support Using Accelerometer Signals from the Carotid

Diogo Jesus[1(✉)], Paulo Carvalho[1], Jens Muehlsteff[2], and Ricardo Couceiro[1]

[1] CISUC, University of Coimbra, Coimbra, Portugal
diogo.abjesus@gmail.com
[2] Philips Research, Eindhoven, The Netherlands

Abstract. The use of accelerometer (ACC) sensors above the carotid artery provides an interesting approach to pulse detection during Cardiopulmonary Resuscitation (CPR) efforts. In order to study the basic feasibility of these ACC sensors in a resuscitation scenario, a protocol was designed with the aim of simulating characteristics present in a real-life scenario under controlled conditions. Using this protocol, a dataset of 12 healthy volunteers' signals was created. For each subject two ACC signals, electrocardiogram (ECG) and photoplethysmography (PPG) were measured synchronously. Additionally, a dataset from a previous study of 5 patients undergoing real-life CPR was available allowing for a comparison between the behavior of the simulated acquired data with real-life signals. Using these two datasets, technical solutions were developed with two different classifiers discriminating artefacts, compressions, pulse and absence of pulse.

Keywords: Accelerometer · Pulse detection · Cardiopulmonary Resuscitation · Feature engineering

1 Introduction

Cardiac arrest is a major health problem accounting for a substantial number of deaths in both Europe [1] and the United States [2]. Despite survival rates of cardiac arrest being extremely low, delivery of CPR has been proven to exert a significant survival benefit [3].

Manual pulse palpation is still the Golden Standard for assessment of pulse presence in unconscious patients for professional rescuers [4]. However, this method takes too long (often 25 s or more [5, 6]) and is very unreliable as well as highly subjective, with a reported sensitivity of 90% and specificity of 55% [7]. Therefore, a need for a reliable, objective and automatic pulse detection and characterization technique for CPR scenarios can be identified. Such a technical solution should also be characterised by ease of application on the patient and use by emergency medical services (EMS) personnel, thus improving the responsiveness and the efficiency of the resuscitation process.

© Springer Nature Switzerland AG 2020
K.-P. Lin et al. (Eds.): ICBHI 2019, IFMBE Proceedings 74, pp. 320–327, 2020.
https://doi.org/10.1007/978-3-030-30636-6_44

Accelerometry presents itself as a technology which offers great interest and promise for this end. Accelerometer sensors are inexpensive and low power. They exhibit high sensitivity and portability, which makes them suitable for pulse detection [8].

2 Methods

2.1 Data Acquisition and Measurement Setup

For this study two datasets were available, one consisting of signals acquired from 12 healthy volunteers for this study and the other consisting of data acquired during 5 real-life CPR scenarios (this dataset was first used in [8]). In the simulated signals dataset two accelerometers were positioned above the carotid artery, whilst in the real CPR dataset only one ACC signal is measured.

Accelerometer signals in a controlled study with subjects mimicking CPR phases were acquired using the SENSATRON device (see Table 1). This multi-parameter

Table 1. Protocol followed during simulated data acquisitions

t_{begin}	t_{end}	Phase	ECG
00:00	00:10	Transition	Yes
00:10	00:40	Lying down	Yes
00:40	00:50	Transition	Yes
00:50	01:20	Neck movements	Yes
01:20	01:30	Transition	Yes
01:30	02:00	Arm movements	Yes
02:00	02:10	Transition	Yes
02:10	02:40	Compressions	Yes
02:40	02:45	Transition	Yes
02:45	03:15	Compressions + Neck movements	Yes
03:15	03:20	Transition	Yes
03:20	04:10	Compressions + Neck and arm movements	Yes
04:10	04:40	Lying down	Unstable
04:40	04:50	Transition	Unstable
04:50	05:20	Neck movements	Unstable
05:20	05:30	Transition	Unstable
05:30	06:00	Arm movements	Unstable
06.00	06:10	Transition	Unstable
06:10	06:40	Compressions	Unstable
06:40	06:45	Transition	Unstable
06:45	07:15	Compressions + Neck movements	Unstable
07:15	07:20	Transition	Unstable
07:20	07:50	Compressions + Neck and arm movements	Unstable
07:50	08:10	Transition	Unstable
08:10	08:40	Lying down	Unstable
08:40	08:50	Transition	Unstable

battery operated device was developed by Philips [9] and allows synchronous measurement of ECG, impedance cardiography, near-infrared PPG, infrared PPG, thoracic inductive plethysmogram, sound signals and up to three tri-axial accelerometers.

In this work, the device was used for measurement of ECG, PPG and two accelerometer signals. Sound signals were also retrieved as during the acquisitions an external loud noise was made to support the annotation of the data. Sampling rates vary with the ECG being extracted at 250 Hz, PPG at 62.5 Hz, sound signals at 4000 Hz and ACC signals at 125 Hz. All signals are acquired with 16 bit ADC resolution. In this work only the accelerometer signal is used. However, emphasis was put on designing a protocol from which the data acquired can be used for future investigation of other hypotheses as well. Data acquisition was performed with the subject lying down on an air mattress, with the two accelerometers positioned above the left external carotid artery. As seen in Fig. 1 one accelerometer was positioned above the other, with pulse being palpable in both positions chosen.

The study was approved by the Ethics Committee of the Faculty of Medicine of the University of Coimbra.

2.2   Feature Engineering

For the development of the classification algorithms it was necessary to extract different features from the accelerometer signal. Pre-processing consisted only of a Butterworth bandpass filter in the range [0.5 30] Hz.

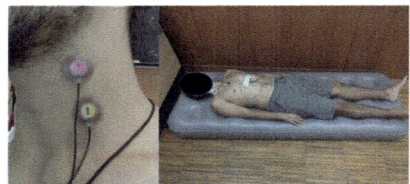

Fig. 1. Setup for the simulated data acquisition

Feature extraction was performed on non-overlapping 3 s windows, with 10 features being extracted directly in the time domain representation and 4 from the Phase Space Reconstruction (PSR) of the signal. The latter approach constitutes a non-linear dynamic signal processing technique and has provided good results on ECG characterisation [10] and Heart Sound Classification [11]. However, its use for accelerometer based pulse detection is a novel contribution.

Feature engineering is usually defined as the process of extracting information from the data source which is able to adequately compress the domain. There are at least the following approaches for feature engineering:

– Extraction of features based on domain knowledge: this process is usually applied in contexts where the processes involved in the signal generation are reasonably known and it is possible to define specific features to capture relevant characteristics of the signal.

- Extraction of features not based on domain knowledge: in this approach the aim is to capture fundamental information which might prove useful, using different feature extraction techniques. Afterwards, feature reduction techniques (such as a feature selection score) are usually applied to simplify the feature sphere.
- Feature learning: In this situation a data-domain approach is followed to automatically identify relevant features using techniques such as auto-encoders or deep learning.

In this work, the first two approaches were used (see Table 2 for a description of the feature set), as commonly techniques related to feature learning require large amounts of data to effectively represent the data. Identified relevant domain knowledge in the context of this thesis are activity level and periodicity. Pulse and No Pulse are usually low amplitude signals, whilst Artefacts and Compression are commonly higher amplitude signals. Pulse and Compression segments are also usually characterised by their periodicity, with the latter presenting common values of periodicity in the interval [60 100] beats per minute and the former in the interval [100 120] compressions per minute.

Table 2. Feature set

Feature	Calculated from
Standard Deviation (STD)	Window signal
Teager Energy (TE)	Window signal
Prominence (PM)	Window signal
Module of the lag of the highest peak in the autocorrelation of the window signal (LHP)	Window signal
Average power of the 4 highest peaks of the window's signal periodogram (P_{4Peaks})	Window signal
Standard Deviation of the cross-correlation ($t_{delay} = 0$) between the ACC's x and z axis (STD_{xz})	Window signal
Standard Deviation of the cross-correlation ($t_{delay} = 0$) between the ACC's y and z axis (STD_{yz})	Window signal
Standard Deviation of the ACC signal derivative ($STD_{acc'}$)	Window signal
Skewness (SK)	Window signal
Kurtosis (KU)	Window signal
Spatial Filling (SF)	PSR
Area of the C-column Average Curve ($AUC_{C-curve}$)	PSR
Entropy (EN)	PSR
Simplicity (SM)	PSR

2.3   Two Classifier Approaches

As depicted in Fig. 2, following pre-processing of the data and extraction of different features, two distinct supervised pulse detection algorithms were developed in this work. The first approach consisted in a two-step cascading classifier similar to the one developed by Dellimore et al. [8]. A first classifier serves to identify a window as *Pulse/No Pulse* or *Compression/Artefact*, with a second and third classifier providing the final classification of each window.

A second approach was developed consisting of a single multiclass classifier. For each algorithm, a different approach to feature selection was taken.

For the cascade classifier, a feature selection score (FSS) was used to determine the features for each individual classifier. This measure combines relevance measured by the Area Under the receiver operating characteristic curve (AUC) and redundancy computed by Spearman's rank correlation coefficient (RCC). Initially only the feature with the highest AUC is present in the subset with subsequent features being added according to the highest FSS in each iteration [12]. The formula for the score is as follows:

$$FSS_i = AUC(f_i) - \frac{\left| \sum_{f_s \in S} RCC(f_i, f_j) \right|}{|S|} \tag{1}$$

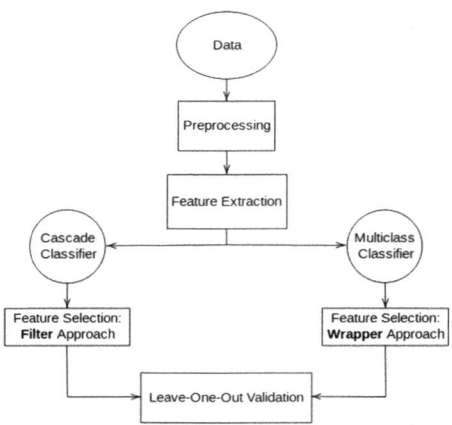

Fig. 2. Diagram of the workflow

with $AUC(f_i)$ representing the AUC of the ith feature, $RCC(f_i, f_j)$ the Spearman's RCC between the two features, S the subset of features at each iteration and $|S|$ its cardinality (Table 3).

Table 3. Selected features for the cascade classifier

Sensor	Classifier 1	Classifier 2	Classifier 3
Top ACC	STD$_{xz}$	SM, TE	–
Bottom ACC	STD	PM, STD$_{xz}$	–
Real life data	STD$_{yz}$, KU	SF, LHP, TE	PM, LHP, STD$_{acc'}$

For the multiclass classifier a wrapper approach was used, meaning all possible feature combinations were tested and the geometric mean was used to select the best combination (Table 4).

Table 4. Selected features for the multiclass classifier

Sensor	Features
Top ACC	STD, PM, STD$_{xz}$, SF, SIM
Bottom ACC	PM, LHP, STD$_{xz}$, KU, SK, STD$_{acc'}$, EN, SIM
Real life data	TE, PM, STDyz, STD$_{acc'}$, SF

3 Results

The metrics used to evaluate performance of the two classifier approaches are the following (Tables 5 and 6):

$$Accu_{final} = \frac{\sum_{class=1}^{n_{class}} TP_{class}}{\sum_{class=1}^{n_{class}} (TP_{class} + FN_{class})} \quad (2)$$

$$Sensitivity_{class} = \frac{TP_{class}}{TP_{class} + FN_{class}} \quad (3)$$

$$Specificity_{class} = \frac{TN_{class}}{TN_{class} + FP_{class}} \quad (4)$$

Table 5. Average results for the simulated datasets with Leave-one-out

Class	ACC sensor	Cascading classifier		Multiclass classifier	
		Top	Bottom	Top	Bottom
	Final accuracy	0.60 ± 0.11	0.75 ± 0.13	0.89 ± 0.06	0.97 ± 0.03
Pulse	Sensitivity	1.00 ± 0.00	1.00 ± 0.00	0.98 ± 0.04	0.99 ± 0.02
	Specificity	0.67 ± 0.19	0.67 ± 0.20	0.97 ± 0.03	0.99 ± 0.01
Compression	Sensitivity	0.78 ± 0.33	0.55 ± 0.36	0.86 ± 0.21	0.97 ± 0.05
	Specificity	0.73 ± 0.09	0.96 ± 0.03	0.94 ± 0.06	0.98 ± 0.02
Artefact	Sensitivity	0.03 ± 0.09	0.66 ± 0.14	0.82 ± 0.14	0.95 ± 0.04
	Specificity	1.00 ± 0.00	0.97 ± 0.03	0.92 ± 0.11	0.98 ± 0.03

Table 6. Average results for the real-life dataset with Leave-one-out

Class	Final accuracy	Cascading classifier	Multiclass classifier
		0.51 ± 0.04	0.57 ± 0.07
Pulse	Sensitivity	0.80 ± 0.19	0.28 ± 0.20
	Specificity	0.61 ± 0.10	0.87 ± 0.09
No Pulse	Sensitivity	0.27 ± 0.20	0.46 ± 0.14
	Specificity	0.84 ± 0.08	0.75 ± 0.10
Compression	Sensitivity	0.94 ± 0.11	0.87 ± 0.11
	Specificity	0.89 ± 0.07	0.98 ± 0.03
Artefact	Sensitivity	0.00 ± 0.00	0.67 ± 0.15
	Specificity	1.00 ± 0.00	0.83 ± 0.08

4   Discussion and Conclusion

It was found that the developed protocol was able to accurately introduce periodic components simulating compression rate. It was possible to infer that sensor positioning at the neck plays an important role in the sensitivity of the measured signal content. The bottom sensor demonstrated having a higher quality, with frequency components being better defined in the signals measured.

Regarding the feature engineering performed, success was achieved in finding new features which accurately characterize the domain space for several of the existent classification problems.

Regarding the use of a cascading classifier in the protocol data, it was found that despite relatively good performance being achieved in the individual steps of the method, the overall performance of this algorithm was relatively low for both sensor positions. Final accuracy averaged 60% and 75% for the top and bottom ACC respectively. The reason for this is that this approach suffers from intrinsic accumulation of error as a window misclassified in the first step will never be correctly classified in the end. Nevertheless, it was possible to observe that the bottom accelerometer signals presented better and less heterogeneous results which corroborates the previous insight on the signal quality of this sensor. When the second approach, i.e., the multiclass classifier was used on this dataset, the effect was drastic with an average final accuracy of 89% in the top accelerometer data and 97% in the bottom accelerometer. Sensitivity and Specificity for each class in the bottom ACC all averaged 95% with standard deviations ±0.05%. However, it is important to note that transitions windows were excluded from training and testing in this dataset, thus possibly improving the results.

Concerning the behaviour of a cascading classifier approach in the real life data it was found that due to the aforementioned source of error in this approach, all of the artefact windows were misclassified either as compressions or pulse absence/presence. This changes when using the multiclass classifier, with the average sensitivity of this class increasing to 67%. However, in this approach average artefact specificity decreased from 100% to 83%, which affected pulse sensitivity which becomes very low, averaging a value of 28%, whilst on the cascade classifier it averaged 89%.

Nevertheless, this approach provided some interesting results and shows classification potential for the problem. Pulse and No Pulse discrimination proved to be a difficult task with its performance in both approaches being fairly poor. However, it is important to note certain limitations faced: (1) there was a lack of data regarding absence of pulse; (2) real-life signals are fairly contaminated with noise; (3) annotation was performed without medical expertise; (4) no windows were excluded from training and testing. Due to all of these, no definitive conclusions can be taken from the results obtained.

Conflict of Interest. The authors declare that they have no conflict of interest.

References

1. Gräsner, J.-T., et al.: EuReCa ONE 27 Nations, ONE Europe, ONE Registry. Resuscitation **105**, 188–195 (2016)
2. Benjamin, E.J., et al.: Heart disease and stroke statistics – 2018 update: a report from the American Heart Association. Circulation **137**(12), e67–e492 (2018)
3. Rea, T.D., Donohoe, R.T., Bloomingdale, M., Eisenberg, M.S.: CPR with chest compression alone or with rescue breathing. N. Engl. J. Med. **363**, 423–433 (2010)
4. Soar, J., Nolan, J.P., Böttiger, B.W., et al.: European resuscitation council guidelines for resuscitation 2015. Resuscitation **95**, 100–147 (2015)
5. Brearley, S., Shearman, C.P., Simms, M.H.: Peripheral pulse palpation: an unreliable physical sign. Ann. R. Coll. Surg. Engl. **74**(3), 169–171 (1992)
6. Lundin, M., et al.: Distal pulse palpation: is it reliable? World J. Surg. **23**(3), 252–255 (1999)
7. Eberle, B., Dick, W.F., Schneider, T., Wisser, G., Doetsch, S., Tzanova, I.: Resuscitation **33**(2), 107–116 (1996)
8. Dellimore, K., et al.: Towards an algorithm for automatic accelerometer-based pulse presence detection during cardiopulmonary resuscitation. In: Conference of the Proceedings of IEEE Engineering in Medicine and Biology Society, pp. 3531–3534 (2016)
9. Muehlsteff, J., Carvalho, P., Henriques, J., Paiva, R.P., Reiter, H.: Cardiac status assessment with a multi-signal device for improved home-based congestive heart failure management. In: Conference of the Proceedings of IEEE Engineering in Medicine and Biology Society, pp. 876–879 (2011)
10. Rocha, T., Paredes, S., Carvalho, P., Henriques, J., Antunes, M.: Phase space reconstruction approach for ventricular arrhythmias characterization. In: Conference of the Proceedings of IEEE Engineering in Medicine and Biology Society, pp. 5470–5473 (2008)
11. Kumar, D.: Automatic heart sound analysis for cardiovascular disease assessment. Ph.D. thesis (2015). http://hdl.handle.net/10316/27015
12. Wang, R., Tang, K.: Feature selection for maximizing the area under the ROC curve. In: IEEE International Conference on Data Mining Workshops, pp. 400–405 (2009)

Input Clinical Parameters for Cardiac Heart Failure Characterization Using Machine Learning

Ernesto Iadanza[1(✉)] and Camilla Chilleri[2]

[1] Department of Information Engineering,
University of Florence, Florence, Italy
ernesto.iadanza@unifi.it
[2] School of Engineering, Degree Course in Mechanical Engineering,
Florence, Italy

Abstract. Congestive Heart Failure (CHF) is a serious chronic cardiac condition that brings high risk of urgent hospitalization and could lead to death. In this work we show how all the input clinical parameters for classifying CHF using Machine Learning can be acquired. The requested input are Blood Pressure, Heart Rate, Brain Natriuretic Peptide, Electrocardiogram, Blood Oxygen Saturation, Height, Weight and Ejection Fraction. The next step will be designing a novel device and connecting it to our Machine Learning classifier. A particular attention will be put to the assessment of electromagnetic compatibility (EMC) with other devices, taking into account that this new device will be used in many different settings (home, outdoor, etc.).

Keywords: Congestive Heart Failure · Machine Learning · Clinical input · Device · Home monitoring · ECG · Blood Pressure · Heart Rate · SpO_2 · BNP · Ejection Fraction · Weight · Height

1 Introduction

In this work it is described how to acquire input features to feed a Machine Learning (ML) Decision Support System (DSS) for Congestive Heart Failure (CHF) aiming at offering an efficient and cost-effective solution to enforce patients' home monitoring, in order to prevent inappropriate hospitalizations while improving the ability of self-diagnosing exacerbations.

This solution is based on the improvement of the multi-sensing device proposed by *Pollonini et al.* [1], together with the machine learning DSS described by *Guidi et al.* [2–4].

The clinical parameters that are needed as input to the selected machine learning classifier, described in [2] are the following:

- 12-Lead ECG
- Systolic Blood Pressure
- Diastolic Blood Pressure
- Ejection Fraction

K.-P. Lin et al. (Eds.): ICBHI 2019, IFMBE Proceedings 74, pp. 328–334, 2020.
https://doi.org/10.1007/978-3-030-30636-6_45

- Height
- Weight
- Oxygen Saturation
- Heart Rate
- BNP (Brain Natriuretic Peptide) or NT-proBNP

Our study started by examining the most recent scientific developments in literature, focused on different wearable health devices and home telemonitoring systems [5]. The purpose of all devices is to be comfortable, small in dimensions, easy-to-use, unobtrusive and interoperable among various computing platforms, in order to provide better health care service and affordable price for aging people.

Flexibility is also a crucial point for wearable devices. *Majumder et al.* presented a review of the development in wearable systems by comparing the most significant contributions in each field [6]. Wearable sensors attracted the attention of many researchers in recent years according to the development in low-power and compact wearables (sensors, actuators, smart textiles). However, the necessity of monitoring a set of physiological parameters with a minimum number of electrodes and sensors that also ensure information privacy and data security needs more research and technology developments. Hence, we will treat each parameter aiming at obtaining an improved multi parameter system that can be adequate for the scope of the ML algorithms.

All the adopted sensors will be based on contactless measurement techniques, thus avoiding the use of gel for the conduction of the signal and possible skin irritation due to contact. Wearable and textile-based sensors are still a new field with opportunities to build innovative products and has become one of the main research avenues in the textile field [7].

2   Methods

2.1   12-Lead ECG

To obtain a full 12-leads Electrocardiogram (ECG), instead of using the typical approach of using 10 electrodes, we consider adopting the EASI model, proposed by *Dower* [8] and further improved by using ML and regression techniques [9]. The EASI-lead monitoring system requires only five, optimally placed, electrodes and it can adequately reconstruct the waveforms of the 12 leads. The signals are derived from four thorax electrodes plus one reference electrode: this reduced number of electrodes improves the comfort and mobility for the patients while reducing the sensitivity to noise. The EASI lead system uses the *Frank* [10] E, A, and I electrode locations, plus an electrode S. The electrode S is positioned at the upper sternum, E at the lower sternum, A and I at the left and right mid-axillary, respectively, while the final electrode can be placed at any positions for ground. In Dower's method paired signals A-I, E-S and A-S are used, derived as a weighted linear sum [8]. This could be a good basis for deriving a 12-leads ECG (Fig. 1).

In a recent research *Kaewfoongrungsi et al.* [9] compared five different ML and regression techniques to find which model was more effective in deriving 12-leads ECG signals. From their experiments they concluded that the best performance was

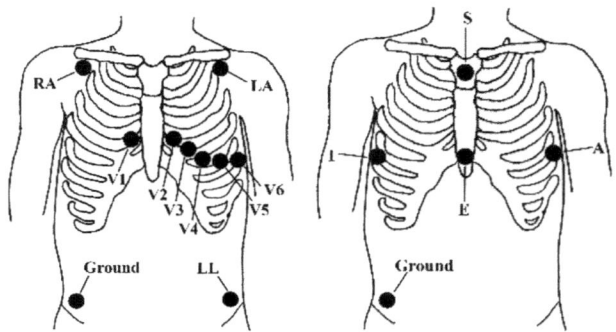

Fig. 1. Standard 12-lead ECG system (left) vs. EASI-lead system (right) [9]

obtained using *Support Vector Regression* (SVR) and *Artificial Neural Network* (ANN). Based on the existing literature, we assume that the accuracy of this solution could be sufficient for the scope of the ML algorithms. Different considerations might be done, should the EASI model be used by a cardiologist for performing his diagnosis, which is not our case [11].

2.2   Systolic Blood Pressure and Diastolic Blood Pressure

Cuffless blood pressure monitoring has been presented in previous researches in which recent efforts in developing next-generation blood pressure monitoring devices with innovative wearable sensors were highlighted [12]. Pulse Wave Velocity (PWV) could be one possible method to estimate noninvasive cuffless blood pressure (BP). It can be obtained using the distance and the Pulse Transit Time (PTT) of the blood between two arterial sites. A common way to measure PWV and PTT is by combining the ECG signal and the photoplethysmography (PPG) acquired at the level of the finger or the toe. Moreover, there are several main measurements that can be applied, such as accelerometers, pressure sensors, and bioimpedance (BI). In case of the PPG sensor, the need for a light-emitting source for the reflection method and the necessity of a direct and tight contact with the skin are drawbacks. It can require higher levels of power and users might feel uncomfortable [13] (Fig. 2).

$$\text{Calculation}: \quad PWV = D/PTT$$

In order to cope with the limitations of the above described methods, *Liu et al.* [14] replaced the PPG signal with the impedance-plethysmography (IPG), used to detect the PTT. Then, they designed an IPG arm ring that could measure an accurate IPG signal. They compared the change of PTT_{PPG} (the PTT from the ECG and the PPG signals) with that of PTT_{IPG} (from the ECG and the IPG signals). Their results showed that the change of the systolic pressure had a better relationship with the change of the PTT_{IPG} compared to the PTT_{PPG} (r = 0.700 vs. r = 0.450). Moreover, the IPG ring with spot electrodes would be more suitable to develop with the wearable cuffless blood pressure monitors. This happens because the electrodes are placed symmetrically and the IPG ring could be rotated around, so they only need to make slight contact with the skin. Soft material would not feel uncomfortable to patients.

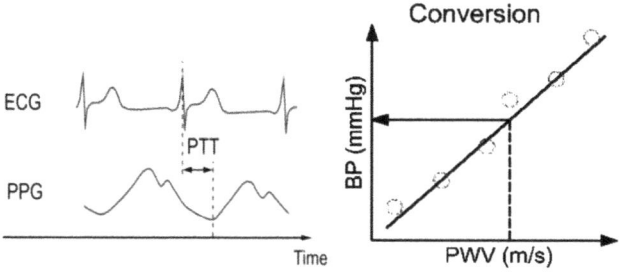

Fig. 2. Methodology of pulse wave velocity (PWV)-based blood pressure (BP) estimation. D is the distance from the arterial sites [13].

Although these approaches are interesting, *Simjanoska et al.* [15] have developed a method for the BP estimation by using only ECG signals. They acquired BP by introducing complexity analysis in the feature extraction process as well as a stack of ML models for more robust predictive models. In the experimental results they obtained that with the use of a calibration, the method can achieve results close to those of a common medical device for BP estimation. This research represents a contribution on the use of ECG sensor without additional devices for detecting BP. It provides with a demonstrable relationship between BP and ML that could be an innovative development in this field.

However, there is still a need for a more in-depth analysis about the most accurate cuffless method.

2.3 Ejection Fraction

Ejection Fraction (EF) refers to the measurement, expressed in percentage, of blood amount pumped out of the ventricles with each contraction. EF measurement requires Echocardiography or Magnetic Resonance Imaging.

Hence, this clinical parameter could not be simply acquired in the proposed device, without requiring external input from these pieces of equipment.

2.4 Weight and Height

This parameter is crucial for diagnosis CHF worsening.

There are some methods for estimating both weight and height using computer vision. Weight measurement using these techniques is currently not accurate enough, therefore it will be acquired using a Bluetooth scale, according to *Pollonini et al.* [1]. Instead Height will be detected with a webcam, using computer vision systems.

2.5 Oxygen Saturation

The blood oxygen saturation level (SpO_2) indicates the percentage of oxygenated hemoglobin molecules in arterial blood. For its detection, a textile-based sensing principle for long term PPG monitoring could be adopted [16]. This photonic textile, using embroidered optical fibers and working in reflection mode, bestows a highly flexibility. It is very versatile for wearable long-term monitoring, allowing the measurements in different parts of the body and enhancing the acceptance of the wearer. SpO_2 was determined by using a modified Beer-Lambert law for measuring the light attenuation at two different wavelengths (632 nm and 894 nm). All the recorded data were imported into MATLAB R2012b for further signal processing (Fig. 3).

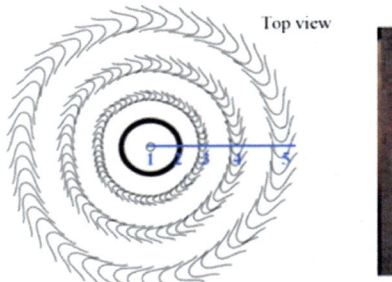 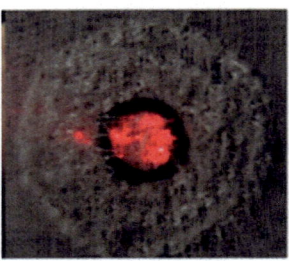

Fig. 3. Sketch presenting embroidered optical fibers. Where (1) optical fibers stitched to couple the light out; (2) three-dimensional embroidered black ring to prevent light short circuit. (3), (4) and (5) represent rings of optical fibers stitched to couple the light in. Each "V"-shaped line in the rings represents a portion of a single optical fiber (left). Top view of the photonic textile: light is delivered by the central fiber, while the black ring prevents "short circuit". A woven textile is used (right) [16].

2.6   Heart Rate

Heart Rate (HR) can be easily extracted from ECG (R-peak) or PPG signals [16, 17]. Although these measurements have two different physiological origins, they contain a similar heart rate information. The PPG monitor is the same used for detecting SpO_2, therefore we could monitor both these parameters using a single device.

Instead, for heart rate detection from ECG the most used algorithm was developed by *Pan and Tompkins* [17] and later improved by many authors. In 2006 *Paoletti et al.* [18] compare it with a new algorithm. They demonstrated that both algorithms showed similar performances in order to detect QRS complexes, but the new one had the advantage of being faster.

2.7   BNP (Brain Natriuretic Peptide) or NT-proBNP

BNP or NT-proBNP are identified as the standard biomarkers for CHF diagnosis and prognosis. *Sarangadharan et al.* [19] developed a hand-held field effect transistor (FET) based biosensor aiming at detecting Brain Natriuretic Peptide (BNP) from a single drop of whole blood, without sample pre-treatments. They created an integrated portable biosensor system that could allow whole blood diagnostics in five minutes. It works by separating the cells from plasma using gravity. The authors also show their device can be used both in a face down or a face up configuration, with no significant differences in performance. Hence its portability and its rapid diagnosis could be a plus for home caring and clinical application.

3 Conclusion

In this paper we showed how all the required parameters for feeding a ML decision support system for CHF can be acquired using simple techniques and sensors that might be engineered in a single hardware device. The next step will be designing this novel device and connecting it to our ML classifier [20]. In previous researches *Guidi et al.* investigated some techniques for classifying CHF, such as Classification And Regression Tree (CART), Random Forest and other algorithms, obtaining good results in severity assessment and in reducing clinical errors [3, 21].

A particular attention should be put in assessing the electromagnetic compatibility (EMC) with other devices (electro medical equipment, personal devices, home devices), taking into account that this new device will be used in many different settings (home, outdoor, etc.) [22].

Conflict of Interest. The authors declare that they have no conflict of interest.

References

1. Pollonini, I., Quadri, S., et al.: Blue scale: a multi-sensing device for remote management of congestive heart failure. In: Annual Meeting of the IEEE Engineering in Medicine and Biology Society (EMBC 2014) (2014)
2. Guidi, G., Pollonini, L., Dafford, C., Iadanza, E.: A multi-layer monitoring system for clinical management of Congestive Heart Failure. BMC Med. Inform. Decis. Mak. **15**(Suppl 3), S5 (2015). https://doi.org/10.1186/1472-6947-15-s3-s5
3. Guidi, G., Iadanza, E., Pettenati, M.C., et al.: Heart failure artificial intelligence-based computer aided diagnosis telecare system. In: Lecture Notes in Computer Science (including subseries Lecture Notes in Artificial Intelligence and Lecture Notes in Bioinformatics). LNCS, vol. 7251, pp. 278–281 (2012). https://doi.org/10.1007/978-3-642-30779-9_44
4. Guidi, G., Pettenati, M.C., Melillo, P., Iadanza, E.: A machine learning system to improve heart failure patient assistance. IEEE J. Biomed. Health Inform. **18**(6), 1750–1756 (2014). https://doi.org/10.1109/jbhi.2014.23377522. Art. no. 6851844
5. Dias, D., Cunha, J.: Wearable health devices—vital sign monitoring, systems and technologies. Sensors (Switzerland) (2018). https://doi.org/10.3390/s18082414
6. Majumder, S., Mondal, T., Deen, M.: Wearable sensors for remote health monitoring. Sensors (Switzerland) (2017). https://doi.org/10.3390/s17010130
7. Gonçalves, C., Ferreira da Silva, A., Gomes, J., et al.: Wearable e-textile technologies: a review on sensors, actuators and control elements. Inventions **3**(1), 14 (2018). https://doi.org/10.3390/inventions3010014
8. Dower, G.E., et al.: Deriving the 12-lead electrocardiogram from four (EASI) electrodes. J. Electrocardiol. **21**(Supplemental issue), S182–S187 (1988)
9. Kaewfoongrungsi, P., Hormdee, D.: Improving EASI model via machine learning and regression techniques. J. Telecommun. Electron. Comput. Eng. **10**(1), 115–120 (2018). ISSN 22898131

10. Frank, E.: An accurate, clinically practical system or spatial vectorcardiography. Circulation **13**, 537 (1956)
11. Holderith, M., Schanze, T.: Cross-correlation based comparison between the conventional 12-lead ECG and an EASI derived 12-lead ECG. Curr. Dir. Biomed. Eng. **4**(1), 621–624 (2018). https://doi.org/10.12693/aphyspola.118.131
12. Arakawa, T.: Recent research and developing trends of wearable sensors for detecting blood pressure. Sensors (Switzerland) (2018). https://doi.org/10.3390/s18092772
13. Huynh T., Jafari R., Chung W.: An accurate bioimpedance measurement system for blood pressure monitoring. Sensors (Switzerland) **18**(7) (2018). https://doi.org/10.3390/s18072095
14. Liu, S., Cheng, D., Su, C.: A cuffless blood pressure measurement based on the impedance plethysmography technique. Sensors (Basel, Switzerland) **17**(5), 1–13 (2017). https://doi.org/10.3390/s17051176
15. Simjanoska, M., Gjoreski, M., Gams, M., et al.: Non-invasive blood pressure estimation from ECG using machine learning techniques. Sensors (Switzerland) **18**(4), 1–20 (2018). https://doi.org/10.3390/s18041160
16. Krehel, M., Wolf, M., Boesel, L., et al.: Development of a luminous textile for reflective pulse oximetry measurements. Biomed. Opt. Express **5**(8), 2537 (2014)
17. Pan, J., Tompkins, W.: A real-time QRS detection algorithm. IEEE Trans. Biomed. Eng. (BME) **32**(3), 230–236 (1985). https://doi.org/10.1109/tbme.1985.325532
18. Paoletti, M., Marchesi, C.: Discovering dangerous patterns in long-term ambulatory ECG recordings using a fast QRS detection algorithm and explorative data analysis. Comput. Methods Programs Biomed. **82**(1), 20–30 (2006). https://doi.org/10.1016/j.cmpb.2006.01.005
19. Sarangadharan, I., Wang, S., Tai, T., et al.: Risk stratification of heart failure from one drop of blood using hand-held biosensor for BNP detection. Biosens. Bioelectron. **107**, 259–265 (2018)
20. Guidi, G., Pettenati, M.C., Miniati, R., Iadanza, E.: Random forest for automatic assessment of heart failure severity in a telemonitoring scenario. In: Proceedings of the Annual International Conference of the IEEE Engineering in Medicine and Biology Society, EMBS, art. no. 6610229, pp. 3230–3233 (2013). https://doi.org/10.1109/embc.2013.6610229
21. Guidi, G., Pettenati, M.C., Miniati, R., Iadanza, E.: Heart failure analysis dashboard for patient's remote monitoring combining multiple artificial intelligence technologies. In: Proceedings of the Annual International Conference of the IEEE Engineering in Medicine and Biology Society, EMBS, art. no. 6346401, pp. 2210–2213 (2012). https://doi.org/10.1109/embc.2012.6346401
22. Iadanza, E., Dori, F., Miniati, R., Corrado, E.: Electromagnetic Interferences (EMI) from active RFId on critical care equipment. In: IFMBE Proceedings, vol. 29, pp. 991–994 (2010). https://doi.org/10.1007/978-3-642-13039-7_251

An Investigation on Phase Characteristics of Galvanic Coupling Human Body Communication

Weikun Chen[1,2], Wenzhu Liu[1,2], Ivana Čuljak[3], Xingguang Chen[1,2], Haibo Zheng[1,4], Yueming Gao[1,2(✉)], Željka Lučev Vasić[3], Mario Cifrek[3], and Min Du[1,2]

[1] College of Physics and Information Engineering,
Fuzhou University, Fuzhou, China
fzugym@gmail.com

[2] Key Lab of Medical Instrumentation and Pharmaceutical Technology of Fujian Province, 2 Xue Yuan Road, University Town, Fuzhou, China

[3] Faculty of Electrical Engineering and Computing, University of Zagreb, Zagreb, Croatia

[4] School of Basic Medical Sciences, Fujian Medical University, Fuzhou, China

Abstract. Human body communication (HBC) has the advantages of low power consumption, low radiation and anti-interference ability, which has broad application prospects in entertainment and health care. Accurate human channel characteristics will contribute to the development of HBC. This paper explores the effect of channel length and electrode size on human body channel phase characteristic. A galvanic coupling human body communication experimental platform was built. The measurement results show that in the low frequency band, the phase transition is less than the high frequency. When the frequency is in the range of 200 kHz to 300 kHz, the phase will oscillate. Increasing the electrode size can improve phase oscillation. This paper provides a reference for the application of human body communication in long channel and the miniaturization design of transceiver.

Keywords: Human body communication (HBC) · Galvanic coupling · Phase characteristic · Channel length

1 Introduction

Human body communication (HBC) is an emerging communication method that uses human body conductivity to transmit information [1]. Because of its low power consumption, low radiation and anti-interference ability, it has been widely used in daily life, entertainment and medical field [2]. In 2012, the IEEE 802.15.6 standard defined three physical layers for wireless body area networks, depending on the operating frequency: narrowband, ultra-wideband, and human body communication [3]. According to signal coupling, HBC is divided into galvanic coupling and capacitive coupling [4]. In capacitive coupling, both transmitter and receiver units use only one signal electrode to connect with the human body, thus reducing the complexity of the

K.-P. Lin et al. (Eds.): ICBHI 2019, IFMBE Proceedings 74, pp. 335–341, 2020.
https://doi.org/10.1007/978-3-030-30636-6_46

device design. However, since the signal return path is closed capacitively through the environment, it is extremely susceptible to environmental factors [5]. In galvanic coupling, the alternating current is injected into the human body through the two electrodes of the transmitter unit. Compared to the capacitive coupling, transmission frequency of the galvanic coupling is lower, and the interference caused by high frequency is avoided [6]. Therefore, galvanic coupling has a strong anti-interference ability.

HBC technology provides a new way for people to prevent and treat diseases. According to the position of the device and the human body, HBC is divided into two groups: wearable [7] and implantable [8] HBC. In-depth research on human channel characteristics contributes to the design and development of HBC equipment. Differences in measurement methods and electrode placement schemes can make measurement results very different. The common ground measurement at the transmitting and the receiving ports causes the measured channel attenuation to be significantly lower, which is because the coupling between the transmitter and receiver ground electrodes increases the coupling of the signal, making the measurement result inaccurate [9]. In the electrode configuration scheme, the size of the electrodes, the distance between the electrodes, and their position on the body may bring different measurement results [10]. The human body is usually equivalent to a four-layer model of skin, fat, muscle, and bone [11]. Studies have found that muscles play a major role in the electrical properties of the human body [4].

The existing research has carried out extensive measurements of the attenuation characteristics of human channels based both on capacitive and galvanic coupling. The current research is mainly divided into two aspects: the first is to conduct the measurement of human channel characteristics using network analyzers and spectrum analyzers [12]. The second is the development of portable device which uses programmable logic chip based on the existing communication theory [13]. Most of the above studies have focused only on the amplitude characteristics of the human channel, and little research has paid attention to the phase characteristics of the human body channel. Lučev Vasić et al measured IBC system amplitude and phase transmission characteristics using three types of galvanic decouplers [14]. In this paper, a galvanic coupling detection platform was built, in order to study the influence of channel length and electrode size on the phase-frequency characteristic of the human body.

2   Methods

2.1   Experimental Setup

In order to study the effects of different channel lengths and different electrode sizes on the galvanic coupling human communication channel, an experimental platform was built, as shown in Fig. 1. The phase-frequency characteristics of the human body were measured using an Agilent E5061B network analyzer. The frequency range was set between 1 kHz and 10 MHz; frequency step was set to 500 Hz between 1 kHz and 2 MHz, and 5 kHz between 2 MHz and 10 MHz. A 0 dBm signal was generated at the port 1 output, which was connected to the right wrist of a test subject through a pair of physiotherapy electrodes (Shanghai Cross Health Biotechnology Co., Ltd. Type: LT-1). The received signal was connected to the input port 2 of the network analyzer through a pair of physiotherapy electrodes and a differential probe (Agilent, 1141A), for eliminating the common ground between the devices. The network analyzer was set to measure the phase difference between port 1 and port 2 signals. Repeated measurements were performed for each test subject, and the data was averaged to obtain the phase frequency response in degrees.

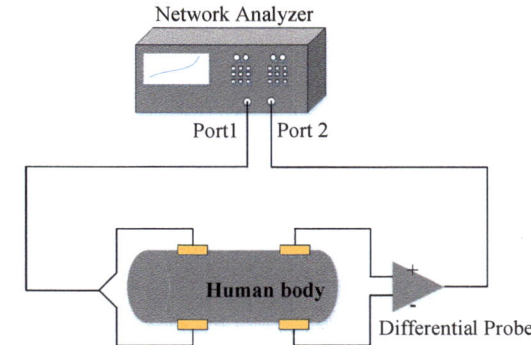

Fig. 1. Experimental platform for studying human channel characteristics.

2.2   Experiment Protocol

In this study, four volunteers aged 23 to 25 were selected to participate in the survey. The measurement parameters are summarized in Table 1, and the anthropometric characteristics of the volunteers, are given in Table 2. In the table, arm length is the distance between the right and left wrist. Before measurement, a through calibration was performed on the network analyzer, to eliminate the errors associated with port 1 and port 2 connecting differential probes and physiotherapy electrodes. The skin of all test subjects was cleaned with an alcohol cotton pad at the positions of the electrodes prior to the measurements. The volunteers were instructed to stand still in front of the test bench.

Table 1. Measurement parameters

Parameters	Value
Test subjects	Two males and two females
Signal transmission power	0 dBm
Frequency range	1 kHz–10 MHz
Electrodes	Physiotherapy electrodes
Electrode size	40×40 mm^2, 20×20 mm^2
Distance between electrodes	9 cm, 15 cm, 28 cm, 92 cm, 112 cm

Table 2. Anthropometrical parameters of volunteers

Volunteer	Sex	Age	BMI	Arm Length (cm)
V1	Male	25	20.2	126
V2	Female	24	19.7	118
V3	Male	25	19.9	130
V4	Female	24	19.0	121

For investigating the influence of channel length on human body phase characteristic, 40×40 mm^2 physiotherapy electrodes were used. Two transmitting electrodes were attached to the right wrist of the subject, and the two receiving electrodes moved towards the left arm side as the distance increased. In the experiment, channel lengths of 9 cm, 15 cm, 28 cm, 92 cm, and 112 cm were tested. For three shorter distances transmitting and receiving electrodes were on the right arm: for 9 cm and 15 cm channel lengths the receiving electrodes were on the right lower arm, and for 28 cm channel length receiving electrodes were on the right upper arm, thus including the elbow joint in the signal path. For the remaining two distances receiving electrodes were set on a left upper arm (92 cm) and left lower arm (120 cm) of a test subject, thus including both shoulder joints for both channel lengths, as well as another elbow joint for 120 cm distance. In these two cases the posture of test subjects' arms also has an influence on the signal path: when the distance between the electrodes through the air is shorter than the distance through the human body (e.g. the arms are parallel in front of the body), most of the signal path will close from the transmitting electrodes to the receiving electrodes through the air [15]. Therefore, the subjects were instructed to keep their arms still and wide spread in line with their shoulders, in order to ensure that the distance between the electrodes along the human body would be equal to the distance through the air.

For investigating the influence of the electrodes size on human body phase characteristics, the distance between transmitting and receiving electrodes was set to 112 cm. The electrode dimensions were 40×40 mm^2, and 20×20 mm^2, respectively. For each case, the test subjects maintained the posture for 10 s, and the data of the network analyzer was saved after being stabilized to ensure the accuracy of the experimental data.

3   Results and Discussions

This section describes the effect of channel length and electrode size on the phase-frequency characteristics of current-coupled human channels. Measurements on each test subject were performed on three different days in the same environment (indoor, temperature 25 C), using the same experimental equipment and protocol. The final results presented in this section were obtained by averaging the three-days measurement results.

3.1   Effect of Channel Length

The relationship between channel length and human phase characteristics of test subjects V1 (male) and V2 (female) is shown in Figs. 2(a) and (b), respectively. The results show that in the low frequency range, the channel length has less influence on the phase, and the frequency and phase change linearly. In the higher frequency range, the phase begins to increase, and for some channel lengths, the change of the phase exceeds 200°.

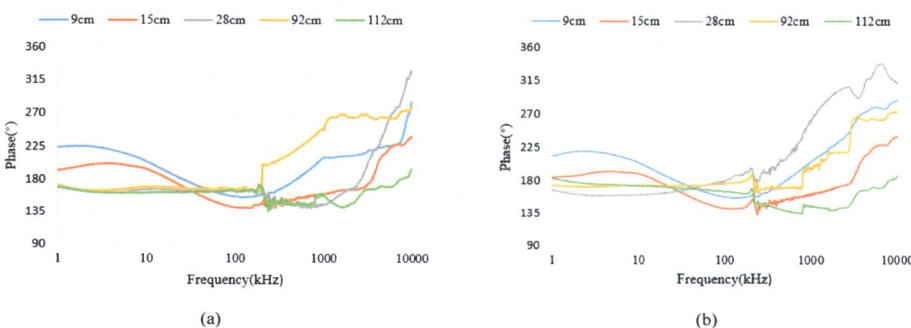

Fig. 2. Phase-frequency characteristic of the human body for different channel lengths and test subjects (a) V1 and (b) V2.

Looking at Fig. 2(a), it can be found that when the frequency is lower than 200 kHz and the channel length is larger than 15 cm, the phase is relatively constant. In particular, when the channel lengths are 28 cm, 92 cm, and 112 cm, the measured phases are between 150° and 200°, and the phase tends to decrease as the channel length increases. For the shorter channel lengths (9 cm and 15 cm) the signal path does not cross any joint, and the phase oscillation is small between in the frequency range of 200 kHz to 300 kHz. When the frequency is between 200 kHz and 300 kHz and the channel length is 28 cm or longer, the phase oscillates. When the frequency is higher than 300 kHz, the phase begins to increase rapidly, and the partial phase change exceeds 200°, which is particularly obvious for 28 cm channel length. In Fig. 2(b), showing measurement results of a female volunteer, we can see a similar regular pattern as in Fig. 2(a). The results show that the phase changes of males and females are similar under different channel lengths in a tested frequency range.

3.2   Effect of Electrode Size

The measurement results of the influence of the electrode size on the phase characteristics are shown in Fig. 3 for volunteers V1 and V2 (a), and V3 and V4 (b). The results show that the effect of electrode size on phase characteristics is consistent in the low frequency range. In the high frequency range, the effect of the electrode size on the phase is disordered. In Fig. 3(a), it is found that when frequency band is below

200 kHz, for both test subjects, the phase of the 40×40 mm^2 electrodes is higher than the phase of size 20×20 mm^2 electrodes. In particular, it is apparent for test subject V2. For V1, the phase with an electrode size of 40×40 mm^2 is only slightly higher than the phase obtained with 20×20 mm^2 electrodes. This consistency is satisfied for both V3 and V4, in Fig. 3(b). In the high frequency range, for V1, V2, and V4, the effect of the electrode size on the phase is exactly opposite to the low frequency range, and higher phase is achieved for smaller electrodes. However, in Fig. 3(b) for volunteer V3, when the frequency is higher than 1 MHz, measured phase is higher for larger electrodes. From Figs. 3(a) and (b), it can be confirmed that in the frequency region where phase changes rapidly, the electrode size of 40×40 mm^2 is always better than that of the electrode of 20×20 mm^2.

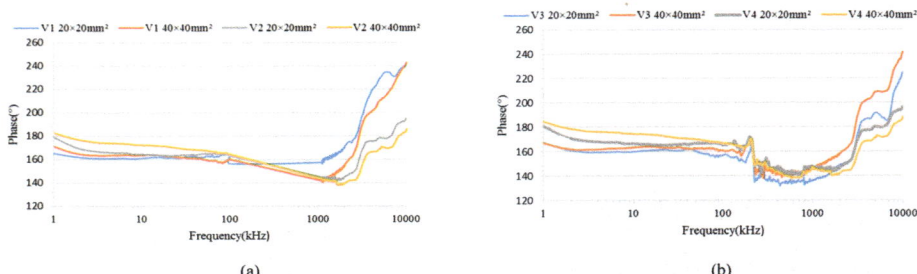

(a)   (b)

Fig. 3. Phase-frequency characteristic of the human body for different electrode sizes and test subjects (a) V1 and V2, (b) V3 and V4.

4   Conclusion

In this paper, the effects of channel length and electrode size on galvanic coupling human body communication are explored. The experimental results show that since each individual's tissue composition is very different, we can't get the phase characteristics common to the whole frequency band, and the human body has phase specificity. But we can find that in the low frequency band, the phase change is smaller than in the high frequency band. When the frequency is in the range of 200 kHz to 300 kHz, the phase will oscillate. Increasing the electrode size can improve phase oscillation. Therefore, this paper provides a reference for transceiver design and human channel research. For galvanic coupling human communication, choosing a lower frequency signal and avoiding frequency bands with rapid change of the phase can reduce the effects of other factors.

Acknowledgment. This work was supported by the National Natural Science Foundation of China U1505251 and 61201397, the Project of Chinese Ministry of Science and Technology 2016YFE0122700, and the S&T Project of Fujian Province 2018I0011.

Conflict of Interest. The authors declare that they have no conflict of interest.

References

1. Callejón, M.A., Naranjo-Hernández, D., Reina-Tosina, J., Roa, L.M.: A comprehensive study into intrabody communication measurements. IEEE Trans. Instrum. Meas. **62**(9), 2446–2455 (2013)
2. Gao, Y.M., Wu, Z.M., Pun, S.H., Mak, P.U., Vai, M.I., Du, M.: A novel field-circuit FEM modeling and channel gain estimation for galvanic coupling real IBC measurements. Sensors **16**(4), 471–486 (2016)
3. Kwak, K.S., Ullah, S., Ullah, N.: An overview of IEEE 802.15.6 standard. In: Proceedings of International Symposium on Applied Sciences in Biomedical and Communication Technologies, ISABEL2010, Rome, Italy, pp. 1–6 (2011)
4. Naranjo-Hernández, D., Callejón-Leblic, M.A., Lučev Vasić, Ž., Seyedi, M., Gao, Y.M.: Past results, present trends, and future challenges in intrabody communication. Wirel. Commun. Mob. Comput. **2018**(4), 1–39 (2018)
5. Pereira, M.D., Alvarez-Botero, G.A., de Sousa, F.R.: Characterization and modeling of the capacitive HBC channel. IEEE Trans. Instrum. Meas. **64**(10), 2626–2635 (2015)
6. ICNIRP: Guidelines for limiting exposure to time-varying electric and magnetic fields (1 Hz to 100 kHz). Health Phys. **99**(6), 818–827 (2010)
7. Maity, S., Das, D., Sen, S.: Wearable health monitoring using capacitive voltage-mode human body communication. In: Conference Proceedings of the IEEE Engineering in Medicine and Biology Society, EMBC 2017, Seogwipo, South Korea, pp. 1–4 (2017)
8. Chow, E.Y., Ouyang, Y.H., Beier, B., et al.: Evaluation of cardiovascular stents as antennas for implantable wireless applications. IEEE Trans. Microw. Theory Tech. **57**(10), 2523–2532 (2009)
9. Lučev Vasić, Ž., Krois, I., Cifrek, M.: A capacitive intrabody communication channel from 100 kHz to 100 MHz. IEEE Trans. Instrum. Meas. **61**(12), 3280–3289 (2012)
10. Bae, J., Yoo, H.J.: The effects of electrode configuration on body channel communication based on analysis of vertical and horizontal electric dipoles. IEEE Trans. Microw. Theory Tech. **63**(4), 1409–1420 (2015)
11. Mao, J., Yang, H., Lian, Y., Zhao, B.: A five-tissue-layer human body communication circuit model tunable to individual characteristics. IEEE Trans. Biomed. Circuits Syst. **12**(2), 303–312 (2018)
12. Bae, J., Cho, H., Song, K., Lee, H., Yoo, H.J.: The signal transmission mechanism on the surface of human body for body channel communication. IEEE Trans. Microw. Theory Tech. **60**(3), 582–593 (2012)
13. Nie, Z., Ma, J., Ivanov, K., Lei, W.: An investigation on dynamic human body communication channel characteristics at 45 MHz in different surrounding environments. IEEE Antennas Wirel. Propag. Lett. **13**(1), 309–312 (2014)
14. Lučev Vasić, Ž., Krois, I., Cifrek, M.: Effect of transformer symmetry on intrabody communication channel measurements using grounded instruments. Automatika **57**(1), 15–26 (2016)
15. Hwang, J.H., Kang, T.W., Kim, Y.T., Park, S.O.: Measurement of transmission properties of HBC channel and its impulse response model. IEEE Trans. Instrum. Meas. **65**(1), 177–188 (2015)

Noise Reduction for Continuous Positive Airway Pressure Machine

Cheng-Yuan Chang$^{(\boxtimes)}$, Sen M. Kuo, and Xiu-Wei Liu

Department of Electrical Engineering, Chung Yuan Christian University,
Jhongli, Taoyuan, Taiwan
ccy@cycu.edu.tw

Abstract. Continuous Positive Airway Pressure (CPAP) machine is a form of positive airway pressure ventilator, which utilizes mild air pressure on a continuous basis to keep the airways continuously open in people who are not able to breathe spontaneously on their own. The CPAP machine is widely used for sleep apnea patients. This paper presents the development of active noise control (ANC) system for reducing the noise from CPAP machine. By integrating loudspeaker and microphones, we develop feedback ANC structure and filtered-X least mean square (FXLMS) algorithm using the Texas Instrument (TI) TMS320C6713 starter kit. Real-time experimental results show that the proposed method reduces the noise of CPAP machine and achieves global cancellation of the noise.

Keywords: CPAP machine · Noise · ANC · FXLMS

1 Introduction

Continuous positive airway pressure (CPAP) machines that are used in therapy of sleep apnea. Patients would wear a face mask that is connected to a centrifugal fan (pump) that provides a natural flow of air into the nasal passages during sleep in order to keep the airway properly opened. The CPAP machines are meant to help patients sleep better. However, CPAP machines make loud noise, resulting in the patients and their bed partners cannot sleep well. This paper uses artificial anti-noise based on the active noise control (ANC) technology [1] to make destructive interference for the fan noise. Figure 1 shows the idea of ANC system. This idea was proposed by Lueg [2] in 1965. With the development of high-speed microprocessors, there are many applications using the ANC systems, such as earphone, helmet, headrest, and pillow, been developed in the past few years. The anti-noise signal, with the same amplitude but opposite phase to the noise, is generated by the ANC system and driven by the secondary source (loudspeaker) to reduce the primary noise. The anti-noise signal is generated to drive the secondary loudspeaker to cancel the noise at error microphone location. Error microphone measures the error signal, which is minimized by adapting the coefficients of the adaptive filter.

Generally, the ANC system can be divided into two types, feedforward and feedback ANC systems. The feedforward ANC system needs reference sensors close to the undesired noise to detect the reference signals. Whereas the feedback type ANC utilizes

© Springer Nature Switzerland AG 2020
K.-P. Lin et al. (Eds.): ICBHI 2019, IFMBE Proceedings 74, pp. 342–348, 2020.
https://doi.org/10.1007/978-3-030-30636-6_47

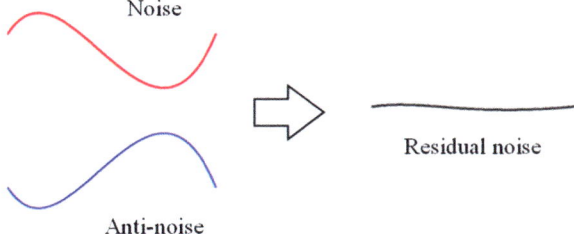

Fig. 1. The idea of ANC

the output signal of the ANC system and error signal to synthesis the reference signal, so the reference sensor is not necessary in a feedback ANC (FBANC) system. The FBANC method saves space and cost, but it can only cancel predictable noise.

Centrifugal fan in CPAP machine generates airflow but makes annoying noise. To the best of our knowledge, there is no study regarding the CPAP machines noise. Suggestions such as re-positioning the CPAP machines, checking the machines for any leak, or even applying additional white noise machines to play masking sounds cannot really solve the noise problems from the CPAP machines. There are some research about reducing noise of centrifugal fans. Most of them discussing the ways to design the blades of centrifugal fans [3, 4]. Besides, some research using ANC methods to achieve fan noise reduction but need large space for the related loudspeakers [5–7], which is not suitable to be realized in a CPAP machine.

In this paper, the feedback ANC technique is used to cancel the noise from a CPAP machine. Since the main noise of a CPAP machine is from the centrifugal fan (pump), which results in narrowband noise regarding to its rotating speed and blades number. Therefore, a feedback ANC scheme is suitable to be applied to cancel the noise of CPAP machine. Besides, the size of general CPAP machine is small; therefore, a small size receiver is utilized to play the anti-noise signal to destructively interfere the CPAP machine noise.

This paper is organized as follows. Section 2 reveals the FBANC algorithm. Experimental setup of the FBANC system in a CPAP machine and the experimental results are given in Sect. 3 to verify the noise reduction performance. The result of global cancellation of the noise is presented too.

2 Feedback ANC Algorithm

The idea of a single channel FBANC system is shown in Fig. 2. Assuming that the noise source is a narrowband noise and estimated; therefore, in Fig. 2, we can apply only error microphone to measure the residual noise and then synthesize the reference signal by the ANC system. The ANC system computes the anti-noise signal, and then drive the secondary loudspeaker to destructively interfere the primary noise. The block diagram can be shown in Fig. 3.

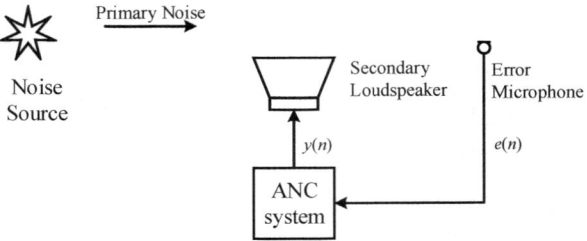

Fig. 2. Idea of a single channel ANC system.

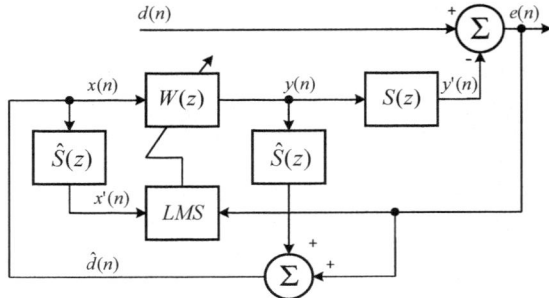

Fig. 3. Block diagram of a single channel ANC system.

Suppose $d(n)$ is the primary noise to be canceled. We derive the anti-noise signal $y(n)$ by the FBANC system. After driving the secondary path $S(z)$, an error microphone is used to measure the residual noise $e(n)$

$$e(n) = d(n) - y'(n) = d(n) - s(n) * y(n), \tag{1}$$

where $s(n)$ is the impulse response of $S(z)$, composed by transfer functions of analog to digital converter, smoothing filter, power amplifier, loudspeaker, acoustic plant information, error microphone, per-amplifier, anti-aliasing filter and analog to digital converter. Usually, we use offline modeling method to identify $S(z)$, obtaining an estimation $\hat{S}(z)$.

The FBANC system synthesizes the reference noise signal by using

$$x(n) = \hat{d}(n) = e(n) + \sum_{m=0}^{M-1} \hat{s}_m y(n-m), \tag{2}$$

where $\hat{s}_m$ denotes the mth coefficient of the Mth order transversal filter $\hat{S}(z)$. Therefore, the anti-noise signal $y(n)$ is

$$y(n) = \sum_{l=0}^{L-1} w_l x(n-l), \tag{3}$$

where w_l is the lth coefficient of the Lth order adaptive filter $W(z)$. Besides, the filtered reference signal is

$$x'(n) = \sum_{m=0}^{M-1} \hat{s}_m x(n-m), \tag{4}$$

and the adaptive algorithm to tune the weights is

$$w_l(n+1) = w_l(n) + \mu x'(n-l)e(n), \tag{5}$$

where μ is the step size and $l = 0, 1, \cdots, L-1$.

The FBANC method, including Eqs. (2)–(4), tunes the weights in (5) to minimize the residual noise $e(n)$ according to the filtered-X least mean square (FXLMS) algorithm [8].

3 Experiments

Experiments are implemented using single channel FBANC technique to cancel the noise at the air inlet part of a CPAP machine (APEX XT). The experimental setup is shown below. Figures 4(a) and (b) show a CPAP machine and its interior. Obviously, a centrifugal fan is installed at the center part (refer to Fig. 4(b)). The function of the centrifugal fan is to suck air from the air inlet and to push the air to patients through the air outlet. The schematic diagram of the CPAP, from air inlet to the air outlet, is shown in Fig. 4(c). Since the noise of the CPAP machine is mainly from the centrifugal fan; therefore, there are two outlets for the fan noise – from the air inlet and the air outlet. In this paper, we only deal with the noise spread from the air inlet. The noise from the air outlet can be reduced using the same way.

In order to reduce the fan noise, an aluminum film speaker was put at the pathway as the secondary loudspeaker and an MEMS microphone (Knowles SPH1642HT5H-1) was set at the rear-end opening of the CPAP machine as the error microphone. Since that loudspeaker and the MEMS microphone are both small, they can be put at the pathway and will not block the airflow.

The FBANC algorithm is implemented using TMS320C6713 DSK with 6713IFB analogue to digital (A/D) and digital to analogue (D/A) conversion card from Heg Co. Ltd. The parameters used for the FBANC algorithm to reduce the CPAP machine noise is shown in Table 1. Experimental results is shown in Fig. 3. We measure 25 noise power, distributed in 50×50 cm^2 area at 20 cm behind the rear end (inlet) of the CPAP machine, shown in Fig. 5. The noise power before and after the activation of the FBANC system are shown in Tables 2 and 3. Obviously, we can see the noise power being reduced when the ANC system is activated. The average noise reduction is 3.7 dB. The noise spectrum before and after the ANC system is shown in Fig. 6.

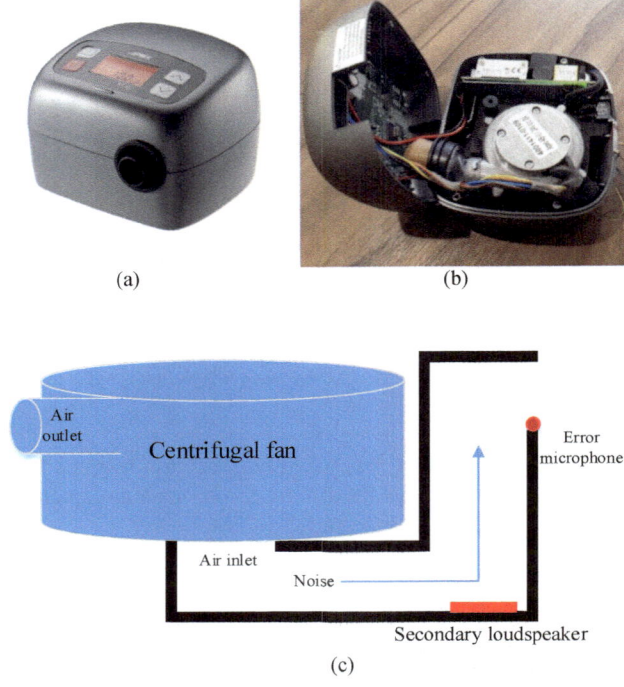

Fig. 4. (a) CPAP machine (b) its interior (c) schematic diagram.

Table 1. Parameters for FBANC algorithm

Parameters	Values
Sampling rate	10 kHz
Cut off frequency	3800 Hz
$\hat{S}(z)$ filter length	128
$W(z)$ filter length	512
Off-line step size	0.005
ANC Step size	0.00005

The noise from the air outlet to the patient can be canceled by using the FBANC algorithm too. For this case, a multi-channel algorithm such as two-by-two FBANC system is suggested to be utilized.

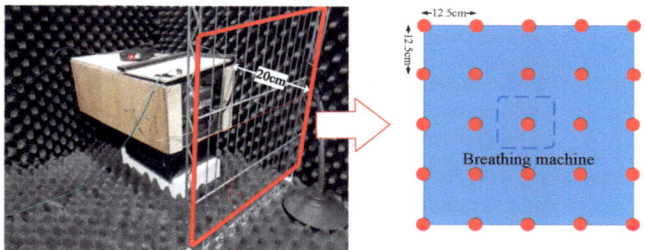

Fig. 5. Noise power spread, left: before ANC, right: after ANC.

Table 2. Noise power (ANC OFF, in dB)

5	−30.95	−28.12	−33.55	−30.35	−29.76
4	−30.09	−30.02	−30.40	−28.09	−32.40
3	−31.63	−25.37	−24.06	−27.24	−28.05
2	−25.34	−24.46	−23.19	−26.80	−28.41
1	−32.09	−27.44	−25.64	−26.67	−30.00
	1	2	3	4	5

Table 3. Noise power (ANC ON, in dB)

5	−32.27	−32.67	−36.16	−35.73	−34.34
4	−30.23	−33.39	−31.76	−32.78	−35.44
3	−32.37	−28.67	−27.58	−28.42	−34.50
2	−32.95	−33.24	−29.76	−31.05	−33.02
1	−33.80	−30.95	−31.07	−29.73	−31.74
	1	2	3	4	5

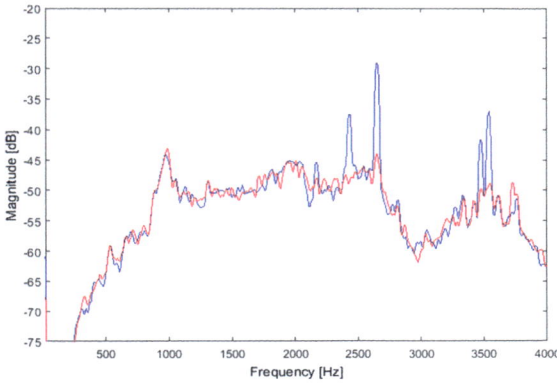

Fig. 6. Noise spectrum, before (blue) and after (red) ANC.

4   Conclusions

A single channel FBANC algorithm is developed to cancel the noise from a CPAP machine. By using small size loudspeaker and MEMS microphone with real-time digital signal processing (DSP) technique, we successfully implemented FBANC technique to cancel noise for the patients using the CPAP machines. More applications related to medical noise cancellation can be developed.

Conflict of Interest. The authors declare that they have no conflict of interest.

References

1. Lueg, P.: Process of silencing sound oscillations, U.S. Patent 2043416 (1936)
2. Kuo, S.M., Morgan, D.R.: Active Noise Control Systems Algorithms and DSP Implementations. Wiley, New York (1996)
3. Lemire, S., Vo, H.D.: Reduction of fan and compressor wake defect using plasma actuation for tonal noise reduction. J. Turbomach. **133**, 11 (2011)
4. Gerard, A., Berry, A., Masson, P., Gervais, Y.: Experimental validation of tonal noise control from subsonic axial fans using flow control obstructions. J. Sound Vib. **321**, 8–25 (2009)
5. Wu, C., Wan, L., Zhao, W., Zhou, Q.: Research on active control of axial flow fan noise using a novel and simplified duct system. In: 2015 International Conference on Control, Automation and Information Sciences (ICCAIS), pp. 153–158 (2015)
6. Cordourier-Maruri, H.A., Orduna-Bustamante, F.: Active control of periodic fan noise in laptops: spectral width requirements in a delayed buffer implementation. J. Biomed. Mater. Res. B **7**, 124–135 (2009)
7. Rust, R.L., Gee, K.L., Sommerfeldt, S.D., Blotter, J.D.: Active noise control of an exhaust-mounted two-fan array. Noise Control Eng. J. **60**, 481–489 (2012)
8. Widrow, B., Stearns, S.D.: Adaptive Signal Processing. Prentice-Hall, Englewood Cliffs (1985)

Dysphonia Measurements Detection Using CQT's and MFCC's Methods

Mario Lopez-Rodríguez[1(✉)], Mireya Sarai García-Vázquez[1(✉)],
Luis Miguel Zamudio-Fuentes[1(✉)], and Alejandro Ramírez-Acosta[2]

[1] Instituto Politécnico Nacional-Centro de Investigación y Desarrollo de Tecnología Digital, Av Instituto Politécnico Nacional 1310, Nueva, Tijuana, Mexico
`mlopez@citedi.mx`, {`msarai,lzamudiof`}`@ipn.mx`
[2] MIRAL R&D&I, San Diego, USA

Abstract. Dysphonia is a vocal impediment that appears as a symptom of Parkinson's disease, and can be used for its diagnosis. Among the important measurements for dysphonia detection are jitter, shimmer, fundamental frequency (F0), Harmonics to noise ratio (HNR) and noise to harmonics ratio (NHR). The frequency space of the speech signal is used to detect these five dysphonia measurements, through this space the acoustic markers jitter, shimmer and F0 are calculated. In this article, an evaluation of the detection of acoustic markers is presented through the mathematical methods of the Constant Q Transform (CQT) and the Mel Frequencies Cepstral Coefficients (MFCC) in speech signals of patients with Parkinson's disease. The classifier method Support Vector Machine (SVM) is used to detect the Biomarkers. According to the results, the CQT method and MFCC method (57% and 62% precision respectively) which is a promising results for Parkinson's disease diagnosis by the detection of Dysphonia measurements.

Keywords: Mel Frequencies Cepstral Coefficients · Support Vector Machine · Constant Q Transform · Parkinson's disease · Voice analysis · Dysphonia measurements

1 Introduction

Parkinson's disease (PD) is one of the most frequent neurodegenerative diseases [1]. The PD occurs when a patient does not produce dopamine in the substantia nigra of the brain [2]. It is known, that 1% of the 65-year-old people has Parkinson's disease [3]. This percentage is going to increase, and it will become a social problem [4]. The Parkinson's disease symptoms are: (1) instability when the patient is resting; (2) bradykinesia (slowness of movement); (3) muscle tremor; (4) vocal impediment [5]. The last symptom is present in 90% of the cases [1]. There are investigations dedicated to analyze and represent the vocal impediment through Dysphonia and Dysarthria, with the objective of the detection and the monitoring of Parkinson's disease, some of the research examples are Little et al. [6, 7], Tsanas et al. [1, 8–10], and Benba et al. [11, 12]. All these authors use features that could be used to represent Dysphonia in the patient's

© Springer Nature Switzerland AG 2020
K.-P. Lin et al. (Eds.): ICBHI 2019, IFMBE Proceedings 74, pp. 349–355, 2020.
https://doi.org/10.1007/978-3-030-30636-6_48

voice. These Dysphonia measurements are jitter, shimmer, harmonicity and their variants. Jitter is the frequency variation between consecutive periods and Shimmer is the variation of the amplitude in consecutive periods [11, 12]. Benba et al. [11] used the Dysphonia measurements to discriminate subjects with Parkinson's disease from the control subjects; Achaf Benba et al presented 82.5% of correct classification, using the K Nearest Neighbor (k-NN) as the classification method. The Mel Frequencies Cepstral Coefficients (MFCC) and the Q Constant transform (CQT) methods, are used for spectral analysis, the MFCC method has been used by A. Tsanas for monitoring and detecting persons with Parkinson's disease [1, 13]. The CQT method has not been used with said purpose; in contrast, the CQT method has been used for audio scene classification by Rakotomamonjy et al. [14] and for sound analysis by Brown [15]. According to Browm [15], the method CQT can produce a better frequency representation of the music audio signals, compared to the Fourier Transformation (FT) used in the MFCC method. In this paper, the CQT method is used to discriminate subjects with Parkinson's disease form the control subjects, also an analysis between the CQT methods and the MFCC is presented to determent which method can be better to obtain the Dysphonia features. The remainder of this paper is organized as follows: section two contains the methodology and information of the databased used for the experiments and the methods used for features extraction and classification; in section three, a discussion of the results of the experiments is presented; the final section contains the conclusions of the experiments.

2   Methodology

For the tests carried out, a database was created from the database used by the working group of Orozco Arroyave [16], for this article the created database will be call DB1. The recordings from database DB1, were captured by the working group of Juan Rafael Orozco, with a sampling frequency of 44.1 kHz and a resolution of 16 bits with an omnidirectional dynamic microphone (Shure, SM 36L), the audio card used in the one captured is M-Audio, Fast Track C400.

The DB1 database consist of four groups, the first group is form by male subjects with Parkinson's disease, the second group consist of male control subjects, the third group represents the female subjects with Parkinson's disease and the final group are the female control subjects, each group contribute with 90 voice recordings of each vowel, making a total of 1800 voice recordings in the DB1 database.

2.1   Data

The Dysphonia measurements used in this paper are: (1) jitter's local value; (2) jitter's local absolute value (jitter$_{LA}$); (3) jitter's relative average perturbation (jitter$_{RAP}$); (4) jitter's five-point period perturbation Quotient (jitter$_{PPQ5}$); (5) jitter's difference of differences of Periods (jitter$_{DDP}$); (6) shimmer's local value; (7) shimmer's local absolute value (shimmer$_{LA}$); (8) shimmer's three point period perturbation (shimmer$_{PPQ3}$); (9) shimmer's five point perturbation period (shimmer$_{PPQ5}$); (10) shimmer's eleven point perturbation period (shimmer$_{PPQ11}$); (11) shimmer DDP (Shimmer$_{DDP}$) [17].

The calculation of the frequency F0, jitter and shimmer measurements are obtained from an analysis of the frequency space of the signal. The Fast Fourier Transform (FFT) is implemented in the MFCC (Fig. 1). The result of the FFT method is a signal that presents different amplitudes; each amplitude corresponds to a frequency (Fig. 2), the highest amplitude is known as the fundamental frequency F0.

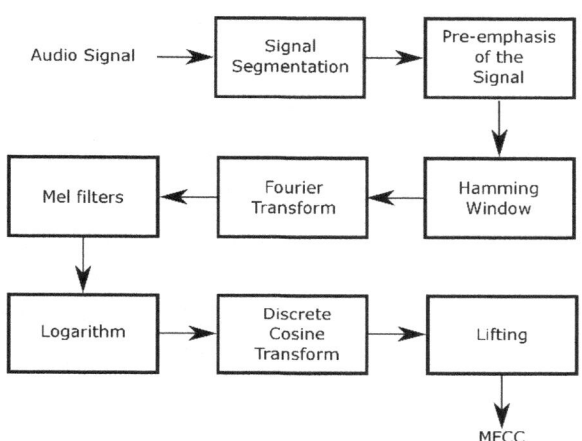

Fig. 1. Process to obtain the Coefficients of the method MFCC

From the F0 it is possible to determine de Period T, because the inverse value of the F0 frequency is the period T that allows retrieving the jitter and the variants of jitter values, as we can see in the equations below:

$$\text{Jitter (Local)} = \frac{\sum_{i-2}^{N} \frac{|T_i - T_{i-1}|}{N-1}}{\sum_{i-1}^{N} \frac{T_i}{N}} \tag{1}$$

$$Shimmer(Local) = \frac{\sum_{1=2}^{N} \frac{|A_i - A_{i-1}|}{N-1}}{\sum_{i=1}^{N} \frac{A_i}{N}} \tag{2}$$

Jitter's local value and shimmer's local value, represent the changes in frequency an amplitude of two consecutive periods respectively, the presence of high values of jitter and shimmer means a pathologic disorder in the voice, meaning the existents of dysphonia in the subject.

The process used with the FFT method in order to obtain the F0, is implemented with the method CQT, since the two methods allows to obtain a representation of the frequency space of the analyzed signal, however, it is necessary to implement the rights

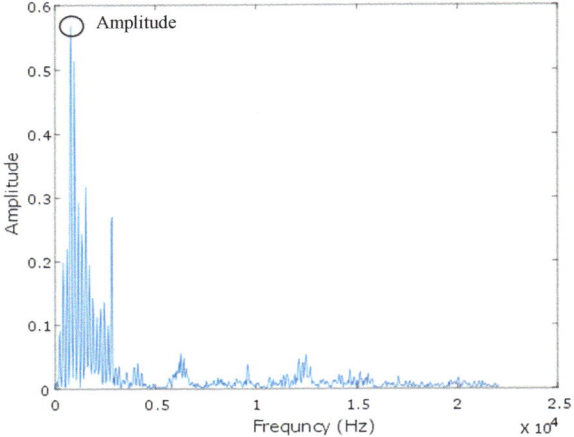

Fig. 2. Resulting signal from FFT implementation.

parameters for the CQT method. The CQT method needs to determent the number of bins per octave of the signal, for the experiments it was used 138 bins that will give 554 samples.

2.2   Classification Method

The Support Vector Machine (SVM) is a learning algorithm use for classification, developed by Vladimir Vapnik. The SVM is binary classifier, with the capacity to determine if an input vector belongs to the class A or the class B [22, 23], in our case the calculated features of dysphonia. The hyperplane is stablished with the purpose of determine the limits of the classes. The optimal hyperplane requires a minimum distance 'd' between the hyperplane and the nearest sample of each class (the letters 'A' and 'B'), as shown in Fig. 3 [23].

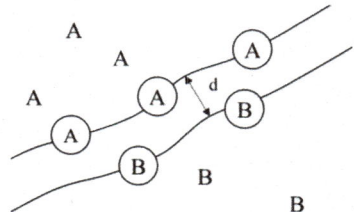

Fig. 3. Example of a hyperplane showing the separation between classes.

3   Results

For each recording from the database, it was calculated the dysphonia features mentioned in the section II, each record represents 2 s, the results obtained were used to build a matrix of features. This matrix becomes the input data for the SVM method, the outputs are shown in the confusion matrix tables below, were Table 1 represents the results from implementing the CQT method. Table 2 contains the results of the implementation of the MFCC method, and in both tables, the numbers inside the parenthesis are the number of recordings that represent percentages values.

Table 1. Results of the CQT method using SVM method.

	PD subjects	Control subjects
PD subjects	55.22% (497)	44.78% (403)
Control subjects	41.67% (375)	58.33% (525)

Table 2. Results of the MFCC method using SVM method.

	PD subjects	Control subjects
PD subjects	51.89% (467)	48.11% (433)
Control subjects	32.44% (292)	67.56% (608)

In this paper, we use the precision and recall to analyze the performance of the methods of MFCC and CQT for calculate the dysphonia measurements.

Precision represents the percentage of the recordings classified correctly as Parkinson's disease, from the total of the recordings classified as Parkinson's disease by the SVM method (see Eq. 3). Recall represents the percentage of the recordings classified correctly as Parkinson's disease, from the totals of the recordings of subjects with Parkinson's disease in the database DB1 (see Eq. 4).

$$Prescision = \frac{true\ positives}{true\ positives + false\ positives} \qquad (3)$$

$$Recall = \frac{true\ positives}{true\ positives + false\ negatives} \qquad (4)$$

The results from the Tables 1 and 2 were used to calculate the precision (Eq. 3) and recall (Eq. 4). The results are presented in Table 3.

Table 3. Results of precision and recall from the methods CQT and MFCC

	MFCC method	CQT method
Precision	61.53%	56.99%
Recall	51.89%	52.22%

3.1 Discussion

According to the Tables 1 and 2 the average of the principal diagonal of each confusion matrix shows that the MFCC method 59.73% is higher than the CQT method 56.78%, due to the resulted spatial separation of frequencies from the CQT method is not the appropriate one, this reduce the detection of the fundamental frequency F0 for each recording.

4 Conclusion

The analysis of the voice for the dysphonia measurements is a method recommended to help the medical doctors. Our proposal provides 61.53% precision in the diagnosis of Parkinson's disease, this could be more comfortable for patients and it is not an invasive procedure.

The Biomarkers for multiresolution spaces is one of the approaches that is being explored, like the CQT method due to its versatility in response to low and high frequency ranges, allowing better representation of the frequency information of the analyzed signal. It is necessary to determine the appropriate parameters to achieve a higher resolution in the frequency space, since in theory with the CQT method should have a better performance than the MFCC method.

Acknowledgment. This research is supported by SIP-IPN-20190139 and CONACYT from Mexico. In addition, thanks to Dr. Juan Rafael Orozco and group PC-GITA for providing the database.

Conflict of Interest. The authors declare that they have no conflict of interest.

References

1. Tsanas, A., Little, M.A., McSharry, P.E., et al.: Novel speech signal processing algorithms for high-accuracy classification of Parkinson's disease. IEEE Trans. Biomed. Eng. **59**(5), 1264–1271 (2012)
2. Hornykiewicz, O.: Biochemical aspects of Parkinson's disease. Neurology **51**(2 Suppl 2), S2–S9 (1998)
3. Frid, A., Kantor, A., Svechin, D., et al.: Diagnosis of Parkinson's disease from continuous speech using deep convolutional networks without manual selection of features. In: IEEE International Conference on the Science of Electrical Engineering (ICSEE). IEEE (1998)
4. Dorsey, E.R., George, B.P., Leff, B., et al.: The coming crisis Obtaining care for the growing burden of neurodegenerative conditions. Neurology 10-1212 (2013)

5. Frid, A., Safra, E.J., Hazan, H., Lokey, L.L., et al.: Computational diagnosis of Parkinson's Disease directly from natural speech using machine learning techniques. In: 2014 IEEE International Conference on Software Science, Technology and Engineering (SWSTE), pp. 50–53. IEEE, June 2014

6. Little, M.A., McSharry, P.E., Hunter, E.J., et al.: Suitability of dysphonia measurements for telemonitoring of Parkinson's disease. IEEE Trans. Biomed. Eng. **56**(4), 1015–1022 (2009)

7. Little, M., McSharry, P., Moroz, I., et al.: Nonlinear, biophysically-informed speech pathology detection. In: IEEE International Conference on Acoustics, Speech and Signal Processing, ICASSP 2006 Proceedings, vol. 2, pp. II–II (2006)

8. Tsanas, A., Little, M.A., Fox, C., et al.: Objective automatic assessment of rehabilitative speech treatment in parkinson's disease. IEEE Trans. Neural Syst. Rehabil. Eng. **22**(1), 181–190 (2014)

9. Tsanas, A., Little, M.A., McSharry, P.E., et al.: Accurate telemonitoring of Parkinson's disease progression by noninvasive speech tests. IEEE Trans. Biomed. Eng. **57**(4), 884–893 (2010)

10. Tsanas, A., Little, M.A., McSharry, P.E., et al.: Enhanced classical dysphonia measures and sparse regression for telemonitoring of Parkinson's disease progression. In: 2010 IEEE International Conference on Acoustics Speech and Signal Processing (ICASSP), pp. 594–597 (2010)

11. Benba, A., Jilbab, A., Hammouch, A.: Voice analysis for detecting persons with Parkinson's disease using MFCC and VQ. J. Theor. Appl. Inf. Technol. **70**(3) (2014)

12. Benba, A., Jilbab, A., Hammouch, A.: Voice analysis for detecting patients with Parkinson's disease using the hybridization of the best acoustic features. Int. J. Electr. Eng. Inf. **8**(1), 108 (2016)

13. Tsanas, A., Little, M.A., McSharry, P.E., et al.: Nonlinear speech analysis algorithms mapped to a standard metric achieve clinically useful quantification of average Parkinson's disease symptom severity. J. Roy. Soc. Interface **8**(59), 842–855 (2011)

14. Rakotomamonjy, A., Gasso, G.: Histogram of gradients of time-frequency representations for audio scene classification. IEEE/ACM Trans. Audio Speech Lang. Process. (TASLP) **23**(1), 142–153 (2015)

15. Brown, J.C.: Calculation of a constant Q spectral transform. J. Acoust. Soc. Am. **89**(1), 425–434 (1991)

16. Orozco-Arroyave, J.R., Arias-Londoño, J.D., Vargas-Bonilla, J.F., et al.: New speech corpus database for the analysis of people suffering from Parkinson's Disease. In: Proceedings of the International Conference on Language Resources and Evaluation (LREC), Reykjavik, Iceland, pp. 342–347 (2014)

17. Praat. http://www.fon.hum.uva.nl/praat/manual/Voice.html

18. Suárez, E.J.C.: Tutorial sobre máquinas de vectores soporte (sVM). Tutorial sobre Máquinas de Vectores Soporte (SVM) (2014)

19. Nalini, N., Palanivel, S.: Music emotion recognition: the combined evidence of MFCC and residual phase. Egypt. Inf. J. **17**(1), 1–10 (2016)

Quantification of Systolic Time Intervals Using Continuous Wavelet Transform of Electrocardiogram and Phonocardiogram Signals

Suparerk Janjarasjitt[(⊠)]

Department of Electrical and Electronic Engineering,
Ubon Ratchathani University, Ubon Ratchathani, Thailand
suparerk.j@ubu.ac.th

Abstract. There are a number of methods and diagnostic tools for assessing the health of the heart. The systolic time intervals (STI) have been clinically useful parameters representing cardiac cycle and measuring the ventricular performance. In this study, a continuous wavelet transform (CWT) based approach for quantifying the systolic time intervals, in particular, the pre-ejection period (PEP) and the left ventricular ejection time (LVET), using electrocardiogram (ECG) and phonocardiogram (PCG) signals are proposed. The proposed CWT-based STI quantification approach is composed of three main stages: ECG signal processing, PCG signal processing, and computation of the systolic time intervals. The proposed CWT-based STI quantification approach is validated using ECG and PCG data recorded from both healthy subjects and subjects suffering from various cardiovascular diseases. The computational results suggest that the proposed CWT-based STI quantification approach has a considerable capability for clinical applications. The means of average absolute errors on PEP and LVET quantifications are, respectively, 13.4251 ms and 27.1348 ms. The best total score achieved is 868.9192.

Keywords: Electrocardiogram · Phonocardiogram ·
Continuous wavelet transform · Systolic time intervals

1 Introduction

Cardiovascular diseases (CVDs) which are associated with the heart and blood vessels are the leading cause of death globally. There are a number of symptoms and forms of cardiovascular diseases. The measurement of systolic time intervals (STIs) derived by Weissler et al. [1] has been applied for evaluating left ventricular systolic function. The measurement of systolic time intervals is a simple and noninvasive method. The left ventricular ejection time (LVET) and the pre-ejection period (PEP) are ones of the systolic time intervals indices. A ratio of PEP/LVET [1, 2] is also another STI index measured which is less heart rate dependent [3].

© Springer Nature Switzerland AG 2020
K.-P. Lin et al. (Eds.): ICBHI 2019, IFMBE Proceedings 74, pp. 356–362, 2020.
https://doi.org/10.1007/978-3-030-30636-6_49

The pre-ejection period (PEP) is measured from the time interval between the depolarization of the left ventricle and the beginning of ventricular ejection while the left ventricular ejection time (LVET) is measured from the time interval of left ventricular ejection [4]. Practically, the PEP is determined from the time interval between the peak of the R wave of ECG and the onset of the opening of the aortic valve. The LVET is determined from the time interval between the opening and the closure of the aortic valve. Echocardiography is used as the gold standard method for evaluating the left ventricular systolic function. Heart sounds recorded using phonocardiography (PCG) are also used to diagnosing the opening and the closure of the aortic valve leading to the evaluation of the systolic time intervals.

In this study, both ECG and PCG signals are applied for identifying timings of cardiac events including the peak of the R wave of ECG, the opening of the aortic valve, and the closure of the aortic valve. Accordingly, the systolic time intervals, in particular, the PEP and the LVET, are quantified. The proposed approach for quantifying the PEP and the LVET is based on the continuous wavelet transform (CWT) of ECG and PCG signals. The CWT of ECG signal is used for identifying the peaks of the R wave of ECG and also segmenting the heart cycle. The events of opening and closure of the aortic valve are identified using the CWT of PCG signal. The ECG and PCG data provided in the ICBHI 2019 Scientific Challenge [4] are used to validate the performance of the proposed CWT-based STI approach.

2   Methods

2.1   The ICBHI 2019 Scientific Challenge Data

The dataset examined in this study contains the synchronized electrocardiogram (ECG), phonocardiogram (PCG), photoplethysmogram (PPG), and echocardiogram data [4, 5]. The data were collected from 68 volunteers (51 male and 17 female) in the Centro Hospitalar da Universidade de Coimbra, Coimbra, Portugal [4, 5] divided into two subject groups: healthy and CVD subject groups. The healthy subject group includes 33 subjects with the average age of 29.72 ± 8.54 years and the average BMI of 24.48 ± 2.41 kg/m^2 while the CVD subject group includes 35 subjects suffering from various cardiovascular diseases with the average age of 58.97 ± 17.22 years and the average BMI of 25.38 ± 3.10 kg/m^2.

For the ICBHI 2019 Scientific Challenge [4], the dataset was divided into two phases referred to as Phase I and Phase II. In the Phase I, there are 37 recordings including 24 recordings from the healthy subject group and 13 recordings from the CVD subject group. There are 35 recordings including 23 recordings from the healthy subject group and 12 recordings from the CVD subject group in the Phase II. The ECG and PCG data were recorded using the sampling frequency of 44,100 Hz. A segment of exemplary ECG and PCG signals associated with the CVD subject group is shown in Fig. 1(a)–(b), respectively.

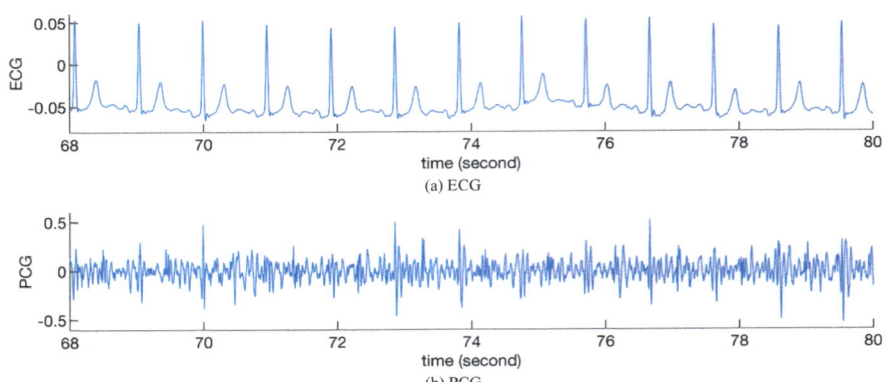

Fig. 1. Exemplary ECG and PCG signals of a subject suffering from a cardiovascular disease

2.2 The Proposed CWT-Based Approach

The CWT-based STI quantification approach is divided into three main stages. In the first stage, the ECG signal is processed using five computational steps as follows.

(1) The CWT [6] is applied to the ECG signal x_{ECG} defined as

$$W_{\text{ECG}}(n, s) = \frac{1}{\sqrt{s}} \int_{-\infty}^{+\infty} \psi^* \left(\frac{\tau - n}{s} \right) x_{\text{ECG}}(\tau) d\tau. \tag{1}$$

(2) A subband power of ECG signal corresponding to a spectral subband $[f_{C_L}, f_{C_U}]$ is obtained by summing the CWT of ECG signal over the range of scales as given by

$$p_{\text{ECG}}(n) = \sum_{s_{C_0} \leq s \leq s_{C_1}} W_{\text{ECG}}(n, s) \tag{2}$$

where the scales s_{C_0} and s_{C_1} correspond to the upper and lower frequencies of the subband of the ECG signal, i.e., f_{C_U} and f_{C_L}, respectively.

(3) Locations of the peaks of the R wave of ECG signal $\{R_k\}$ are then detected from the subband power of ECG signal p_{ECG} where its peaks correspond to the locations of the peaks of the R wave of ECG signal.

(4) The derivative of subband power of ECG signal p_{ECG} is obtained using a backward difference given by

$$\Delta p_{\text{ECG}}(n) = p_{\text{ECG}}(n) - p_{\text{ECG}}(n - 1). \tag{3}$$

(5) For each cycle of heartbeat, i.e., an interval between two consecutive R waves of ECG signal (namely, an interval between R_k and R_{k+1}), a peak and a valley of the derivative of subband power of ECG signal Δp_{PCG} denoted, respectively, by u_k and v_k are detected.

In the second stage, a PCG signal is processed using four computational steps as follows:

(1) The CWT [6] is applied to the PCG signal x_{PCG} defined as

$$W_{\text{PCG}}(n, s) = \frac{1}{\sqrt{s}} \int\limits_{-\infty}^{+\infty} \psi^* \left(\frac{\tau - n}{s} \right) x_{\text{PCG}}(\tau) d\tau. \tag{4}$$

(2) A subband power of PCG signal corresponding to a spectral subband $[f_{S_L}, f_{S_U}]$ is obtained by summing the CWT of PCG signal over the range of scales as given by

$$p_{\text{PCG}}(n) = \sum_{s_{S_0} \leq s \leq s_{S_1}} W_{\text{PCG}}(n, s) \tag{5}$$

where the scales s_{S_0} and s_{S_1} correspond to the upper and lower frequencies of the subband power of PCG signal, i.e., f_{S_U} and f_{S_L}, respectively.
(3) A timing of the opening of the aortic valve A_k^{open} is determined from peak of the subband power of PCG signal p_{PCG} within the interval between the consecutive valley v_{k-1} and peak u_k.
(4) A timing of the closure of the aortic valve A_k^{close} is determined from the peak of the subband power of PCG signal p_{PCG} within the interval between the consecutive peak u_k and valley v_k.

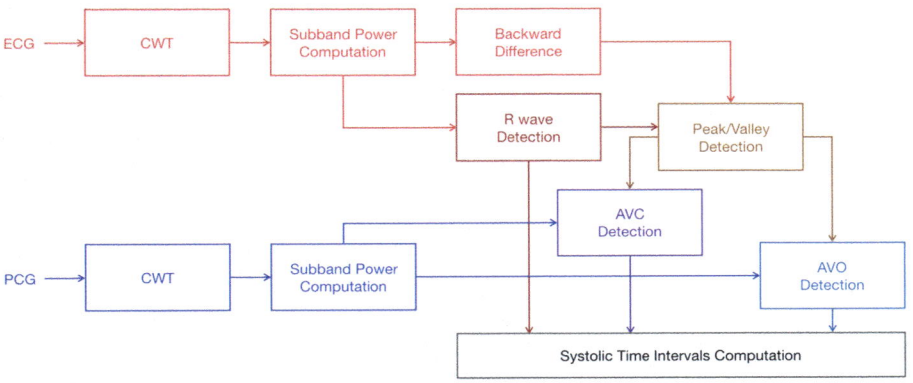

Fig. 2. A block diagram of the proposed CWT-based STI quantification approach

In the last stage, the systolic time intervals including the PEP and the LVET are determined from the timings of R waves of ECG signal $\{R_k\}$ and their corresponding opening and closure of the aortic valve, $\{A_k^{\text{open}}\}$ and $\{A_k^{\text{close}}\}$. Thus, the PEP and the LVET are, respectively, given by $PEP_k = R_k - A_k^{\text{open}}$ and $LVET = A_k^{\text{open}} - A_k^{\text{close}}$.

Figure 2 illustrates a block diagram of the proposed CWT-based STI quantification approach.

2.3   Performance Evaluation

The performance on PEP and LVET quantifications is evaluated using the overall score that is defined as [4]

$$
score = \frac{100}{2} \times \left(\frac{\sum_{k=1}^{N} \left| PEP_k - PEP_k^R \right|}{\sum_{k=1}^{N} PEP_k^R} + \frac{\sum_{k=1}^{N} \left| LVET_k - LVET_k^R \right|}{\sum_{k=1}^{N} LVET_k^R} \right) \tag{6}
$$

where PEP_k^R and $LVET_k^R$ denote the pre-ejection period and the left ventricular ejection time measured using the echocardiography, respectively, and N denote the total number of valid cardiac cycles of all recordings contained in the dataset.

3   Results

3.1   Detection of Cardiac Events

The subband power of exemplary ECG signal shown in Fig. 1(a) and its derivative are shown in Fig. 3(a)–(b), respectively. In Fig. 3(a), the peaks of subband power indicating the locations of detected R waves plotted in a magenta '×' mark are compared to the locations of actual R waves plotted in a black 'o' mark. The peaks and the valleys of derivative of subband power of ECG signal are plotted in magenta '+' and '×' marks, respectively, in Fig. 3(b). The mean and the standard deviation of average absolute errors on R wave detection are 7.0764 ± 5.4783 ms.

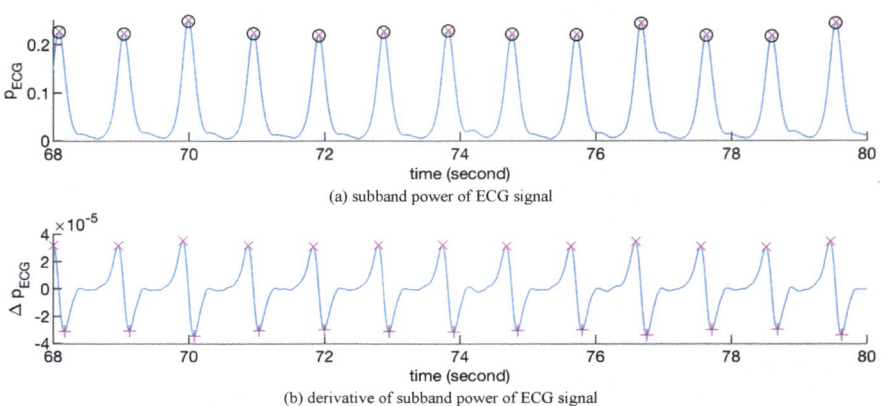

(a) subband power of ECG signal

(b) derivative of subband power of ECG signal

Fig. 3. Processed exemplary ECG signal shown in Fig. 1(a)

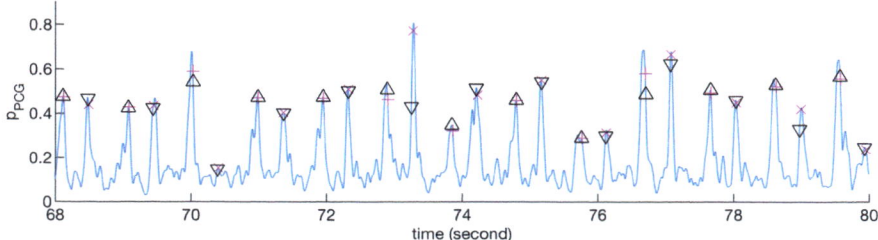

Fig. 4. Subband power of exemplary PCG signal shown in Fig. 1(b)

The subband power of exemplary PCG signal shown in Fig. 1(b) is shown in Fig. 4. The locations of detected AVO events plotted in a magenta '+' mark are compared to the locations of actual AVO events plotted in a black 'Δ' mark. The locations of detected AVC events plotted in a magenta '×' mark are also compared to the locations of actual AVC events plotted in a black '∇' mark. The mean and the standard deviation of average absolute error on AVO detection are 12.9275 ± 9.5918 ms while the mean and the standard deviation of average absolute error on AVC detection are 21.0777 ± 27.2347 ms, respectively.

3.2   Performance on the PEP and LVET Quantification

The mean and the standard deviation of average absolute errors on PEP and LVET quantifications are, respectively, 13.4251 ± 11.3458 ms and 27.1348 ± 33.4267 ms. The best total score, i.e., the minimum total score, achieved and officially obtained using the CWT-based STI quantification approach for the Phase II of the ICBHI 2019 Scientific Challenge is 868.9192. Accordingly, the best average score for the Phase II of the ICBHI 2019 Scientific Challenge is 24.8263 (23.5918 for the healthy subject group and 27.1923 for the CVD subject group).

4   Conclusions

In this study, the systolic time intervals, in particular, the PEP and the LVET, are quantified using the proposed CWT-based approach applied to the ECG and PCG data provided in the ICBHI 2019 Scientific Challenge. From the computational results, it is shown that the means of average absolute errors on R wave, AVO, and AVC detections are, respectively, 7.0764 ms, 12.9275 ms, and 21.0777 ms. Furthermore, the best total score achieved using the proposed CWT-based STI quantification approach for the Phase II is 868.9192. This results in the average score of 24.8263.

Conflict of Interest. The author declares that he has no conflict of interest.

References

1. Weissler, A.M., Harris, W.S., Schoenfeld, C.D.: Systolic time intervals in heart failure in man. Circulation **37**, 149–159 (1968)
2. Weissler, A.M., Harris, W.S., Schoenfeld, C.D.: Bedside technics for the evaluation of ventricular function in man. Am. J. Cardiol. **23**, 577–583 (1969)
3. Oh, J.K., Tajik, J.: The return of cardiac time intervals. J. Am. Coll. Cardiol. **42**, 1471–1474 (2003)
4. Scientific Challenge. https://www.icbhi2019.com/call-for-sc
5. Carvalho, P., et al.: Assessing systolic time-intervals from heart sound: a feasibility study. In: Proceedings of the 31st Annual International Conference of the IEEE EMBS, Minnesota, USA (2009). https://doi.org/10.1109/iembs.2009.5332565
6. Lilly, J.M., Olhede, S.C.: Generalized Morse wavelets as a superfamily of analytic wavelets. IEEE Trans. Signal Process. **60**, 6036–6041 (2012)

PEP and LVET Detection from PCG and ECG

Yi-Fang Yang[✉], Yu-Sheng Chou, and Jia-Yin Wang

Department of Electrical Engineering, Chung Yuan Christian University,
No. 200, Zhongbei Road, ZhongLi District, Taoyuan, Taiwan
mf7811@gmail.com, {s10428105,jyw}@cycu.edu.tw

Abstract. The systolic time intervals of hearts are related to health. People with myocardial dysfunction will have a longer pre-ejection period (PEP) and a shorter left ventricle ejection time (LVET) than healthy people. The purpose of this paper is intended to detect PEP and LVET accurately from electrocardiography (ECG) and phonocardiogram (PCG). Generally, there are several kinds of noises from environment or breathing in PCG. It is necessary but difficult to extract the best signals we want. Our approach is to use a simple DSP-based method in PCG to detect aortic valve opening (AVO) and aortic valve closure (AVC) times as well as R-peak time in ECG. Then, the PEP and LVET can be calculated. We evaluated PEP and LVET of 72 files from 46 people. To the annotated data, the PEP range is around 5 ms to 100 ms; the LVET range is around 170 ms to 380 ms. Our PEP results have 63.96% accuracy within 20 ms absolute error and 91.74% accuracy within 40 ms absolute error; LVET have 75.48% accuracy within 40 ms absolute error and 93.53% accuracy within 80 ms absolute error.

Keywords: Pre-ejection period (PEP) · Left ventricle ejection time (LVET) · Phonocardiogram (PCG) · Electrocardiography (ECG)

1 Introduction

The systolic time intervals of hearts are directly related to the health of heart cells. From [1], the ratio of PEP and LVET is an index to the health of heart. The ratio of PEP and LVET can be used as a judgment of cardiovascular diseases (CVDs), such as arrhythmia, hypertension, coronary artery disease, and aortic stenosis. A subject with myocardial dysfunction prolongs PEP and shortens LVET. PEP is the time interval of R-peak (or Q) in ECG to the time of AVO in PCG; LVET is the time interval of AVO to AVC in PCG.

In general, the heart rate is between 50 beats to 100 beats per minute. It means that the heartbeat intervals are around 0.6 s to 1.2 s. It is very important to accurately measure every R-peak in ECG.

The first heart sound (S1) is a complex wave composed of vibrations of the atrioventricular valve closing and the semilunar valve opening. The frequency range of S1 is around 40 Hz to 60 Hz. The amplitude peak of S1 is related to the closure of the atrioventricular valves like the mitral and tricuspid valves. The event of semilunar valve opening (like AVO) can be detected, but it is not so obvious as atrioventricular valve closing. The aortic valve opening usually occurs after atrioventricular valve

K.-P. Lin et al. (Eds.): ICBHI 2019, IFMBE Proceedings 74, pp. 363–370, 2020.
https://doi.org/10.1007/978-3-030-30636-6_50

closing. The second heart sound (S2) is generated by the event of aortic valve closing, so the highest peak of S2 is considered as AVC. The frequency range of S2 is around 60 Hz to 100 Hz.

The S1 and S2 can also be detected without ECG [2], and the PEP and LVET can be estimated accurately from PCG using the Bayesian approach [3]. However, there were still many ways to detect PEP and LVET instead of using PCG. In [4], LVET were detected from the photoplethysmogram (PPG) by using Gaussian functions. In [5, 6], the PEP and LVET were obtained from seismocardiogram (SCG). In [7], the authors used impedance cardiogram (ICG) and ECG to calculate PEP and LVET.

In this paper, PEP and LVET were estimated by using a simple DSP approach. The data were collected from 68 volunteers in the "Centro Hospitalar da Universidade de Coimbra", Coimbra, Portugal [8]. The volunteers were divided into two groups, 33 healthy subjects and 35 subjects suffering from CVDs. The annotated data were collected using PCG, ECG, photoplethysmogram (PPG), and echocardiography (Doppler mode). The PEP and LVET were manually annotated by a clinical technician.

2   Material and Method

The information of the data evaluating in this study are collected from 51 males and 17 females. The characteristics of population are shown in Table 1 (mean $\pm$ std):

Table 1. Characteristics of population

	Healthy subjects	CVD subjects
Age	29.72 ± 8.54	58.97 ± 17.22
BMI	24.48 ± 2.41	25.38 ± 3.10

The proposed method can be divided into several procedures. First, pre-process the signal. Second, detect R-peaks. Third, detect S1 and S2. Fourth, detect AVO and AVC. Finally, the PEP and LVET are estimated.

2.1   Pre-processing

First, original ECG and PCG signals were pre-processed. To reduce processing complexity, the sampling frequency of ECG and PCG is resampled from 44100 Hz to 4410 Hz. Compared to the annotated data, the error of each R-peak is small enough in the acceptable range (less than 0.3 ms). Then, band-pass filters were used to reduce the noises of ECG and PCG signals. In ECG, the frequencies between 10 Hz to 20 Hz were preserved and other frequencies were removed to obtain a signal for detecting R-peaks. In PCG, the frequencies between 30 Hz to 150 Hz were preserved and other frequencies were removed. After the signal were filtered, S1 and S2 could be found obviously, as shown in Fig. 1. From the figure, most of the S1 have larger amplitudes compared to the S2.

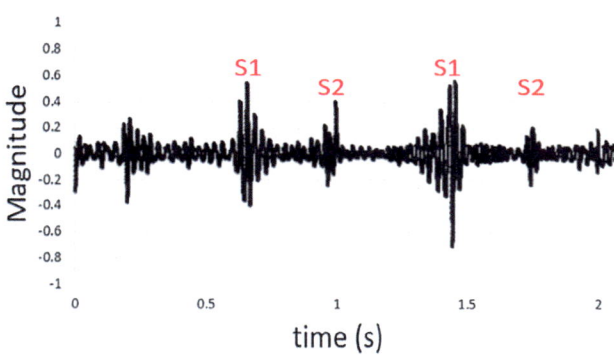

Fig. 1. Processed PCG (C028001)

After filtering, the noise frequencies within the band-pass filter are not removed, so the processed PCG still contains some noises. However, the processed PCG is still good enough for preserving the features of S1 and S2. It is quite normal that processed PCG contains some noises after filtering.

2.2 Detecting R-Peak

Most of the R-peaks can be easily detected in the original ECG signal without filtering. The obvious peaks in the measured interval are considered as R-peaks. However, since noises existed in ECG, sometimes it is difficult to identify the real R-peaks. Hence, the ECG signal should be band-pass filtered before detecting R-peaks to improve the performances. Here we used a 10–20 Hz band-passed filter which was good enough. The filtered ECG was then used to estimate the R-peaks, and together with the filtered PCG to estimate S1, S2 regions and AVO, AVC times.

Here we proposed two methods. In the first method, the R-peaks were estimated as follows. (1) All local maximum points in whole ECG signal were identified as R-peak candidates. (2) For a candidate point, if its next candidate point is within 0.2 s and has larger value, then this candidate point was removed. (3) For a candidate point, if its previous candidate point occurs before 1.2 s, then we added the mid-point of these two candidate points as an extra candidate point.

In the second method, the R-peaks were estimated as follows. (1) The signal was divided into segments of 10 s length. (2) All local maximum points in every segment were identified as R-peak candidates. (3) The candidate points with values below 0.8 times of average value of the candidate points were removed. This step was repeated until stable, that is, no more candidate points were removed again. (4) The average time interval between all candidate points were calculated. (5) The candidate points of step 4 with adjacent time intervals less than half of the average value were removed. (6) All the candidate points were considered as R-peaks.

2.3   Detecting S1 and S2

After removing noises from the PCG, the S1 region contains the R-peak time, the atrioventricular valve closure time, and the AVO occurrence time; the S2 region contains the AVC time. Figure 2 shows a sample of a processed PCG signal with annotated data.

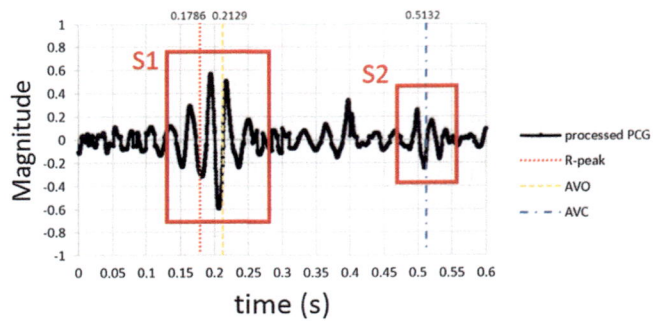

Fig. 2. Processed PCG with annotated data

2.4   Detecting AVO and AVC

According to the statistics from the annotated data, the PEP range is from 5 ms to 100 ms; the LVET range is from 160 ms to 360 ms. Therefore, these values were set as the time ranges of AVO and AVC starting from the time of R-peak.

In the first method, the maximum point (the peak) of S1 was considered as AVO; the maximum point (the peak) of S2 was considered as AVC.

Compared to the annotated data, the AVO estimated by the first method are 5 ms to 25 ms earlier than those of annotated data. Hence in the second method, we adjusted the AVO as the points with 20 ms delay from the maximum point (the peak) of S1.

3   Results

We used the two proposed methods to estimate the PEP and LVET from ECG and PCG signals. After PEP and LVET were estimated, a score was calculated by using the following formula:

$$
score = \frac{\left[\frac{\sum_{i=1}^{N}\left|PEP_i - PEP_i^R\right|}{\sum_{i=1}^{N} PEP_i^R} \times 100 + \frac{\sum_{i=1}^{N}\left|LVET_i - LVET_i^R\right|}{\sum_{i=1}^{N} LVET_i^R} \times 100\right]}{2} \tag{1}
$$

For the first method, the total score for 37 cases in the annotated database 1 is 2,181.337, or in average 58.955 for each case. For the annotated data, the PEP range is around from 6 ms to 70 ms; the LVET range is around from 170 ms to 360 ms.

Compared to the annotated data, our PEP results got 66.80% accuracy within 20 ms absolute error and 85.07% accuracy within 40 ms absolute error; the LVET results got 67.32% accuracy within 40 ms absolute error and 87.54% accuracy within 80 ms absolute error. For the people with cardiovascular diseases, the average and standard deviation of PEP were 55.73 ms and 52.81 ms; the average and standard deviation of LVET were 302.08 ms and 77.55 ms. For the healthy people, the average and standard deviation of PEP were 31.83 ms and 32.21 ms, the average and standard deviation of LVET were 269.29 ms and 51.14 ms. The comparison of the results (average ± std) for the first method is shown in Table 2.

Table 2. Comparison of PEP and LVET using method 1 (DB1)

	The annotated data	The first method
PEP (CVDs)	38.99 ± 18.88	55.73 ± 52.81
PEP (healthy)	35.33 ± 21.15	31.83 ± 32.21
LVET (CVDs)	302.47 ± 37.41	302.08 ± 77.55
LVET (healthy)	251.25 ± 35.31	269.29 ± 51.14

For the second method, the total score for 35 cases in database 2 is 1574.938, or in average 44.99 for each case. For the annotated data, the PEP range is around from 3 ms to 103 ms; the LVET range is around from 170 ms to 385 ms. Our PEP results got 61.64% accuracy within 20 ms absolute error and 87.66% accuracy within 40 ms absolute error; the LVET results got 73.75% accuracy within 40 ms absolute error and 93.98% accuracy within 80 ms absolute error. For the people with cardiovascular diseases, the average and standard deviation of PEP were 55.70 ms and 21.92 ms; the average and standard deviation of LVET were 287.75 ms and 52.37 ms. For the healthy people, the average and standard deviation of PEP were 45.15 ms and 16.16 ms, the average error and standard deviation of LVET were 242.69 ms and 44.88 ms. The comparison of the results (average ± std) for the second method is shown in Table 3.

Table 3. Comparison of PEP and LVET using method 2 (DB2)

	The annotated data	The second method
PEP (CVDs)	44.34 ± 21.32	55.70 ± 21.92
PEP (healthy)	32.12 ± 13.46	45.15 ± 16.16
LVET (CVDs)	302.26 ± 43.86	287.75 ± 52.37
LVET (healthy)	252.83 ± 27.94	242.69 ± 44.88

The accuracies within specific error intervals of PEP and LVET for the two methods are shown in Table 4. The accuracies of the second method are shown in Table 5.

Table 4. Accuracy of the methods

	The first method (DB1)	The second method (DB1)
PEP (20 ms error)	66.80%	66.35%
PEP (40 ms error)	85.07%	95.11%
LVET (40 ms error)	67.32%	77.30%
LVET (80 ms error)	87.54%	93.54%

Table 5. Accuracy of the improved methods

	DB1	DB2	DB1+DB2
PEP (20 ms error)	66.35%	61.71%	63.96%
PEP (40 ms error)	95.11%	88.55%	91.74%
LVET (40 ms error)	77.30%	73.75%	75.48%
LVET (80 ms error)	93.54%	93.98%	93.53%

Table 6. Comparison of PEP and LVET (DB1+DB2)

	The annotated data	The second method
PEP (CVDs)	41.80 ± 20.36	51.79 ± 20.68
PEP (healthy)	33.66 ± 17.66	43.19 ± 14.99
LVET (CVDs)	302.36 ± 40.93	285.76 ± 54.55
LVET (healthy)	252.07 ± 31.71	246.09 ± 41.85

The comparison (average ± std) of people with CVDs and healthy heart is shown in Table 6. It's the results of DB1 and DB2 using the improved program.

The PEP with CVDs compared to the PEP of healthy hearts are longer. However, the LVET are related to heart rate, mentioned in [1, 9, 10]. If the heart rate is high, the LVET is lower.

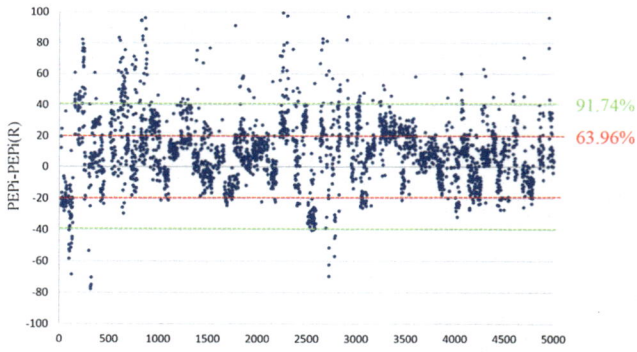

Fig. 3. Error of PEP

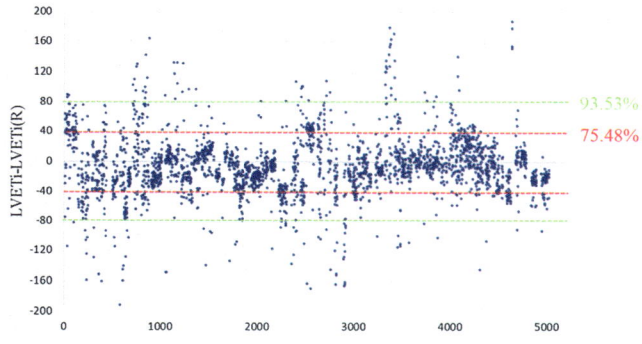

Fig. 4. Error of LVET

By using the improved method, the error of PEP is shown in Fig. 3; the error of LVET is shown in Fig. 4. The standard deviation of PEP and LVET are about 20 ms and 40 ms, as shown in Table 6. The subjects between red dotted lines, in Figs. 3 and 4, are the results within one standard deviation; the subjects between green dotted lines are the results within two standard deviations.

4   Conclusions and Discussion

In this study, the authors proposed two simple DSP-based methods to estimate the PEP and LVET from ECG and PCG signals. The second method is an improved version of the first method. The PCG and ECG signals were first down-sampled and band-pass filtered to reduce the complexities and noises. Then the two methods were conducted to estimate the PEP and LVET.

The accuracy of PEP in method 2 is 63.96% within 20 ms absolute error and 91.74% within 40 ms absolute error; the accuracy of LVET is 75.48% within 40 ms absolute error and 93.53% within 80 ms absolute error. The proposed method can be used in the initial healthy judgment of hearts. If it detected something wrong, then the Echocardiography measurement can be further used to find the problem accurately.

Acknowledgment. The authors would like to thank ICBHI and the volunteers from Centro Hospitalar da Universidade de Coimbra who provided the data for this study.

Conflict of Interest. The authors declare that they have no conflict of interest.

References

1. Weissler, A.M., et al.: Systolic time intervals in heart failure in man. Circulation **37**, 149–159 (1968). South, J., Blass, B.: The Future of Modern Genomics. Blackwell, London (2001)

2. Kumar, D., Carvalho, P., Antunes, M., Henriques, J., Eugenio, L., Schmidt, R., Habetha, J.: Detection of S1 and S2 heart sounds by high frequency signatures. In: Proceedings of the 28th Annual International Conference of the IEEE EMBS, pp. 1410–1416 (2006)

3. Paiva, R., Carvalho, P., Aubert, X., Muehlsteff, J., Henriques, J., Antunes, M.: Assessing PEP and LVET from heart sounds: algorithms and evaluation. In: IEEE-EMBS (2009)

4. Couceiro, R., Carvalho, P., Paiva, R., Henriques, J., Antunes, M., Quintal, I., et al.: Multi-Gaussian fitting for the assessment of left ventricular ejection time from the Photoplethys-mogram. In: IEEE-EMBS (2012)

5. Di Rienzo, M., Vaini, E., Castiglioni, P., Lombardi, P., Meriggi, P., Rizzo, F.: A textile-based wearable system for the prolonged assessment of cardiac mechanics in daily life. In: 36th Annual International Conference of the IEEE Engineering in Medicine and Biology Society, Chicago, pp. 6896–6898 (2014)

6. Tavakolian, K., Blaber, A.P., Ngai, B., Kaminska, B.: Estimation of hemodynamic parameters from seismocardiogram. In: Computing in Cardiology, pp. 1055–1058 (2010)

7. Javaid, A.Q., Ashouri, H., Inan, O.T.: Estimating systolic time intervals during walking using wearable ballistocardiography. In: IEEE-EMBS International Conference on Biomedical and Health Informatics (BHI), Las Vegas, pp. 549–552 (2016)

8. Carvalho, P., Paiva, R., Couceiro, R., Henriques, J., Quintal, I., Muehlsteff, J., Aubert, X., Antunes, M.: Assessing systolic time-intervals from heart sound: a feasibility study. In: IEEE-EMBS (2009)

9. Jilek, J., Stork, M.: Assessing left ventricular ejection time from wrist cuff pulse waveforms: Algorithm and evaluation. In: International Conference on Applied Electronics (AE), Pilsen, pp. 1–4 (2017)

10. Hahn, J.-O., McCombie, D., Asada, H.H., Reisner, A., Hojman, H., Mukkamala, R.: Adaptive left ventricular ejection time estimation using multiple peripheral pressure waveforms. In: IEEE Engineering in Medicine and Biology 27th Annual Conference, Shanghai, pp. 2383–2386 (2005)

To Determinate PEP and LVET Through Analyzing LPC of Heart Sounds

Jin-Hao Ou, Ming-Hao Yang, Ming-Hsien Yu,
and Wen-Chien Chen[✉]

Department of Electrical Engineering, Chung Yuan Christian University,
Taoyuan, Taiwan
smpss91276@gmail.com

Abstract. To determine the pre-ejection period (PEP) and the left ventricular ejection time (LVET) thorough heart sounds and ECG are major tasks in this paper. The first step was to determine the event time of PEP, which detected the feature point of the first heart sound (S1) of PCG about 0.02–0.07 s after the R-peak of the ECG, and then obtained the prominent peaks of PCG during changes of signal slope with drastic change of peak value. The second step was taking R-peak to define a period of sound signal, making LPC and FFT, and moving certain few points to make another section, which was repeated to find out changes from the coefficient and frequency. Taking the sections with changes occurred, and FFT results as references got the time of PEP and LVET. Comparing the proposed results to the annotations, the average error of PEP detection is approximately 36.4 ms, and that of LVET is approximately 6.95 ms. With the error of the PEP, 83.4% and 33.9% accuracy are achieved within the time of 40 ms and 20 ms. With the error of the LVET, 94.2% and 25.8% accuracy are achieved at the time of 80 ms and 60 ms. The advantage of this method is that although the signals are very small, finding out the peak value of PCG, and analyzing the PEP and LVET are not hard tasks. Another advantage is that if the noise of the signal is not big enough to affect the original characteristic, the ECG signal could be applied to find out the peak value perfectly, and could be cut into piece by piece. The "NaN" point is hard to be defined in the testing data. Some issues are required to be improved or verified by other methods.

Keywords: Pre-ejection period (PEP) · Left ventricular ejection time (LVET) · Electrocardiography (ECG) · Heart sound · RPEAK · Linear predictive coding (LPC)

1 Introduction

The correlations between Electrocardiography (ECG) and Phonocardiogram (PCG) signals have been studied in many researches. It is found that the first and second heart sound corresponds to the systolic and diastolic activity of the heart. The first heart sound (S1) usually occurs during systole, and is longer with lower pitch. This is caused by blood rushing into the blood vessels, and sudden closure of the atrioventricular valve. The reverberation effect in the blood of the first heart sound is related to the sudden blockage of blood flow by the valve. The second heart sound (S2)

© Springer Nature Switzerland AG 2020
K.-P. Lin et al. (Eds.): ICBHI 2019, IFMBE Proceedings 74, pp. 371–380, 2020.
https://doi.org/10.1007/978-3-030-30636-6_51

is the sound of early stage of ventricular diastole, when the valve of the aorta, which is also called aortic semilunar valve, pulmonary valve and half-moon valve, is closed. In ECG, S1 usually occurs in QRS. It mainly happened in the segment of R-peak in ECG to the time when aortic valve opening (avo) in PCG, and is known for pre-ejection period (PEP). As for S2, a study mentioned that there are some similarities between heart sounds and QRS in ECG signals, such as S2 and T-waves. It can be found in the segment of R-peak in ECG to the time when aortic valve closing (avc) in PCG, and is considered to be the period of left ventricular ejection time (LVET) [1–6].

A sound signal with environmental noise and the heart sound are a combination of much different frequency. Many medical studies show that the frequency range of heart sound is low between 20 and 150 Hz [7]. Moreover, S1 is approximately about 60–80 Hz and S2 is about 100–150 Hz, so the first thing to process the signal is to filter it. Setting a low-pass filter at 200 Hz, and a high-pass filter at 0.5 Hz reserve the characteristic of the signal. In order to make the signal more clearly and to analyze it much easier, down-sampling is one of the methods to make it. The original signal is 44.1 kHz and trying to down to 8 kHz.

The linear predictive coding (LPC) was used to analyze the filtered sound signal. This method includes autocorrelation and Levinson Recursion which may get a coefficient in result [8]. Then, fast-Fourier Transform was used to sketch the spectrum. R-peak was used as the start of the periodic signal, and every thousand signal point is a section. Hundred points were moved on the start point of the next section [9, 10] for 1–2 s which means 8000–16000 signal points.

The LPC method was used to analyze sound signals, to define PEP and LVET, and to find out whether different order may cause alternative results in this paper (Fig. 1).

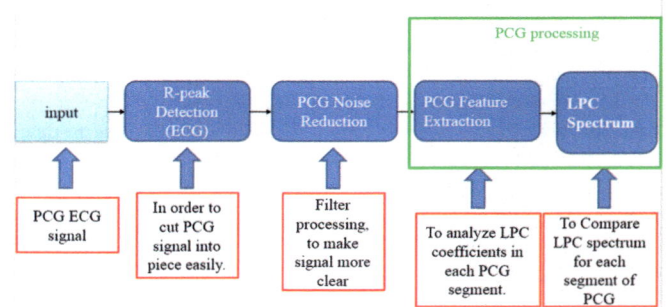

Fig. 1. The process chart for defining the PEP and LVET in this research.

2 Method

2.1 Find QRS

Researches related to detect QRS in ECG signal show that QRS could be found in a period of heart sound by the use of algorithm to adjust the thresholds [11]. In this paper, our way to detect QRS is as accurate as that of the former researches and is easier. QRS is detected during changes of signal slope at different time (Fig. 2).

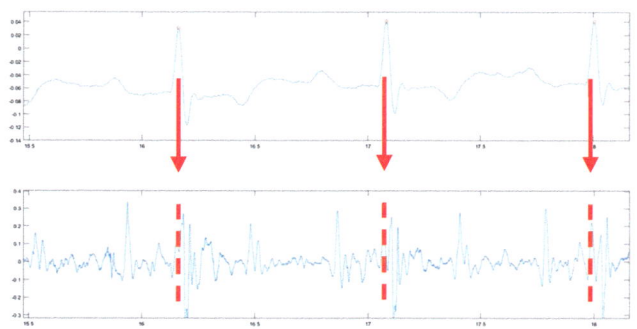

Fig. 2. R-peak found in ECG signal. [11]

The slope of T-wave would never be sharper than QRS. The QRS was detected by calculating the slope of QRS and T-wave and defining a limit slope. If a period of signal slope was larger than a certain value, we tagged it and kept detecting the QRS until the whole signal finished.

2.2 Elliptic Filter for PCG

In order to make the signal more clearly, the band-pass filter was used to process it. Elliptic filter was set about 50 Hz–200 Hz, because the frequency of the first and second heart sounds were from different researches [12]. However, this filter may let some important section disappear, so enlarge the band-pass frequency to 20 Hz–500 Hz from 50 Hz–200 Hz.

The magnitude squared frequency responding to the normalized low-pass elliptic filter of order n is defined by

$$|H_n(j\omega)|^2 = \frac{1}{1 + \varepsilon^2 R_n^2(\omega)} \tag{1}$$

where $R_n(\omega)$ is a Chebyshev rational function of ω determined from the specified ripple characteristics [13] (Fig. 3).

2.3 Linear Predictive Coding (LPC)

Linear predictive coding is a latest tool [14] used mostly in audio signal processing to represent the spectral envelope of a digital signal of speech in compressed form by the information of a linear predictive model. It is one of the most powerful signal analysis techniques, and one of the most useful methods for encoding good quality speech at a low bit rate, and provides extremely accurate estimates of speech parameters. To predict next point as linear combination of previous values:

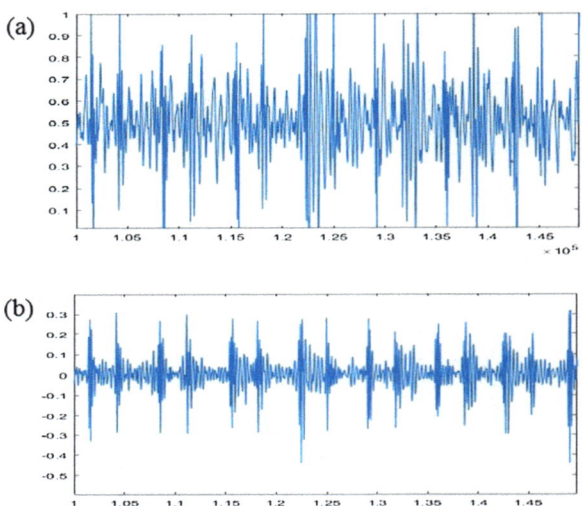

Fig. 3. Filtered heart sound signal by using elliptic filter. (a) the original PCG signal (b) filtered PCG signal.

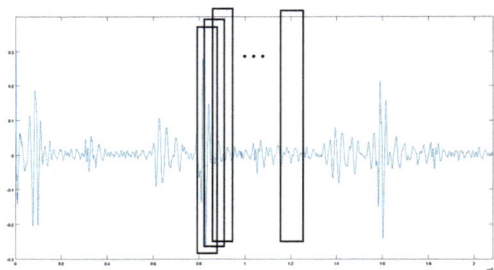

Fig. 4. Each segment for LPC analysis is 1000 sample points in PCG signal and each shifting interval is 100 sample points in PCG signal.

$$x(t) = \sum_{k=1}^{N} a_k x(t - k),$$ (2)

where N is the order of LPC, a_k are the Nth order of linear predictor coefficients.

The basic idea of LPC is that the current value of a speech sample can be approximated by a weighted linear combination of several speech samples of past values.

The weighting coefficients in the linear combination are called predictor coefficients. Linear prediction (LP) is used by most voice codecs to model short time spectrum of speech signal. Usually LPC is calculated for 10 ÷ 30 ms duration of speech signal segments (frames) [15]. An unique set of predictor coefficients can be determined by minimizing the sum when the squares of differences are between the actual speech samples and the linear prediction ones.

The numbers showing the intensity and frequency of the peak sound, the resonance peak, and the residual signal can be saved. The LPC synthesizes a sound signal by a reverse process where a source signal is generated by a buzzer parameter and a residual signal. At the same time, a formant is used to generate a filter representing a channel, and a signal is obtained by processing the source signal through a filter.

Since the heart sound signal is non-stationary and time-varying signal with short-term stationary, it is processed in a segment of the signal frame. Typically, 30 to 50 frames per second can compress well-understood signals. In this paper, R-peak was used as the start of the periodic signal and every thousand signal points was a section. Hundred points were moved on the start point of the next section for 1–2 s, which means 8000–16000 signal points.

Because the direct transmission filter coefficients are very sensitive to errors, it is not desirable to directly transmit the filter coefficients. In other words, a small error does not distort the entire spectrum or degrade the overall spectral quality, but a small error can make the prediction filter unstable.

When the frequency of the signal has changed, the changing coefficients are more and more obvious, like the section three to five in Fig. 5. The LPC coefficients can be determined when the first sound occurred.

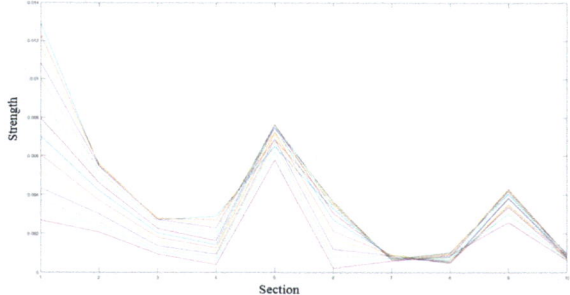

Fig. 5. The LPC coefficient results plotted by 14 segments of PCG signal.

2.4   Frequency Response/Spectrum for LPC Coefficients

Frequency response/spectrum, which is made after a signal from FFT, shows a composition of a signal. The stronger the certain frequency takes up, the larger the amplitude shows on the spectrum (Fig. 6).

Because of the figure shown upon, the largest amplitude in data 1 to 2 is 40 Hz. The 40 Hz signal in composition of data 3 is smaller. The characteristic of signal has changed, which means that something disappears after the period of section moving out of a certain signal.

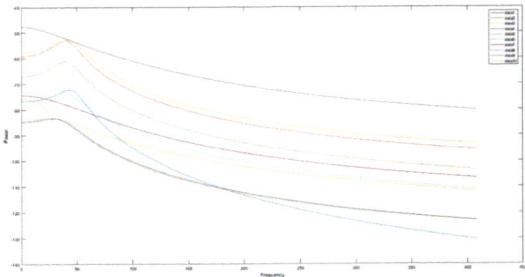

Fig. 6. 14 spectrums of LPC coefficients related to 14 segments of PCG signal in Fig. 5.

3 Result

3.1 Comparing Coefficient and Spectrum

Comparing Figs. 4 and 5, something happened in the same section of both 2 figures. To make sure that data 5 and 6 are where S1 or S2 occurs, the signal between data 5 and 6 was cut, and LPC and FFT were applied repeatedly to let the time more precisely with less error.

3.2 Verify to the Annotation

After the use of LPC and FFT, the answer found by LPC coefficients and spectrum was verified. The answer was re-checked, referring to the answer data and calculate the average time (T_{ave}) of ($T_{avo}-T_{QRS}$). QRS finding in method 1 was used to add with T_{ave} and to verify the differences between two values. The time of LVET was verified in the same way (Figs. 7, 8 and 9).

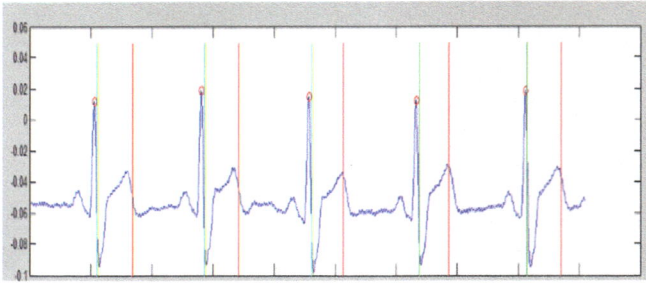

Fig. 7. The PEP and LVET. The line near Rpeak is the time when avo occurs, and the further one is the time when avc occurs.

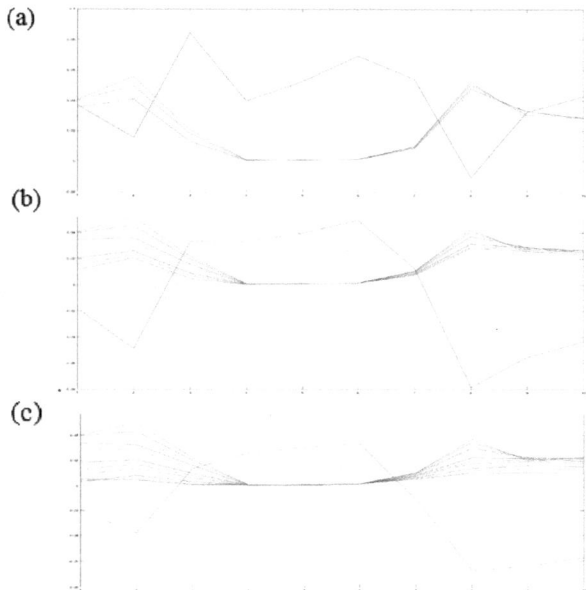

Fig. 8. The LPC coefficient within different order (a) N = 8 (b) N = 12 (c) N = 16

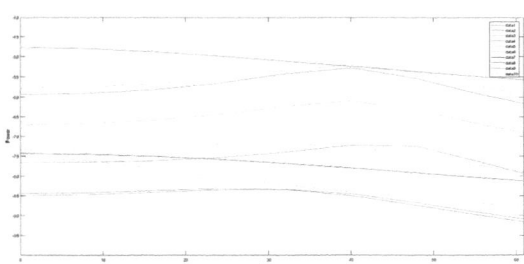

Fig. 9. LPC performed unregularly and poorly on some data. It is hard to define which segment the PEP and LVET appear.

3.3   Statistical Analysis

See Tables 1, 2 and 3.

Table 1. The error of 7 testing cases from LPC analysis.

Case	PEP	LVET
1	−14.365 ms	38.913 ms
2	−10.497 ms	23.520 ms
3	−30.506 ms	19.649 ms
4	−15.755 ms	10.045 ms
5	−14.022 ms	36.872 ms
6	8.331 ms	153.394 ms
7	5.337 ms	104.046 ms
8	−17.695 ms	28.844 ms

Table 2. The value of error between standard test data and experience data for PEP and LVET. (the amount of testing data: 7)

	PEP error	LVET error
MAX	32.34 ms	461.43 ms
Min	−41.34 ms	−61.50 ms
Average	−10.04 ms	55.52 ms
Mean square error	13.77 ms	84.59 ms

Table 3. Calculating the accuracy of the PEP and LVET of testing data in certain error range from the annotation data.

	PEP		LVET	
Error	40 ms	20 ms	80 ms	60 ms
Accuracy	83.4%	33.9%	94.2%	25.8%

4   Discussion and Conclusion

The changes within LPC coefficient through different order (N) are measured to know whether it will get further information.

There are some difficulties to use LPC. First, we cannot define a certain rule to know when the PEP and LVET would appear. Second, LPC performs poorly and weakly on the data obtained from unhealthy subjects. The last is that LPC is disturbed by the surrounding noise, which makes significant influence on the original heart sound.

Because of the poor performance from the use of LPC for some cases, the verification method was chosen repeatedly to make our final answer. It is not accurate enough. With 83.4% and 33.9% accuracy within the time of 40 ms and 20 ms. As for LVET, it has 94.2% and 25.8% accuracy within the time of 80 ms and 60 ms.

The advantage of this method is that although the signal is very small, finding out the peak value in PCG and analyzing the PEP and LVET are not hard tasks. Another advantage is that if the noise of the signal is not big enough to affect the original characteristic, the ECG signal can find the peak value perfectly and cut into piece by piece. The "NaN" point is hard to be defined in the testing data. The smaller the signal it gets, the greater error it might be. There are some issues required to be improved or verified by other methods.

Reference

1. Gamero, L.G., Watrous, R.: Detection of the first and second heart sound using probabilistic models. In: Proceedings of the 25th Annual International Conference of the IEEE Engineering in Medicine and Biology Society (IEEE Cat. No. 03CH37439), Cancun, vol. 3, pp. 2877–2880 (2003). https://doi.org/10.1109/iembs.2003.1280519
2. Jane, R., Laguna, P., Thakor, N.V., Caminal, P.: Adaptive Baseline Wander Removal in the ECG: Comparative Analysis With Cubic Spline Technique. Institut de Cibernetica (UPC-CSIC), Spain. Centro Politecnico Superior, University of Zaragoza, Spain. Johns Hopkins University, USA (1992)
3. Rangayyan, R.M., Lehner, R.J.: Phonocardiogram signal analysis: a review. Crit. Rev. Biomed. Eng. 5(3), 211–236 (1987)
4. Obaidat, M.S.: Phonocardiogram signal analysis: techniques and performance comparison. J. Med. Eng. Technol. 17(6), 221 (1993)
5. Durand, L.G., Pibarot, P.: Digital signal processing of the phonocardiogram: review of the most recent advancements. Crit. Rev. Biomed. Eng. 23(3–4), 163–219 (1995)
6. Lubaib, P., Ahammed Muneer, K.V.: The heart defect analysis based on PCG signals using pattern recognition techniques. Procedia Technol. 24, 1024–1031 (2016)
7. Phua, K., Chen, J., Dat, T., Shue, L.: Heart sound as a biometric. Pattern Recogn. 41(3), 906–919 (2008)
8. Mohseni, E., Shoeibi, A., Mahdi Moghaddasi, S., Mehrshad, N.: Classification ECG of cardiac signals using LPC features and support vector machine. In: 2nd International Conference on Knowledge-Based Research in Computer Engineering & Information Technology, September 2017
9. Redlarski, G., Gradolewski, D., Pałkowski, A.: A system for heart sounds classification. PLoS ONE 9, e112673 (2014). https://doi.org/10.1371/journal.pone.0112673
10. Phanphaisarn, W., Roeksabutr, A., Wardkein, P., Koseeyaporn, J., Yupapin, P.P.: Heart detection and diagnosis based on ECG and EPCG relationships. Med. Devices (Auckl). 4, 133–144 (2011)
11. Pan, J., Tompkins, W.J.: A real-time QRS detection algorithm. IEEE Trans. Biomed. Eng. BME-32(3), 230–236 (1985)
12. Stein, P.D., Sabbah, H.N., Lakier, J.B., Magilligan, D.J., Goldstein, D.: Frequency of the first heart sound in the assessment of stiffening of mitral bioprosthetic valves. Circulation 63(1), 200–203 (1981)

13. Orfanidis, S.J.: Lecture Notes on Elliptic Filter Design. Department of Electrical & Computer Engineering, Rutgers University, 20 November 2006
14. Erkelens, J.S., Broersen, P.M.T.: LPC interpolation by approximation of the sample autocorrelation function. IEEE Trans. Audio Speech Process. **6**(6), 569–573 (1998)
15. Islam, T., Kabal, P.: Partial-energy weighted interpolation of linear prediction coefficients. In: Proceedings of the IEEE Workshop Speech Coding (Delavan, WI), September 2000, pp. 105–107. Electrical & Computer Engineering McGill University, Montreal (2000)

Improvement of Environment and Camera Setting on Extraction of Heart Rate Using Eulerian Video Magnification

Bo-Yu Huang[✉] and Chi-Lun Lin

Mechanical Engineering Department, National Cheng Kung University,
Daxue Road, East District, Tainan, Taiwan
112231tn@gmail.com, chilun.lin@gmail.com

Abstract. Non-contact heart rate measurement has been widely utilized in multiple applications. The Eulerian Video Magnification algorithm proposed by MIT CSAIL group in 2012 can be used to magnify the subtle color variation and small motion in videos and can be used to extract cardio-features through photoplethysmography method. In this study, we intend to improve the accuracy of heart rate prediction for the Eulerian Video Magnification method. With the selected region of interest and the peak detection algorithm, we found out that the signal of the Y component in YIQ color spectrum is more consistent than that of the I component in terms of heart rate estimation. The result also demonstrated that the heart rate extracted under 30 frames per second (fps) was more accurate than which extracted under 60 fps. With an illumination level higher than 1500 lx and a frame rate of 30 fps, the error of heart rate extraction compared to oximeter measurement was 5% while using GoPro Hero 6 for recording. Further data processing and false peak detection are necessary for accurate heart rate variability characterization.

Keywords: Eulerian video magnification · Photoplethysmography · Non-contact heart rate measurement · Heart rate video · Mental fatigue

1 Introduction

Photoplethysmography (PPG), a non-contact heart rate measurement method, has gained its popularity since Poh et al. published two crucial articles [1, 2]. The team used a webcam to record the frontal face of the subject and extracted the color channel signals from the video over a period of time.

In 2012, a new method named Eulerian Video Magnification (EVM) was published [3]. The method reveals low-amplitude motion in everyday life caused by blood flow, such as face color variation, heart-beat of neonatal. Another paper [4] suggested that proportionally selecting the forehead or cheek is essential to successful prediction of heart rate.

Non-contact heart rate measurement is widely used in many occasions. In order to acquire reliable estimations of heart rate and heart rate variability (HRV) through the EVM method, a more robust system should be developed.

© Springer Nature Switzerland AG 2020
K.-P. Lin et al. (Eds.): ICBHI 2019, IFMBE Proceedings 74, pp. 381–388, 2020.
https://doi.org/10.1007/978-3-030-30636-6_52

2 Methods

2.1 Face Detection and Region of Interest

Before the video processing of EVM, the face detection method developed by Viola and Jones [5] was used to crop out the redundant area of the video. Also, focusing only on the face region lessened the computational time of the image processing. Three regions of interests (ROIs) were highlighted, including forehead, right cheek and left cheek as Fig. 1.

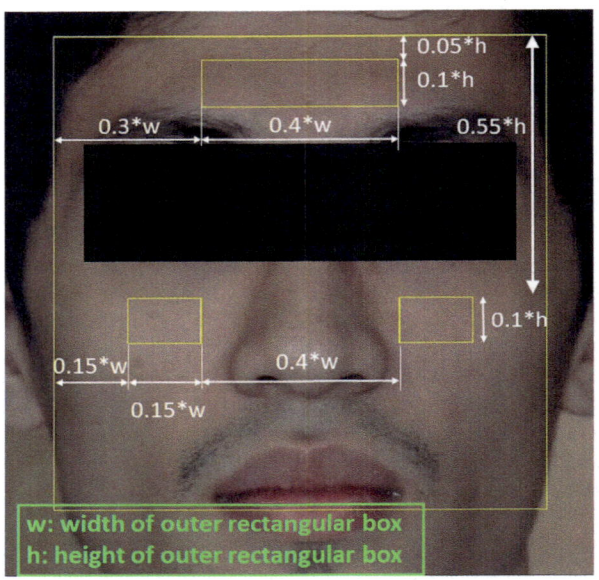

Fig. 1. The regions of interest on the forehead and both side of cheeks, where 'h' and 'w' represent the height and width of the outer yellow rectangular box, respectively

The representing intensity value of each region was calculated by averaging the magnified Eulerian-values in Y and I components of YIQ color spectrum inside the ROI as demonstrated in Eq. (1).

$$I = \frac{1}{w \times h} \sum_1^w \sum_1^h I_i, i = Y, I \tag{1}$$

After acquiring the component value of each frame, we performed data normalization as displayed in Eq. (2). I_m and σ were the mean and standard deviations of I in each video clip. I_N was the normalized data which would be utilized in next section.

$$I_N = \frac{(I - I_m)}{\sigma} \qquad (2)$$

2.2   Peak to Peak Calculation

The local maximum of consecutive component values was detected and recognized as a heartbeat. An identified example is shown in Fig. 2. By recording the frame interval between peaks, we acquired an average frame interval and calculated the corresponding heart rate by using Eq. (3).

$$Heart\ rate = \frac{Sampling\ Rate\ of\ camera}{mean\ (frame\ interval)} \times 60 \qquad (3)$$

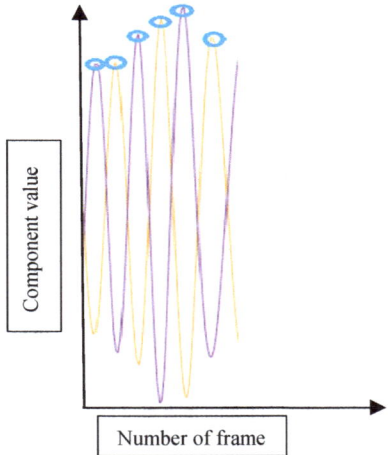

Fig. 2. An example of peaks detected in continuous signal waves

2.3   Experimental Settings

We used GODOX SL-100W as a consistent light source to provide flicker-free filming environment. By changing the output capacity, we could adjust the illumination level. The subject sat in front of a table where the GoPro Hero 6 was set on to record the video of subject, as shown in Fig. 3.

Table 1 shows the detailed settings of the experiment. Part 1 focused on different frame rates and recording durations. Part 2 focused on different illumination level. The oximeter measurement and camera filming were performed simultaneously (Fig. 4) for validation of our method. Hence, oximeter served as the ground truth for both parts of the experiment.

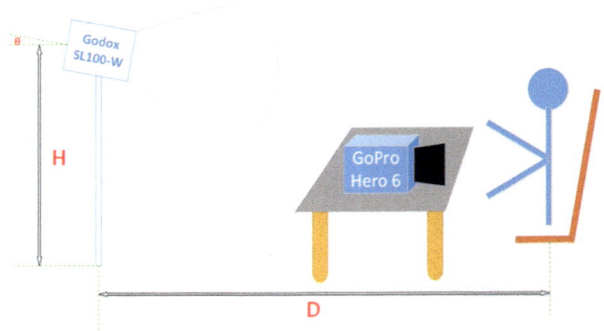

Fig. 3. A schematic diagram of experimental settings

Table 1. Environment setting and variance in two experiments

Part 1		Part 2	
θ (degree)	10–20	θ (degree)	10
H (cm)	140	H (cm)	140
GODOX capacity (%)	70	Recording time (s)	30
D (cm)	140	Frames per second	30
Recording time (s)	15,30	GODOX capacity (%)	30,50,70
Frames per second	30,60	D (cm)	140

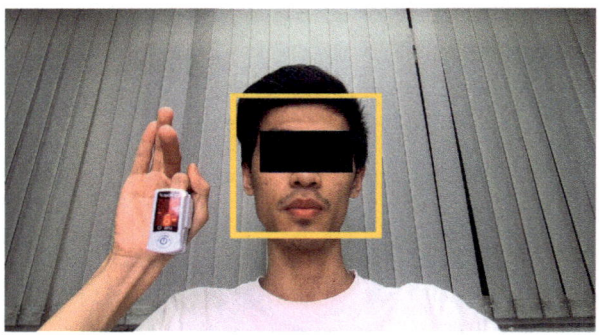

Fig. 4. Performing oximeter measurement while recording

3 Results

3.1 Different Frame Rates and Recording Durations

This sub-section is corresponding to the Part 1 in Table 1. With the same illumination level, different filming durations and frame rates of the camera were tested. The extracted heart rate was compared with that measured by the oximeter. Sample results of comparison are shown in Table 2.

Table 2. Sample results computed from the video output

	Y	I	Oximeter
Forehead	63.35	63.6	63
Right cheek	63.83	65.7	63
Left cheek	64.75	68.98	63

We then used the collected data to calculate the average error between our method and the oximeter. The results of Y and I components are shown in Fig. 5. The prediction of heart rate with 30 fps and 30 s was the most accurate result. Overall, the prediction of the Y component outperformed the I component's.

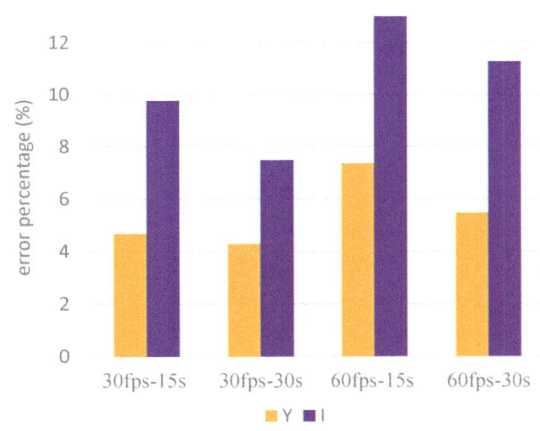

Fig. 5. Average errors of predicted heart beats per minute in Y and I components

3.2 Different Illumination Levels

This sub-section is corresponding to the Part 2 in Table 1. With the same filming duration and frame rate which were 30 s and 30 fps, different illumination levels were tested. Sample PPG raw data is presented in Fig. 6. The extracted heart rate was

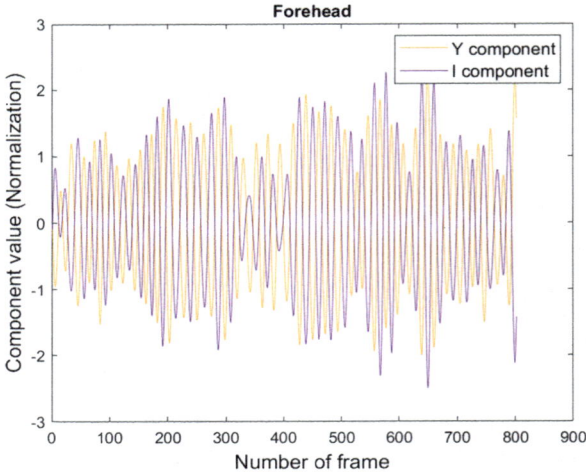

Fig. 6. The waveform of Y and I components from YIQ color spectrum in the forehead region of consecutive video frames

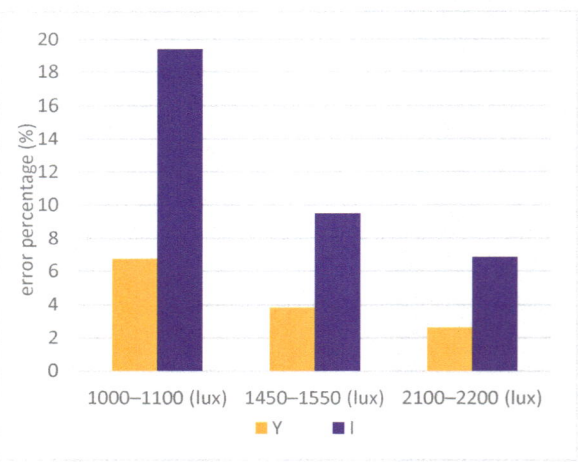

Fig. 7. Average errors of predicted heart beats per minute in Y and I components

compared with that measured by the oximeter. The results of Y and I components are shown in Fig. 7. The prediction of heart rate with illumination level between 2100 to 2200 lx was the most accurate result. Overall, the prediction of the Y component outperformed the I component's.

4   Discussion

First, 30 fps and 30 s of filming duration acquired the most accurate heart rate. We suspect that a higher frame rate could easily capture the involuntary movement from the subject which increased the noise in the video. Therefore, lower fps might lessen the noise effect. On the other hand, the longer the filming duration, the more accurate the heart rate prediction was. We found out that, by averaging the RR-interval, the false peak detection was compensated by much longer recording and consequently had less influence on HR prediction. Also, if the amount of consecutive RR-interval data is large enough, deleting a data point that is too far away from the median of the whole serial data might seem plausible. In terms of heart rate variability measurement, up-sampling using cubic spline interpolation may help solve the lower temporal resolution issue since we only got 30 frames in a second.

Secondly, the higher the illumination level, the more accurate the heart rate prediction was. A more complete reflection of subtle color changes from the facial region can be obtained in a better and consistent lighting condition. It seems obvious but it is difficult and nearly impractical to have same kind of consistent environment in real life scenario. Also, human eyes probably can't withstand the high illumination level for a period of time. Therefore, we argue that the most appropriate scenario to utilize the method is when subject is inside the building, for example, sitting in front of a computer and doing office work. The normal indoor illumination level is under 300 lx because the fluorescent light is from the ceiling. More reasonable illumination level should be around 900 to 1000 lx.

5   Conclusions and Future Work

We have tested both same illumination level with different frame rates and filming duration, and same frame rate and filming duration with different illumination level using GoPro Hero 6 camera. Overall, the Y component outperformed the I component in terms of heart rate estimation in all circumstances. Also, the illumination level should be higher than 1500 lx to acquire reliable heart rate estimation. If the environment is stable and the illumination level is at least 1500 lx, the error percentage of heart rate prediction using Eulerian Video Magnification can achieve 5%. In the future, improvement of HRV and heart beat interval accuracy are our primary task.

Acknowledgment. This research was supported by the Ministry of Science and Technology, Taiwan, R.O.C. under Grants No. MOST 106-2221-E-006-049 and No. MOST 107-2221-E-006-067-MY2. The authors would like to thank our colleagues from Medical Device Innovation and Design Laboratory in the Department of Mechanical Engineering, National Cheng Kung University who provided their insights and expertise that greatly assisted the research.

Conflict of Interest. The authors declare that they have no conflict of interest.

References

1. Poh, M.-Z., McDuff, D.J., Picard, R.W.: Non-contact, automated cardiac pulse measurements using video imaging and blind source separation. Opt. Exp. **18**(10), 10762–10774 (2010)
2. Poh, M.-Z., McDuff, D.J., Picard, R.W.: Advancements in noncontact, multiparameter physiological measurements using a webcam. IEEE Trans. Biomed. Eng. **58**(1), 7–11 (2011)
3. Wu, H.-Y., et al.: Eulerian video magnification for revealing subtle changes in the world (2012)
4. Gambi, E., et al.: Heart rate detection using Microsoft Kinect: validation and comparison to wearable devices. Sensors **17**(8), 1776 (2017)
5. Viola, P., Jones, M.: Rapid object detection using a boosted cascade of simple features. In: Proceedings of the 2001 IEEE Computer Society Conference on Computer Vision and Pattern Recognition, CVPR 2001, vol. 1. IEEE (2001)

Deep Learning Method to Detect Plaques in IVOCT Images

Grigorios-Aris Cheimariotis[1(✉)], Maria Riga[2],
Konstantinos Toutouzas[2], Dimitris Tousoulis[2], Aggelos Katsaggelos[3],
and Nikolaos Maglaveras[1,3,4]

[1] Lab of Computing, Medical Informatics and Biomedical Imaging
Technologies, Aristotle University of Thessaloniki, Thessaloniki, Greece
ncheimar@gmail.com
[2] 1st Department of Cardiology, Athens University, Hippokration Hospital,
Athens, Greece
[3] Department of Electrical Engineering and Computer Science, Northwestern
University, Evanston, IL, USA
[4] Department of Industrial Engineering and Management Sciences,
Northwestern University, Evanston, IL, USA

Abstract. Intravascular Optical Coherence Tomography (IVOCT) is a modality which gives in vivo insight of coronaries' artery morphology. Thus, it helps diagnosis and prevention of atherosclerosis. About 100–300 cross-sectional OCT images are obtained for each artery. Therefore, it is important to facilitate and objectify the process of detecting regions of interest, which otherwise demand a lot of time and effort from medical experts. We propose a processing pipeline to automatically detect parts of the arterial wall which are not normal and possibly consist of plaque. The first step of the processing is transforming OCT images to polar coordinates and to detect the arterial wall. After binarization of the image and removal of the catheter, the arterial wall is detected in each axial line from the first white pixel to a depth of 80 pixels which is equal to 1.5 mm. Then, the arterial wall is split to orthogonal patches which undergo OCT-specific transformations and are labelled as plaque (4 distinct kinds: fibrous, calcified, lipid and mixed) or normal tissue. OCT-specific transformations include enhancing the more reflective parts of the image and rendering patches independent of the arterial wall curvature. The patches are input to AlexNet which is fine-tuned to learn to classify them. Fine-tuning is performed by retraining an already trained AlexNet with a learning rate which is 20 times larger for the last 3 fully-connected layers than for the initial 5 convolutional layers. 114 cross-sectional images were randomly selected to fine-tune AlexNet while 6 were selected to validate the results. Training accuracy was 100% while validation accuracy was 86%. Drop in validation accuracy rate is attributed mainly to false negatives which concern only calcified plaque. Thus, there is potential in this method especially in detecting the 3 other classes of plaque.

Keywords: Segmentation · Intravascular OCT ·
Convolutional Neural Networks · Deep learning

© Springer Nature Switzerland AG 2020
K.-P. Lin et al. (Eds.): ICBHI 2019, IFMBE Proceedings 74, pp. 389–395, 2020.
https://doi.org/10.1007/978-3-030-30636-6_53

1 Introduction

Intravascular Optical Coherence Tomography (IVOCT) is an imaging modality that allows, due to its very high resolution (10 μm), to look closely at the morphological and pathological features of the coronary artery. Particularly in the case of atherosclerotic disease, it enables to look at the various microstructures associated with the formation, progression and thrombotic complications of the atherosclerotic plaque. INOCT is an invasive technology that is constantly improving and has become a very useful tool for the diagnosis and monitoring of treatment of atherosclerotic disease.

The use of this technique involves the collection of a large amount of imaging data (e.g. 100–300 cross-sectional images are collected for each artery), the examination of which requires a lot of time and great effort from a skilled medical specialist. Therefore, an automated classification method is needed to identify and categorize the microstructures of interest.

For this reason, methods have been proposed recently to make lumen segmentation and tissue characterization automatic and faster. Athanasiou et al. [1] proposed various machine learning techniques to classify 4 kinds of tissue. Shalev et al. [2] proposed SVM to classify plaques based mainly on statistical properties of the images. Xu et al. [3] proposed Support Vector Machine to classify tissue using as feature among other Fisher vector, histogram of oriented gradients and local binary pattern.

Abdolmanafi et al. [4] proposed to extract features from OCT images using Alexnet [5]. These features are then used to classify media and intima using AlexNet or other machine learning classifiers. Alexnet is a specific convolutional neural network (CNN), very successful to classify images of the large database ImageNet which is used to compare computer vision algorithms performance. In general, CNNs are neural networks that have commonly convolutional layers along with the fully connected layers that neural networks have and they outperform other algorithms in computer vision tasks. AlexNet consists of five convolutional layers with rectified linear unit (ReLU) activations, some of which are followed by max-pooling layers, and three dense layers. The network was trained with stochastic gradient descent.

In our previous work [6] we propose a multi-step framework based on Convolutional Neural Networks (CNN) for the textural analysis and classification of the lumen wall in order to classify the kind of plaque if it is present. The classification is implemented by an AlexNet version re-trained on bigger patches of images artificially constructed to depict the core of the plaque region.

In the present work we propose a deep learning processing pipeline to automatically detect parts of the arterial wall which are not normal and consist of atherosclerotic plaque (4 different kinds of tissue: fibrous, calcified, lipid and mixed).

2 Materials

The dataset consisted of 120 FD-IVOCT cross-sectional images where a medical expert delineated the different kinds of plaque according to the published expert consensus [7]. Examples of the appearance of the types of tissue are depicted in Figs. 1, 2, 3 and 4.

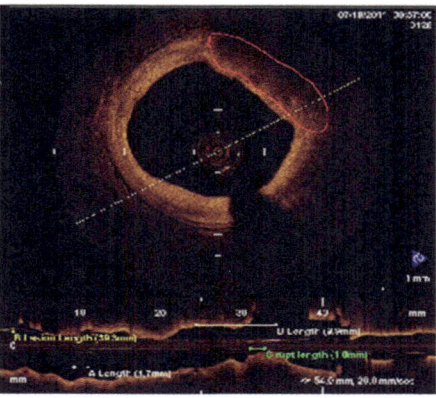

Fig. 1. OCT image with lipid plaque (red contour)

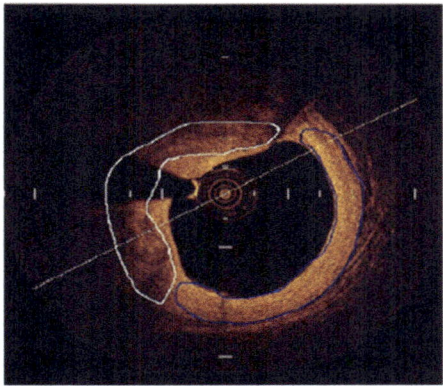

Fig. 2. OCT image with calcified plaque (white contour) and fibrous plaque (blue contour)

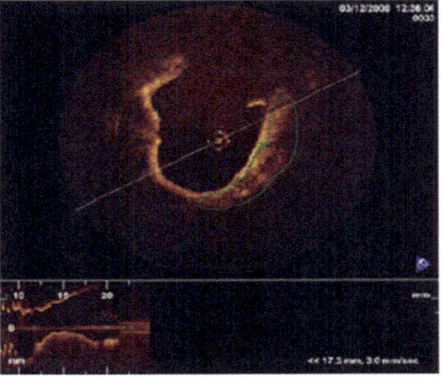

Fig. 3. OCT image with mixed plaque (green contour)

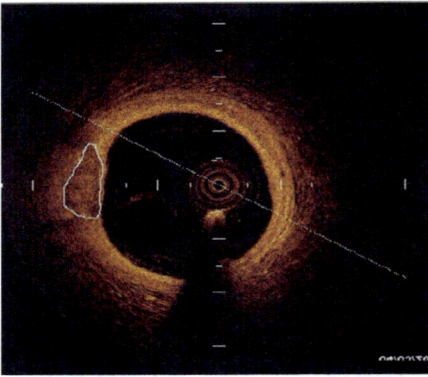

Fig. 4. OCT image with calcified plaque (white contour)

3 Methods

In order to extract patches from the OCT images that are characteristic of the type of tissue, we firstly transformed images to polar coordinates and then we detected the arterial wall. This processing is depicted in Fig. 5 and is applied both for training and for testing of the convolutional neural network and is described below. The OCT images are mainly intensity images; therefore, we kept the grayscale equivalent of them without loss of information. Afterwards a very low threshold (5% of the maximum intensity) was applied to highlight (in white color) only the high reflective parts of the image which are potentially part of the arterial wall while intensities of the image below the threshold were rendered black and were considered background. The catheter part was removed from the images and then morphological opening was applied to smooth the contour of lumen-wall border and to remove small irrelevant objects that are possibly artifacts and not parts of the wall. In addition to that, small objects with fewer pixels than a threshold were removed for the same purpose. The outcome of this procedure is considered arterial wall.

Then, the arterial wall is split to orthogonal patches which undergo OCT-specific transformations and are labelled as plaque (4 distinct kinds: fibrous, calcified, lipid and mixed) or normal tissue Fig. 6. OCT-specific transformations include enhancing the more reflective parts of the image and rendering patches independent of the arterial wall curvature. The first transformation is given by the equation:

$$Iref(\rho, \theta) = Ireg(\rho, \theta) * \left(\sum_{i=1}^{i=\rho} Ireg(i, \theta) / \sum_{i=1}^{\iota=N} Ireg(i, \theta) \right) \tag{1}$$

where Ireg is the initial intensity in the patch and Iref is the transformed. These transformations were chosen because the experimental results show that they significantly enhance accuracy. The size of the patches was chosen because they had better classification results after experiments with different sizes. The patches are resized to be input to AlexNet which, is fine-tuned to learn to classify them. Fine-tuning is

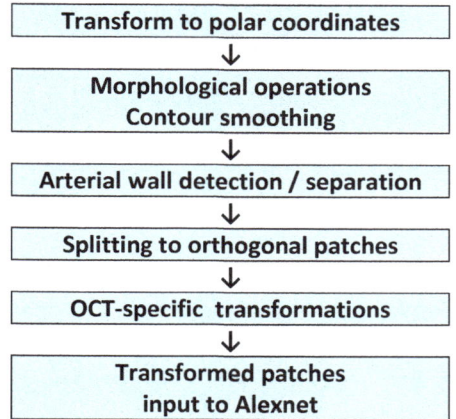

Fig. 5. Flowchart of the processing to create the input to AlexNet

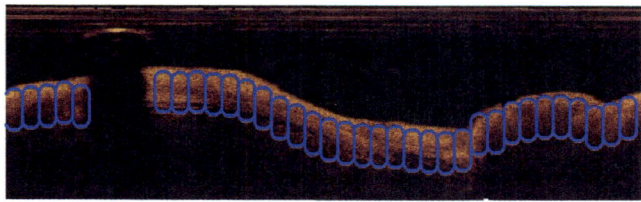

Fig. 6. OCT image in polar domain. The arterial wall is split into orthogonal patches.

performed by retraining an already trained AlexNet with a learning rate which is 20 times larger for the last 3 fully-connected layers than for the initial 5 convolutional layers.

4   Results

114 cross-sectional images were randomly selected to fine-tune AlexNet while 6 were selected to validate the results. Training accuracy was 100% while validation accuracy was 86%. In Figs. 7, 8, 9 and 10 there are 4 examples where it is observed that lipid plaque and mixed plaques are accurately detected as not normal. Calcified plaque is accurately detected in one example, but it is not detected in the last one where fibrous plaque is detected accurately.

Therefore, drop in validation accuracy rate is attributed mainly to false negatives which concern only calcified plaques.

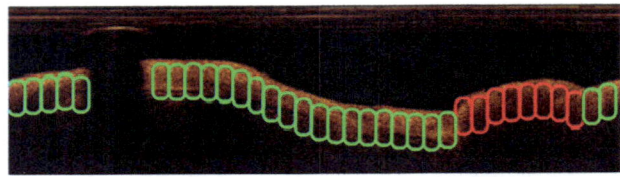

Fig. 7. Polar image of Fig. 1 (lipid plaque) where with red are the patches which are classified as not normal

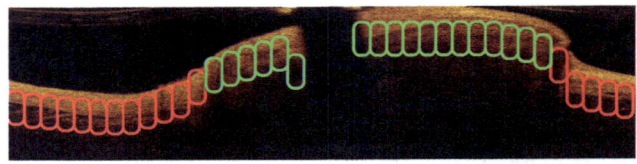

Fig. 8. Polar image of Fig. 2. Fibrous plaque is detected (red patches) but calcified plaque is not detected

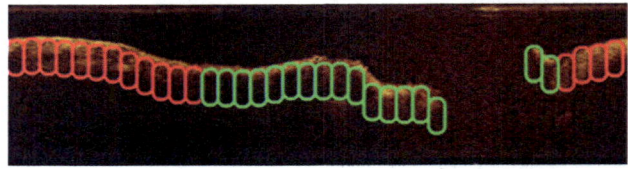

Fig. 9. Polar Image of Fig. 3. Mixed plaque is detected as not normal (red patches)

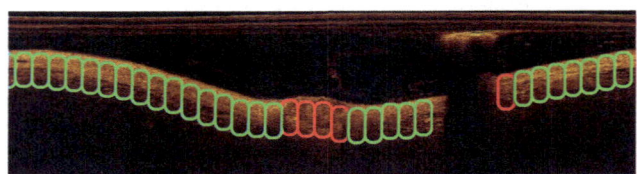

Fig. 10. Polar image of Fig. 4. Calcified plaque is detected while only one patch of normal tissue is characterized as not normal

5   Discussion

This work is part of a project where the goal is to semantically segment OCT images. In our previous work, we classified plaques if they were already detected. In this work we focus on detecting parts of the arterial wall which are not normal. The combination of these methods with some alterations and enhancements should give us the desired results.

An enhancement to this method may be the exhaustive use of other CNN architectures which are known to be effective in similar tasks or the construction of prototype CNN architectures. Another enhancement which we will try out is the use of data augmentation techniques and alter the preprocessing steps. Finally, the input to the CNN may be diferant.

6 Conclusions

We presented a method to detect parts of the arterial wall that are not normal. There is potential in this method especially in characterizing lipid, mixed and fibrous plaque as not normal.

Acknowledgment. This research is funded by the Greek State Scholarships Foundation and European Social Fund.

Conflict of Interest. The authors declare that they have no conflict of interest.

References

1. Athanasiou, L., Bourantas, C., Rigas, G., et al.: Methodology for fully automated segmentation and plaque characterization in intracoronary optical coherence tomography images. J. Biomed. Opt. (2014). https://doi.org/10.1117/1.JBO.19.2.026009
2. Shalev, R., Nakamura, D., Nishino, S., et al.: Automated volumetric intravascular plaque classification using Optical Coherence Tomography (OCT). In: Twenty-Eighth IAAI Conference on Innovative Applications (2016)
3. Xu, M., Cheng, J., Wong, D.W.K.: Automatic image classification in intravascular region. In: 2016 IEEE 10 Conference (TENCON) (2016). https://doi.org/10.1109/TENCON.2016.7848275
4. Abdolmanafi, A., Duong, L., Dahdah, M., et al.: Deep feature learning for automatic tissue classification of coronary artery using optical coherence tomography. Biomed. Opt. Exp. **8**(2), 1203–1220 (2017). https://doi.org/10.1364/BOE.8.001203
5. Krizhevsky, A., Sutskever, I., Hinton, G.: ImageNet classification with deep convolutional neural networks. In: Advances in Neural Information Processing Systems, p. 9 (2012)
6. Cheimariotis, G.A., Riga, M., Toutouzas, K., et al.: Automatic characterization of plaques and tissue in IVOCT images using a multi-step convolutional neural network framework. IFMBE Proceedings, vol. **68**(1), pp. 261–265. https://doi.org/10.1007/978-981-10-9035-6_4
7. Toutouzas, K., Chatzizisis, Y.S., Riga, M., et al.: Accurate and reproducible reconstruction of coronary arteries and endothelial shear stress calculation using 3D OCT: comparative study to 3D IVUS and 3D QCA. Atherosclerosis **240**(2), 510–519 (2015)

Fall Risk Assessment in Older Adults with Diabetic Peripheral Neuropathy

Jhonathan Sora Cárdenas$^{(\boxtimes)}$, Martha Zequera Díaz,
and Francisco Calderón Bocanegra

Electronics Department, School of Engineering,
BASPI/FootLab (Bioengineering, Signal Analysis and Image Processing
Research Group), Pontificia Universidad Javeriana, Bogotá, Colombia
{J_sora,mzequera,calderonf}@javeriana.edu.co

Abstract. Diabetic peripheral neuropathy DPN is the most frequent complication with people with diabetes and affects approximately half of this population. This is reflected in the reduction of the transmission of vibratory sensitivity, proprioceptive and of reflexes osteotendinous, affecting sensory and motor skills. People with DPN are up to 23 times more likely to have falls and 15 times more likely to report an injury compared to healthy older adults. Falls have significant consequences, such as temporary or permanent physical disability, which decreases the quality of life of the elderly and represents an increase in mortality. Therefore, a pilot study is proposed to assess the risk of falls in older adults with DPN by implementing a predictive system based on the clinical information of the AGS/BGS guidelines, the oscillation of the pressure center (CoP) at rest and the Timed up and Go test (TUG) with the use of inertial sensors. A sample of convenience of 19 participants (13 control group and 6 with DPN) older than 45 years, were cited to perform data acquisition, which were used as inputs to evaluate four fall risk classification techniques: K-means, support vector machines, K nearest neighbors and neural networks, obtaining a precision = 90.9%, sensitivity = 80% and specificity = 100%. Therefore, this study suggests that it is possible to evaluate the risk of falls in older adults with DPN through the clinical information of the AGS/BGS guidelines, the oscillation of the CoP at rest and the TUG test with the use of inertial sensors and it also has the potential to be implemented in future studies with larger populations.

Keywords: Diabetic peripheral neuropathy · Fall risk assessment ·
Center of pressure · Instrumented timed up and go · Older adults ·
Pattern recognition

1 Introduction

Diabetes Mellitus (DM) is a chronic metabolic disorder that has a prevalence of 8.8% (425 million) of the world population in 2017 [1], with Diabetic Peripheral Neuropathy (DPN) being one of the most common complications that can affect up to 50% of this population [2]. DPN is associated with physical impairments such as decreased strength, restriction of ankle mobility and retardation of peripheral nerve conduction

© Springer Nature Switzerland AG 2020
K.-P. Lin et al. (Eds.): ICBHI 2019, IFMBE Proceedings 74, pp. 396–404, 2020.
https://doi.org/10.1007/978-3-030-30636-6_54

[3]; On the other hand, it can also be evidenced the reduction of the transmission of vibratory sensitivity, proprioceptive and of reflexes osteotendinous affecting sensory and motor skills [4], all the above leads to greater postural instability, altered patterns of walking and control of altered balance [5], which represents an increase in the risk of falls [6], especially in older adults [7]. Considering that people with DPN are up to 23 times more likely to fall and 15 times more likely to report an injury compared to healthy older adults [8], the assessment of the risk of falling in this specific population is a tool for prevention important and effective, which helps determine the most appropriate interventions to reduce or eliminate falls [9].

In the clinical area, the use of a variety of methods and instruments to assess instability in older adults is carried out in the form of questionnaires and physical tests. Among them are the Functional Reach Test (FRT) [10], the Berg Balance Scale (BBS) [11] and the timed "Up & Go" test (TUG) [12], however, most of these Methods are subjective [13]. Therefore, we have carried out several studies with inertial sensors and these have been reliable for evaluating the balance and characteristics of the gait [14–16]. As the TUG test with inertial sensors has been applied, the TUG test with inertial sensors has been implemented, a robust method has been implemented to evaluate the risk of possible falls.

However, the equilibrium measures identified with the inertial sensors do not evaluate all the systems that intervene in the equilibrium. This is one of the following reasons. with inertial sensors achieving better results with a combined approach of these two methods. On the other hand, the pressure center or CoP is the most used quantitative parameter to assess stability. Studies such as the one carried out by Toloza [18], showed that in the subjects with DPN a greater corporal intensity was obtained in the balance, therefore, this is a vital response now of being able to evaluate the risk of fall in the population with DPN.

There have been several studies evaluating the risk of falling in older adults, but studies conducted with assessment methods in populations of diseases with high risk of falling as the DPN [15, 16]. For the foregoing and with the desire to give continuity to the efforts that are carried out in the BASPI (Bioengineering, Signal Analysis and Image Procedures) research group, from the laboratory Footlab of the Department of Electronics of the Pontificia Universidad Javeriana Bogota, Colombia, in the prevention section and early detection of complications in the line of research in the alterations of balance control in people with neuropathy, a pilot study was proposed in which the risk of falls is sought in older adults with DPN through the implementation of a system predictive from the clinical information of the AGS/BGS guidelines, the oscillation of CoP at rest and the TUG test with the use of inertial sensors.

2   Materials and Methods

2.1   Data Acquisition

A protocol was developed for data acquisition, which was implemented in a convenience sample of 19 participants (13 control group and 6 with DPN) over 45 years, the protocol has four steps, the first step is the acquisition The clinical information is based on the information in the AGS/BGS clinical guide [19]; The data are detailed in the main risk factors of the fall in older adults and from which the following data were obtained: gender, age, height, weight, presence or absence of polypharmacy, orthostatic hypotension, uncorrected vision problems, duration of Diabetes and DPN.

In a second step, the data of the oscillation of the pressure center CoP are acquired; since according to Fortaleza et al. [20] subjects with DPN show a greater fluctuation of the CoP when they are in a static position, they are shown in the middle of the Ecowalk pressure platform with a sampling frequency of 30 Hz, in the Take The data is explained to the contrary. We made 3 replicas, 10 s interspersed by 30 s of rest. From this second step the oscillation data were obtained in the directions (mm): upper, lower left and right. For the left foot, right foot and body. The percentages and the area of the anteroposterior contact surface of each foot have also been acquired under conditions of open eyes and closed eyes.

The third stage corresponds to the Timed Up and Go test (TUG) with inertial sensors, it is the clinical evaluation that has the highest diagnostic accuracy for the assessment of the risk of falls in people with DPN [21]. In addition, the use of a system of inertial sensors in this test, make the measurements reliable for the evaluation of the balance and the characteristics of the gait [14–16]. Three inertial sensors PocKetLab of Myriad Sensors were used, at a sampling frequency of 30 Hz, which were fixed in the lower part of the back, on the vertebrae L3 to L5, this location was chosen by the approximation to the location of the center of Mass [22], the other two sensors are located at the mid-front point of the left and right leg respectively [17]. To this end, the anatomical measurements of each patient were taken, and markers were used to ensure the placement of the sensors at the desired points, as shown in Fig. 1.

The implementation of the iTUG test begins with the participant sitting in a standard chair with armrests, the person must stand up, walk straight by 3 m at their normal pace, turn around, walk towards the chair and sit down again. The time of the test starts at the moment when the order to "go" and stops at the moment when the participant's back touches the back of the seat. The participant was shown how the test was performed by a researcher and a test exercise was carried out by the participant, in order to become familiar with the test. The test had 3 replicas per participant and a 1-minute rest between the tests. The data collected from this test were: the angular velocity (RPM) and the linear acceleration (m/s^2) of the three inertial sensors on the X axes for the anteroposterior direction, Y axis for the mid-lateral direction and the Z axis for the vertical direction.

Finally, to obtain labels for the risk of falls, an evaluation survey of the AGS/BGS clinical guide was carried out [19], which were collected through a survey of "auto" data reported with the following questions: Have you had two (2) or more falls in the last twelve (12) months? Did you present an acute fall? and do you have difficulty walking or maintaining balance? Any affirmative answer to the above questions places the participant in the high-risk group and the results of this survey are used as the classification labels of the participants. The labels were defined as: Class 0: Low fall risk, Class 1: High fall risk, belonging to the control group and Class 2: High fall risk, belonging to the group with DPN.

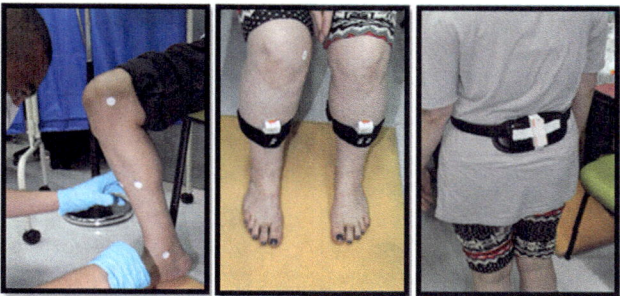

Fig. 1. Location of the markers for the sensors position base on the COP protocol implemented at FootLab.

2.2 Data Processing

Once the data acquisition was done, these were used as inputs for four machine learning techniques, starting with the unsupervised classification method of K-means, with k = 3 using the Euclidean distance, using this technique we wanted to group the data by the characteristics entered For vector support machines (SVM), they were evaluated with the kernel functions: linear, polynomial of order 2 and 3, and the function of radial base (RBF) fine, medium and coarse. For the KNN technique, they used the techniques: fine, medium, coarse, cubic, cosine and weighted. For SVM and KNN, cross-validation with 5 divisions was used. For the neural networks were implemented with three training functions, Levenberg-Marquardt, Bayesian regularization and conjugate gradient scale, for which 2 hidden layers, sigmoid transfer function and the predetermined training parameters were used. They were evaluated with the combinations of 5, 10, 15, 20 and 25 neurons for each of their hidden layers. There was a total of 5 runs in training for each technique. Subsequently, the results of each technique are averaged, the values of the precision for each combination of neurons were averaged, taking the highest value of the average and that had the least number of neurons, both in layer one and layer two was selected. And the best of each technique was used to test the data set.

The performance of the classifier for each fall risk assessment algorithm was evaluated using standard classifier performance measures, accuracy, sensitivity, specificity. The evaluation is carried out independently for the clinical data, the data of the pressure center, the data of the inertial sensors and finally the combined data. Expecting that the combination of these techniques has a higher performance than the techniques individually, when classifying the risk of falling of people with diabetic neuropathy.

3 Result

Performance of the Risk Assessment of Fall Based on Clinical Factors: The classification accuracies of the five runs were averaged and the highest values were taken to evaluate them with the test sets, yielding 34.7% for K-means, 84.0% for linear SVM,

80.0% for KNN Medium and 94.6% for ANN with Bayesian regularization (BR) and 5 neurons in the hidden layer 1 and 10 neurons in the hidden layer 2, of which the K-means is discarded because it is implemented as a point of comparison to evaluate the separability of the characteristics. Following this the test stage was performed with 20% of the data (n = 5), the test results for the best classifier of the SVM, KNN and ANN of the clinical factors was with neural networks with performance with an accuracy 55%.

Performance of the Fall Risk Assessment Based on CoP Data: The classification accuracies of the five runs were averaged and the highest values were taken, yielding 42.7% for K-means, 73.30% for SVM Gaussian Croase, 74.4% for KNN Medium and 88.0% for ANN with the scale of conjugate gradient (GC) and 15 neurons in hidden layer 1 and 20 neurons in hidden layer 2, of which K-means is discarded. the test stage was performed with 20% of the data (n = 5), the test results for CoP data delivered 50% accuracy for the SVM and KNN and 55% for the ANNs.

Fall Risk Assessment Based on Inertial Sensors: The classification accuracies of the five runs were averaged and the highest values were taken, yielding 41.8% for K-means, 90.9% for Cubic SVM, 92.7% for KNN Fine and 98.2% for ANN with Levenberg-Marguart (LM). and 15 neurons in the hidden layer 1 and 15 neurons in the hidden layer, from which the K-means is discarded. The test stage was performed with 20% of the data, the test results (n = 11) for iTUG data yields 90.9% accuracy for the SVM, KNN and ANN.

Fall Risk Assessment Based on Combined Factors: The classification accuracies of the five runs were averaged and the highest values were taken, yielding 36.7% for K-means, 95.0% for SVM Cubic, 96.4% for KNN Fine and 98.6% for ANN with the gradient scale conjugate (GC) and 15 neurons in the hidden layer 1 and 15 neurons in the hidden layer, from which the K-means was discarded and the test stage was performed with 20% of the data, the test results (n = 11) for complete data deliver 90.9% accuracy for the SVM, KNN and ANN.

4   Discussion

Four basic techniques of pattern recognition were evaluated, the first technique K-means was used exploratorily, looking to group the data according to their similarity according to the groups of interest, this technique obtained the lowest performance of the 4 evaluated, which shows that it is necessary to use a non-linear segmentation space to separate the characteristics so that the implementation of the other evaluated techniques becomes necessary and pertinent.

On the other hand, the results obtained using only the clinical risk factors were 50% for SVM and KNN and 55% accuracy with ANN, when classifying the participants in the test set; These results are similar to those reported by Greene et al. [14] with a classifier model based on the clinical risk factors used with a 68.84% pressure, taking into account that the number of study participants was 293. Reaffirming the found by Shirota et al. [23], where they conclude that in individuals with neurological disorders or with mobility problems, accurate and effective measurements of gait and balance are difficult to achieve using only clinical assessment tools.

The results of the second test, where the CoP oscillation was evaluated were: 50% for SVM and KNN and 55% with ANN, when classifying the participants; Although the results in training were 88%, in the tests they had a significant reduction as expected, this may be because the number of data available for the test (n = 4) is not enough. As shown by Saripalle et al. [24] with classification models that use CoP feature sets reporting a precision of 93.5% for the test set, since in this study it was obtained a good value of the precision in training, the performance of the Classification model could be increased using data from more participants.

The results of the third test, which was carried out using the iTUG, showed an accuracy of 90.9%, sensitivity of 80% and specificity of 100% for the three SVM, KNN and ANN techniques when classifying the classifiers. participants; the study conducted by Greene et al. [14] which implemented the iTUG test with a total of 292 participants, showed a pressure of 73.63%, sensitivity of 72.82 and specificity of 74.02%, additionally, a study carried out by Howcroft [22], where they obtain a pressure of 77.8%, sensitivity of 57.1 and specificity of 91.7%, with a total of 75 participants and performing clinical assessment methods such as single task and dual task, to assess risk of falls in older adults.

The combination of fall risk assessment data based on inertial sensors, CoP data and clinical fall risk factor data, led to a classification accuracy of 90.9%, which were equal for the iTUG test data This may be due to the fact that a greater number of data is needed in order to make a significant distinction between the iTUG methods and the totality of the data, since in the study carried out by Greene et al. [14] the pressure of the data was better at the time of making the classification with the clinical data set and iTUG, than separately.

5 Conclusions

Based on the results of this study, it may possible to evaluate the risk of falling in older adults with DPN by implementing a potential predictive system based on the clinical information of the AGS/BGS guidelines, and the oscillation of the CoP at rest and the TUG test with the use of inertial sensors. The assessment of the risk of falls in the group of elderly with DPN, by combining information from clinical factors, CoP and tug test, showed results with an accuracy of 90.9%, sensitivity of 80% and specificity of 100% in SVM methods, KNN and ANN, being a good result in the evaluation of this method compared to that reported by authors with Greene and Howcroft. Even so, it is not possible to define if there is a significant difference between the iTUG methods and the complete data, since the test set (n = 11) is not enough to differentiate them. But reviewing the training results could suggest the possibility of a better performance of the complete data compared with the tug test, which should be confirmed by the implementation of the study with a larger number of participants.

Acknowledgment. The authors acknowledge Pontificia Universidad Javeriana, BASPI-FootLab, Research on assessment of the COP in neuropathy diabetes project.

Conflict of Interest. The authors declare that they have no conflict of interest.

Attached

An example of the angular velocity signal of the three sensors, anteroposterior (AP), medio-lateral (ML) and manual synchronization.

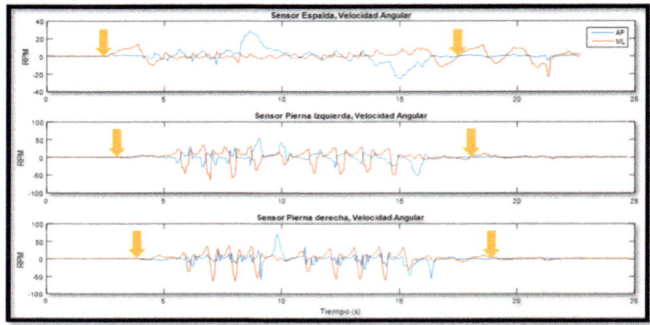

Test results with complete data. Accuracy for SVM (Gauss Coarse) KNN (Medium) ANN (GC)

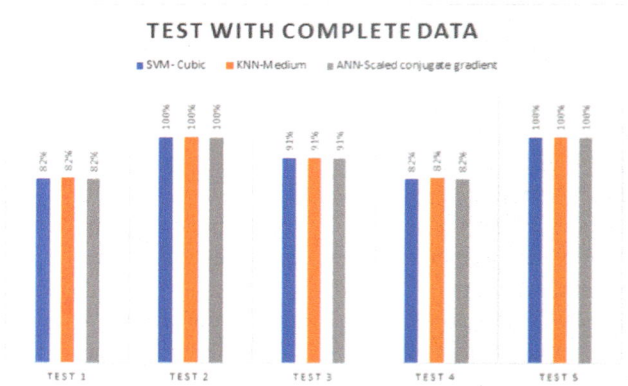

References

1. International Diabetes Federation: Diabetes atlas de la FID, 8. ed., repr. edn. International Diabetes Federation, Executive Office, Brussels (2017)
2. Young, M., Boulton, A., Macleod, A., et al.: A multicentre study of the prevalence of diabetic peripheral neuropathy in the United Kingdom hospital clinic population. Diabetologia **36**(2), 150–154 (1993). https://doi.org/10.1007/BF00400697
3. Shehab Mahmoud, A.E., Salah, E.M.: Ankle Dorsiflexors strength improves balance performance in elderly: a corelational study. Eur. J. Gener. Med. **11**(2), 60–65 (2014). https://doi.org/10.15197/sabad.1.11.40
4. Resnick, H.E., Stansberry, K.B., Harris, T.B., et al.: Diabetes, peripheral, neuropathy, and old age disability. Muscle Nerve **25**(1), 43–50 (2002)
5. Lin, S.I., Chen, Y.R., Liao, C.F., et al.: Association between sensorimotor function and forward reach in patients with diabetes. Gait Posture **32**, 581–585 (2010). https://doi.org/10.1016/j.gaitpost.2010.08.006
6. Brown, S.J., Handsaker, J.C., Bowling, F.L., et al.: Diabetic peripheral neuropath compromises balance during daily activities. Diabetes Care **38**(6), 1116 (2015)
7. Champagne, A., Prince, F., Bouffard, V., et al.: Balance, falls-related self-efficacy, and psychological factors amongst older women with chronic low back pain: a preliminary case-control study. Rehabil. Res. Pract., 1–8 (2012). https://doi.org/10.1155/2012/430374
8. Cavanagh, P.R., Derr, J.A., Ulbrecht, J.S., et al.: Problems with gait and posture in neuropathic patients with insulin-dependent diabetes mellitus. Diabet. Med. **9**(5), 469–474 (1992)
9. Pan, X., Bai, J.: Balance training in the intervention of fall risk in elderly with diabetic peripheral neuropathy: a review. Int. J. Nurs. Sci. **1**(4), 441–445 (2014). https://doi.org/10.1016/j.ijnss.2014.09.001
10. Duncan, P.W., Weiner, D.K., Chandler, J., et al.: Functional reach: a new clinical measure of balance. J. Gerontol. **6**, 192 (1990)
11. Vaz, M.M., Costa, G.C., Reis, J.G., et al.: Original article: Postural Control and Functional Strength in Patients with Type 2 Diabetes Mellitus with and Without Peripheral Neuropathy. Arch. Phys. Med. Rehabil. **94**, 2465–2470 (2013). https://doi.org/10.1016/j.apmr.2013.06.007
12. Diane, P., Sandra, R.: The timed "Up & Go": a test of basic functional mobility for frail elderly persons. J. Am. Geriatr. Soc. **39**(2), 142–148 (1991). https://doi.org/10.1111/j.1532-5415.1991.tb01616.x
13. Lorena Cerda, A.: Manejo del trastorno de marcha del adulto mayor. Rev. Méd. Clín. Las Condes **25**(2), 265–275 (2014). https://doi.org/10.1016/S0716-8640(14)70037-9
14. Greene, B.R., Redmond, S.J., Caulfield, B.: Fall risk assessment through automatic combination of clinical fall risk factors and body-worn sensor data. IEEE J. Biomed. Health Informat., 1 (2016). https://doi.org/10.1109/jbhi.2016.2539098
15. Montesinos, L., Castaldo, R., Pecchia, L.: Wearable inertial sensors for fall risk assessment and prediction in older adults: a systematic review and meta-analysis. TNSRE **PP**(99), 1. https://doi.org/10.1109/TNSRE.2017.2771383
16. Howcroft, J., Kofman, J., Lemaire, E.D.: Review of fall risk assessment in geriatric populations using inertial sensors. J. Neuroeng. Rehabil. **10**(1), 91 (2013). https://doi.org/10.1186/1743-0003-10-91
17. Greene, B.R., Doheny, E.P., Walsh, C., et al.: Evaluation of falls risk in community-dwelling older adults using body-worn sensors (2012). https://doi.org/10.1159/000337259

18. Cano, D.C.T.: Evaluation of the anteroposterior center of pressure in peripheral diabetic neuropathy. Vision Electronica (2017)
19. American Geriatrics Society, Geriatrics Society, American Academy of Orthopaedic Surgeons Panel on Falls Prevention: Guideline for the prevention of falls in older persons. J. Am. Geriatr. Soc. **49**(5), 664–672 (2001). https://doi.org/10.1046/j.1532-5415.2001. 49115.x
20. de Souza Fortaleza, A.C., Chagas, E.F., Ferreira, D.M.A., et al.: Postural control and functional balance in individuals with diabetic peripheral neuropathy. Rev. Bras. Cineantropometria Desempenho Hum. **15**(3), 305–314 (2013)
21. Jernigan, S.D., Pohl, P.S., Mahnken, J.D., et al.: Diagnostic accuracy of fall risk assessment tools in people with diabetic peripheral neuropathy. Phys. Ther. **92**(11), 1461–1470 (2012). https://doi.org/10.2522/ptj.20120070
22. Howcroft, J., Kofman, J., Lemaire, E.D.: Prospective fall-risk prediction models for older adults based on wearable sensors. TNSRE **25**(10), 1812–1820 (2017). https://doi.org/10. 1109/TNSRE.2017.268710
23. Shirota, C., Van Asseldonk, E., Matjačić, Z., et al.: Robot-supported assessment of balance in standing and walking. J. Neuro Eng. Rehabil. **14**(1), 80 (2017)
24. Saripalle, S.K., Vemulapalli, S., King, G.W., et al.: Machine learning methods for credibility assessment of interviewees based on posturographic data. In: Anonymous, United States, p. 6708. IEEE, August 2015
25. Godfrey, A., Lara, J., Del Din, S., et al.: iCap: instrumented assessment of physical capability. Maturitas **82**(1), 116–122 (2015). https://doi.org/10.1016/j.maturitas.2015.04.003

COP Analysis in Type 2 Diabetics with Peripheral Diabetic Neuropathy

(Open Data May Contribute with Prognosis and Intervention in Early Stages to Reduce a Risk of Falling)

Daissy Carola Toloza, Martha Zequera$^{(\boxtimes)}$, and Gustavo Castro

Electronics Department, School of Engineering,
BASPI/FootLab (Bioengineering, Signal Analysis and Image Processing
Research Group), Pontificia Universidad Javeriana, Bogotá, Colombia
{dtoloza, mzequera, dtoloza}@javeriana.edu.co

Abstract. Peripheral Diabetic Neuropathy (PDN) produces nerve damage in lower limps and foot, and therefore, a decrease of information by the proprioceptive system to maintain postural stability denoting greater body sway. Due to postural stability pilot study was develop by using the anteroposterior center of pressure in 60 participants from Bogota, Colombia: 30 diabetics (19 female and 11 male) with PDN and 30 healthy controls (19 female and 11 male) matched by gender, age, height and weight. Wilcoxon test ($p < 0.05$) was used to find significant differences in linear parameters such as: excursion, velocity, Root mean square RMS, maximum and minimum amplitude. Plantar sensitivity was evaluated with the monofilament test of Semmes-Weinstein 5.0. All Diabetic Peripheral Patient DPN participants showed higher values in all parameters with maximum in excursion and RMS values and all DPN presented at least one insensitive zone at the plantar level. In static position DPN participants showed higher body sway and tends to stay on the anterior axis to maintain postural stability. This pilot study stablished what other previous literature have report that DPN disease directly impacts in postural stability becoming an important risk factor for falls.

Keywords: Peripheral Diabetic Neuropathy · Center of pressure ·
Postural stability · Diabetes · Pedar System

1 Introduction

Peripheral Diabetic Neuropathy (PDN) is the most common complication of diabetes that may be present in as many as 70% with diabetes type 2 and is leading the cause of foot amputation. PDN is nerve damage caused by chronically high blood sugar and diabetes [1].

DPN affects the proximal and distal peripheral sensory and motor nerves. Numbness, tingling, and pain are the most common symptoms. Steadily, DPN affect distal muscle strength and deteriorates normal walking function [2]. Alteration of the peripheral nerve due to DPN is the main contributor to postural instability and high gait

© Springer Nature Switzerland AG 2020
K.-P. Lin et al. (Eds.): ICBHI 2019, IFMBE Proceedings 74, pp. 405–412, 2020.
https://doi.org/10.1007/978-3-030-30636-6_55

variability that may increase the likelihood of fall incidence [3, 4]. Therefore, the deterioration of the balance, decreased ability to optimally control stability, which is essential for mobility and reducing the independence of these people.

That postural instability had been analyzed by center of pressure (COP), which is the result of force vertical ground reaction forces and product torques ankle to keep the COP on stability limits [5]. The result of these torques causes a continuous oscillation of the body around the vertical position, and it is achieved through feedback mechanisms detected by visual, vestibular and proprioceptive sensory systems [6].

The COP trajectory in anterior-posterior (AP) direction reflects ankle plantar/dorsiflexion is used because represents the neuromuscular control of the ankle during postural control and could analyzed the postural stability. The data obtained from COP during static standing position have been used to calculate different parameters to analyze body stability behavior. In this sense, the research proposes the analysis using the COP in a pilot population with Diabetes Type 2 and PDN in the Bogotá, Colombia.

2   Methods

2.1   Participants (DPN and Healthy Control)

Sixty individuals participated in this study (age 56.17 ± 9.95 yrs). Individuals were distributed into 2 groups: PDN (PDN; n = 30), and Healthy control matched by gender, age, height and weight (C; n = 30). Both groups have each 19 women and 11 men, in total 38 women and 22 men (Table 1).

Table 1. Characteristics of study subjects

	PDN group	C group
Gender (women/men)	19/11	19/11
Age (years $\pm$ SD)	55.67 ± 9.58	56.67 ± 10.33
Weight (kg)	67.93 ± 16.32	69.28 ± 11.25
Height (m)	1.62 ± 1.1	1.61 ± 1.0
Foot sensibility, 30		
Good	4/30	30/30
Reduced	23/30	0/30
Abscence	3/30	0/30
Diabetes time (years)	11.27 ± 7.79	–
DPN presence	30/30	0/30

Participants have been provided informed consent prior to inclusion to the pilot study after the Pontifical Xaverian University – Ethic Committee gave the approval.

Exclusion criteria included: foot ulcerations, biomechanics alterations and peripheral neuropathy produced by a cause other than diabetes. Inclusion criteria included: diagnosis of diabetes type 2 greater than 4 years, older than 39 years old and be able to stand without any help for more than two minutes.

2.2   Experimental Design

Participants attended two laboratory testing sessions. In the first session, clinical screening was performed. This included PDN evaluation: Semmes-Weinstein 5.07 monofilament and 128 Hz vibration tests. These elements were combined to cause a total neuropathy score. The protocols used was the International Working Group on the Diabetic Foot. This evaluation was made by neurologist specialist in diabetes (Fig. 1).

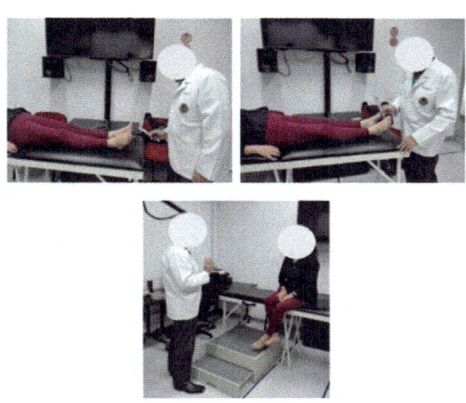

Fig. 1. Clinical assessment by medical specialist in neurology

During session two, COP-AP was performed using Pedar System - Novel GMbH (Table 2). The Pedar is an accurate and reliable plantar pressure distribution measuring system for monitoring local loads between the foot and the shoe. The pedar® offers the ultimate versatility with its multiple standard features and operating modes (Fig. 2).

Table 2. Pedar Technical Requirements

Characteristics	
Number of sensors	99
Pressure range (kPa)	15–600
Hysteresis (%)	7
Resolution (kPa)	2.5
Sensor	Capacitive
Sampling frequency (Hz)	50

The protocol used was The Romberg Test. The Romberg test was performed on a rigid and soft surface (foam) in five different conditions in order to eliminate either alter the proprioceptive, vestibular and visual systems involved in the maintenance of postural stability of the body. Each individual completed six 60 s trials for the following conditions:

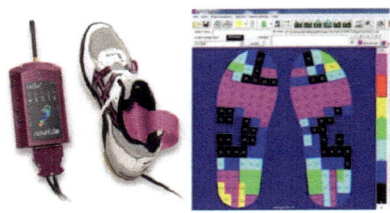

Fig. 2. Pedar system, (http://novel.de/novelcontent/pedar)

1. Eyes open, firm surface, head on Straight.
2. Eyes open, firm surface, head back.
3. Eyes closed, firm surface, head on Straight.
4. Eyes open, foam surface.
5. Eyes closed, foam surface.

The foam surface was 15-cm-thick and of medium density. COP data were filtered using a second-order low-pass Butterworth filter (Cutoff frequency 50 Hz). COP analyses were performed using Matlab (Mathworks R14).

The dependent measures determined for COP-AP (Fig. 3) motion included; excursion, mean velocity, range and RMS value.

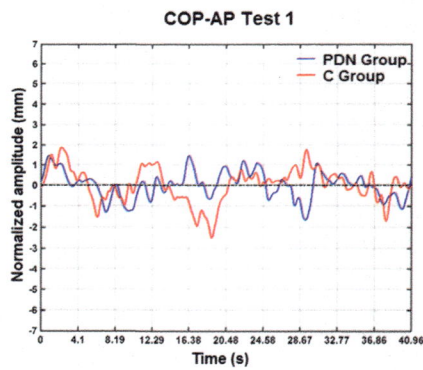

Fig. 3. COP-AP test. Motion parameter (excursion, mean velocity, range and RMS value)

2.3 Statistical Analysis

All analyses were performed in STATA (Version 11, STATA Corporation, College Station, TX, USA), and p-values $p < 0.05$ were considered statistically significant. All analyses were performed using repeated measures, Wilcoxon text.

3   Results

ll parameters evaluated had statistical differences (excursion, mean velocity, range and RMS value) with higher values in DPN Group with respect to Control Group (Fig. 4). The greatest differences were found in the parameters of the Excursion.

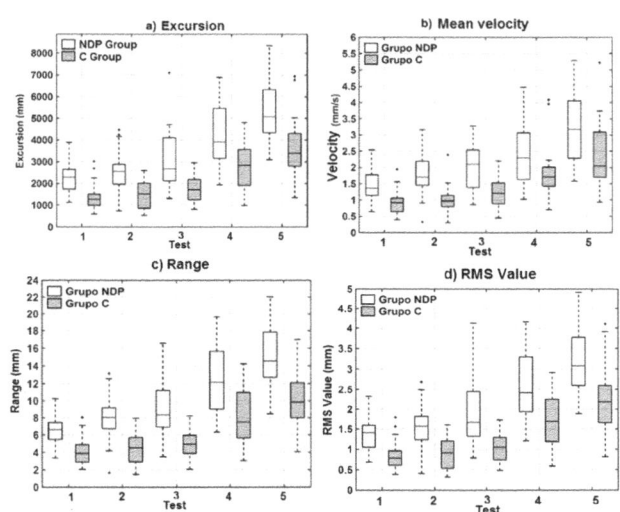

Fig. 4. COP-AP parameters (The COP trajectory in anterior-posterior (AP) direction)

Then, it was evaluated independently the five test conditions to found statistically significant differences by each group. Friedman Test was used ($p < 0.05$) and a post hoc analysis was performed in pairs with the Wilcoxon Test with a value of 0.0125 to control the error global. For both groups founded $p < 0.0001$, this indicates that there are differences between the five tests performed, this is the reason to proceeded and perform the post-hoc analysis in pairs with the Wilcoxon Test for each group independently:

1. Test 1 vs Test 2: founded statistically significant differences in range and mean velocity when altered vestibular system.
2. Test 1 vs Test 3: founded statistically significant differences in all parameters when eliminated visual system.
3. Test 2 vs Test 3: do not founded statistically significant differences in all parameters when visual system eliminated and altered vestibular system.
4. Test 4 vs Test 5: founded statistically significant differences in all parameters when eliminated visual system and altered proprioceptive system.

4 Discussion

It is well known that COP signal in diabetes type 2 with or without DPN, in comparison with control group have a greater range in signal displacement, sway, acceleration, some other parameters, and this increase occurs without import the tests conditions. The same results were obtained in the present investigation, the DPN Group in all the calculated parameters of the COP-AP signal. Situations that were also reported by Dixit et al. [7], Fahmy et al. [8], de Souza Fortaleza et al. [9] and Palma et al. [10].

This may indicate that this group has a less stable posture body in bipedal position either when the participant has all the sensory systems active (visual, vestibular and proprioceptive) or when some are altered (vestibular and proprioceptive) either eliminated (visual).

Horak et al. [11] found that in the DPN, COP displacement increase by 52% with close eyes and velocity by 33% and in this research, DPN Group showed an increase in the COP-AP excursion was 39% and velocity 47%.

Therefore, it could be suggested that this increase in displacement in all COP-AP parameters is due to affectation of somatosensory system, tactile sensation and the motor output produced by the DPN, which affects the reaction time and muscle strength that contribute to the deterioration of postural control [11]. This indicates that the group of people with DT2 and DPN to maintain postural stability in the bipedal position should displace the COP-AP in greater proportion with respect to the control group.

Once it was identified that the participants of the pilot population of the DPN Group presented a greater oscillation with respect to matched Group C, a pairwise analysis of tests (exactly 4) is carried out in the DPN and C Group in order to observe the changes in COP-AP parameters when the sensory systems are active in contrast when are eliminated either altered.

Test 1 vs Test 2, could indicate that vestibular system altered impact less in postural stability than visual system, obtaining higher values in velocity and range. Vestibular system alteration generates a greater displacement in the posterior direction because the person forces its body to sway looking for balance, Salsabili et al. [12] indicated the same result.

Test 1 vs Test 3 suggested that DPN Group used in major proportion visual system than proprioceptive and vestibular as suggested by Turcot et al. [13] and Bonnet et al. [14].

Test 2 vs Test 3, DPN group showed major usability of proprioceptive system when visual and vestibular system were altered.

Test 4 vs Test 5, showed statistically significant differences in all parameters, that confirm the importance of visual system in DPN group, since without this system COP-AP displacement increase significantly, either on a rigid surface or foam.

These results suggest that proprioceptive system alteration not could be compensated by visual and vestibular systems in DPN group evaluating this pilot study.

5 Conclusions

The results obtained from pilot study indicates that the population of DT2 with NDP reported a greater amplitude in the displacement of the COP-AP in bipedal position in all test conditions implemented, which suggests that the study group must produce large displacements of the body to maintain the position bipedal, situation that makes that displacement is near the limits of stability, presenting a risk of falling. It is necessary a greater study with a larger population to conclude the result.

Likewise, the tests reported that the COP-AP variable is significantly affected with the alteration and/or elimination of the proprioceptive and visual systems.

The PDN present in the study group of Diabetes Type 2 is one of the main causes of the alteration of the postural oscillation that was reflected in the variations of the COP-AP. The deterioration of the balance, decreased ability to optimally control stability, which is essential for mobility and reducing the independence of these people. The importance to the access to Open Data in this field may improve diagnosis and intervention in early stages to reduce a risk of falling.

Conflict of Interest

No potential conflicts of interest relevant to this article were reported. Acknowledgment to Electronic Department of Pontificia Universidad Javeriana and FootLab/BASPI research group.

References

1. Martin, C.L., Albers, J.W., Pop-Busui, R.: Neuropathy and related findings in the diabetes control and complications trial/epidemiology of diabetes interventions and complications study. Diabetes Care **37**, 31–38 (2014)
2. Rani, P.K., Raman, R., Rachapalli, S.R., Pal, S.S., Kulothungan, V., Sharma, T.: Prevalence and risk factors for severity of diabetic neuropathy in type 2 diabetes mellitus. Indian J. Med. Sci. **64**(2), 51–57 (2010)
3. El Bardawil, M.M., Abd El Hamid, M.M., et al.: Postural control and central motor pathway involvement in type 2 diabetes mellitus: dynamic posturographic and electrophysiologic studies. Alexandria J. Med. **49**(4), 299–307 (2013). https://doi.org/10.1016/j.ajme.2013.03. 009
4. Dingwell, J.B., Cavanagh, P.R.: Increased variability of continuous overground walking in neuropathic patients is only indirectly related to sensory loss. Gait Posture **14**(1), 1–10 (2001)
5. Ruhe, A., Fejer, R., Walker, B.: The test-retest reliability of centre of pressure measures in bipedal static task conditions - a systematic review of the literature. Gait Posture **32**(4), 436–445 (2010)
6. Peterka, R.J.: Sensorimotor integration in human postural control. J. Neurophysiol. **88**(3), 1097–1118 (2002)
7. Dixit, S., Maiya, A., Shastry, B., Guddattu, V.: Analysis of postural control during quiet standing in a population with diabetic peripheral neuropathy undergoing moderate intensity aerobic exercise training. Am. J. Phys. Med. Rehabil. **95**(7), 1 (2016)
8. Fahmy, I., Ramzy, G., Salem, N., et al.: Balance disturbance in patients with diabetic sensory polyneuropathy. Egypt. J. Neurol. Psychiatry Neurosurg. **51**(1), 21–29 (2014)

9. de Souza, F.A., et al.: Postural control and functional balance in individuals with diabetic peripheral neuropathy. Braz. J. Kinanthropometry Hum. Perform. **15**(3), 305–314 (2013)

10. Palma, F., et al.: Static balance in patients presenting diabetes mellitus type 2 with and without diabetic polyneuropathy. Arq. Bras. Endocrinol. Metabol. **57**(9), 722–726 (2013)

11. Horak, F., Dickstein, R., Peterka, R.: Diabetic neuropathy and surface sway-referencing disrupt somatosensory information for postural stability in stance. Somatosens. Mot. Res. **19** (4), 316–326 (2002)

12. Salsabili, H., Bahrpeyma, F., et al.: Spectral characteristics of postural sway in diabetic neuropathy patients participating in balance training. J. Diabetes Metab. Disord. **12**, 29 (2013)

13. Turcot, K., Allet, L., Golay, A., et al.: Investigation of standing balance in diabetic patients with and without peripheral neuropathy using accelerometers. Clin. Biomech. **24**(9), 716–721 (2009)

14. Bonnet, C., Ray, C.: Peripheral neuropathy may not be the only fundamental reason explaining increased sway in diabetic individuals. Clin. Biomech. **26**(7), 699–706 (2011)

Comparison of Human Fall Acceleration Signals Among Different Datasets

Goran Šeketa[✉], Lovro Pavlaković, Sara Žulj, Dominik Džaja,
Igor Lacković, and Ratko Magjarević

Faculty of Electrical Engineering and Computing,
University of Zagreb, Unska 3, Zagreb, Croatia
goran.seketa@fer.hr

Abstract. Falls can have a major impact on physical and psychological health on elderly people who experience them. To reduce the negative consequences of a fall event, automatic fall detection systems are being developed to correctly identify when a person falls and alert the caregivers to provide assistance on time. Performance of fall detection algorithms is tested with datasets containing measurements of falls and regular activities of daily living. In this work we acquired fall signals with accelerometer sensors and compared them with digitized fall signal records from 6 different datasets. Additionally, three threshold-based algorithms for fall detection were implemented and their performance was tested with the analyzed datasets. The results suggest that a heterogeneity among the fall data in distinct datasets exist and that it affects the performance measures of tested datasets.

Keywords: Fall detection · Datasets · Accelerometer

1 Introduction

As people get older, their bodies experience various physical changes that make them more fragile and more endangered to experience harmful falls. Statistically, one third of the elderly people fall at least once per year [1].

Besides of physical injuries afflicted by the impact, subsequent long lie period after a fall also have a detrimental effect on physical and psychological health of the faller. To tackle the problem of long lies after a fall, various automatic fall detection systems have been developed. Their goal is to detect when a person experiences a fall and to inform caregivers so they could provide help on time.

Different technologies for fall detection have been investigated including use of vision based, ambient and inertial sensors [2] Wearable systems with inertial sensors (accelerometers, gyroscopes) are generally small in size, lightweight and have small power consumption that makes them unobtrusive and suitable for prolonged use [3]. In the current study, we focus on such acceleration-based fall detection systems.

In fall detection systems, algorithms are used to process the information captured by sensors and to decide whether a fall event happened or not. The performance of these algorithms is mainly tested with data recorded from simulated falls and activities of daily living (ADL) performed by young people. There are still very few available

© Springer Nature Switzerland AG 2020
K.-P. Lin et al. (Eds.): ICBHI 2019, IFMBE Proceedings 74, pp. 413–419, 2020.
https://doi.org/10.1007/978-3-030-30636-6_56

data from falls of elderly people captured during real life situation with acceleration sensors. The FARSEEING consortium [4] have made one of the first attempts to collect such data and currently only a limited dataset of 22 signals is available for interested researchers. Until more data is available from real life falls in the elderly population, researchers use data from simulated falls and ADL.

When proposing a new fall detection algorithm, researchers test its performance on a single dataset, either created by simulating falls in their lab or by using one of the open datasets [5]. These datasets of fall signals created by different research groups and in different conditions should contain data with mutually similar features to enable unbiased comparison of various algorithm performances.

The goal of this work is to compare features of fall signals in various datasets and to explore whether fall detection algorithms performance measures are affected by using distinct datasets.

2   Methods

2.1   Public Datasets

Three publicly available datasets with acceleration measurements of falls and ADL were used in this study: TST Fall Detection [6], UmaFall [7] and UR Fall Detection [8]. These datasets contain measurements from a waist mounted sensor worn by young healthy subjects performing simulated falls and ADL in controlled conditions. They were created by different research groups using different experimental protocols.

TST Fall Detection dataset (TST) was developed by the TST Group from Universita Politecnica delle Marche. The dataset contains data from 11 subjects (age range: 22–39). Participants performed 4 types of ADL and 4 types of simulated falls, which were repeated three times by each subject. A Shimmer sensor (Shimmer Sensing, Ireland) was used to collect the data at 100 Hz and with the accelerometer range set at least to ±4 g.

UmaFall dataset (UMA) was created by Dpto. Tecnologia Electronica from University of Malaga. Seventeen healthy subjects (age: 14–55) were recruited for the study. Every subject executed three trials of 7 predetermined ADLs and 3 types of falls (excluded subjects older than 50 years). Data were recorded with a TI SensorTag unit (Texas Instruments, USA) at 20 Hz and with the accelerometer range set at ±16 g.

UR Fall Detection dataset (UR) was made by Interdisciplinary Centre for Computational Modelling, University of Rzeszow. An x-IMU sensor was worn by 5 subjects and in total 30 simulated falls and 40 ADLs were recorded. Each subject performed at least three types of falls. Data were recorded at 256 Hz and the accelerometer range was set to ±8 g.

A summary of the public datasets information can be found in Table 1.

2.2   FER Datasets

Three datasets acquired in our previous studies were used along with the public datasets: FER1, FER2 and FER3 [9]. These datasets were acquired in the same

Table 1. Overview of dataset characteristics

	Number of subjects	Sensor device	Accelerometer range	Number of ADL/Falls
FER1	16	Shimmer	±8 g	680/186
FER2	12	Shimmer	±16 g	264/96
FER3	12	MUHA	±16 g	264/96
TST	11	Shimmer	±4 g	132/132
UMA	17	Sensor Tag	±16 g	322/209
UR	6	x-IMU	±8 g	40/30

experimental setting and with the same protocol: participants performed 3 types of falls on a 2 cm thick tatami mat (forward fall, sideways fall, backward fall) and 12 ADLs: walking, fast walking, running, fast running, jumping, high jumping, sitting, standing up, lying down, getting up from lying position, walking down the stairs and walking up the stairs. The experiment setting is shown in Fig. 1.

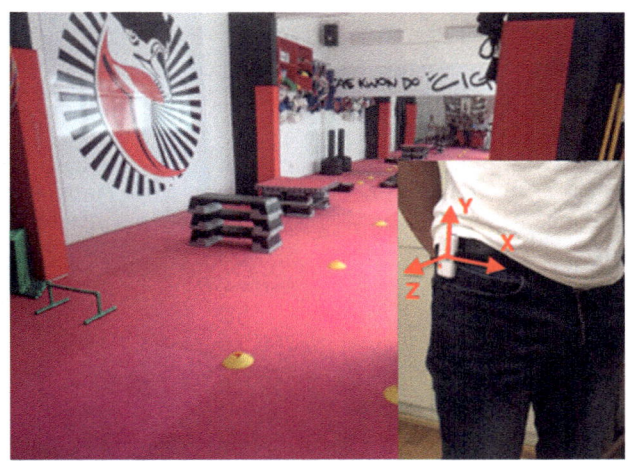

Fig. 1. Experimental setup for FER datasets. Subjects wore sensors attached to their waist and performed a set of ADL and simulated falls on a tatami mat.

For the FER1 dataset, 16 subjects were recruited (age range 15–44). A Shimmer sensor attached to the waist of the subjects was used to acquire the acceleration signals during ADLs and simulated falls. Data was recorded with a frequency of 204.8 Hz and the accelerometer range was set to ±8 g.

For the FER2 and FER3 datasets, 12 volunteers (age range: 21–28) agreed to perform the experimental protocol. Two sensors attached to the waist of the participants were used to simultaneously measure the accelerations during the experiments. For the FER2 dataset, a Shimmer sensor (sampling frequency 204.8 Hz, accelerometer range ±16 g) was used and for the FER3 dataset, a MUHA sensor [10] (sampling frequency 50 Hz, accelerometer range ±16 g) was used.

2.3   Fall Features

From the acceleration measurements of fall events contained in the datasets, features were calculated that are used in two threshold-based fall detection algorithms proposed by Kangas et al. [11]:

- *Kangas impact (KI)* – highest value of the total sum vector (SV_{tot}) in a fall signal calculated from median filtered accelerations;
- *Kangas velocity (KV)* – integrated area of SV_{tot} from the beginning of the fall until the impact;
- *Kangas posture (KP)* – average of low pass filtered vertical acceleration in a 04 s time frame chosen 2 s after the impact.

SV_{tot} is thereby calculated from the following expression:

$$SV_{tot}(n) = \sqrt{a_x(n)^2 + a_y(n)^2 + a_z(n)^2} \tag{1}$$

and for *theta* the following equation is used:

$$theta(n) = \operatorname{atan2}\left(\frac{\sqrt{a_x(n)^2 + a_z(n)^2}}{a_y(n)}\right) \tag{2}$$

where $a_x(n)$, $a_y(n)$, $a_z(n)$ represent x, y and z acceleration components of the n-th measurement sample. A four-quadrant inverse tangent function atan2 was used to calculate the *theta* value.

2.4   Algorithms

From the Kangas et al. [11], the following fall detection algorithms were implemented: KangasIP, KangasSIP and KangasSVIP.

KangasIP algorithm detects a fall if an impact is detected followed by a lying posture. Impact is registered if the KI value is larger than 2 g and lying posture is assumed for KP values lower than 0.5 g.

KangasSIP algorithm first detects the start of the fall when the SV_{tot} value drops under 0.6 g. If this is followed by an impact in 1 s time frame and a lying posture (as in KangasIP), then a fall is detected.

KangasSVIP algorithm works similar to the KangasSIP, but adds the detection of velocity after the start of the fall. For a fall to be detected, the KV feature value has to exceed 0.7 g (along with other conditions described in Kangas SIP).

Implemented algorithms were tested with the ADL and fall measurements from the datasets and contingency tables were created containing the number of true positive (TP; fall happens, device detects), true negative (TN; no fall, not detected), false positive (FP; no fall, device detects) and false negative events (FN; no fall, device detects). Based on these results, algorithm's performance metrics were calculated as:

$$sensitivity = \frac{TP}{(TP + FN)} \tag{3}$$

$$specificity = \frac{TN}{(TN + FP)} \tag{4}$$

$$geometric\_mean = \sqrt{sensitivity * specificity} \tag{5}$$

3   Results

For the fall measurements contained in the analysed datasets, fall features were calculated. Table 2 contains median values and standard deviations of the feature values. For the feature KV, boxplot with the corresponding threshold value used for it in the corresponding algorithm is shown in Fig. 2. Finally, performance of the implemented algorithms was tested on all datasets and the resulting sensitivities and specificities are shown in Table 3.

Table 2. Median values and standard deviations of features calculated on fall measurements from different datasets

	Kangas impact (g)	Kangas velocity (m/s)	Kangas posture (g)
FER1	4.02/1.40	1.19/0.47	0.44/2.28
FER2	3.60/1.33	1.50/0.58	0.70/2.56
FER3	2.40/0.80	0.49/0.19	2.58/3.31
TST	3.20/0.62	3.39/1.46	2.84/2.38
UMA	4.38/1.71	1.27/0.57	0.62/2.39
UR	4.84/1.90	1.06/0.88	−0.51/3.15

Table 3. Performance of fall detection algorithms tested on different datasets expressed as sensitivity (sn), specificity (sp) and geometric_mean (gm)

	KangasIP			KangasSIP			KangasSVIP		
	sn	sp	gm	sn	sp	gm	sn	sp	gm
FER1	97%	95%	96%	84%	98%	90%	71%	99%	84%
FER2	97%	99%	98%	89%	99%	94%	76%	99%	87%
FER3	57%	100%	76%	32%	100%	57%	8%	100%	29%
TST	80%	98%	89%	63%	98%	79%	64%	98%	79%
UMA	94%	99%	96%	89%	100%	94%	76%	100%	87%
UR	93%	75%	84%	83%	88%	85%	47%	88%	64%
Mean	**86%**	**94%**	**90%**	**73%**	**97%**	**83%**	**57%**	**97%**	**72%**

4   Discussion

Overall the best performance in terms of a balance between *sensitivity* and *specificity* had the KangasIP algorithm with a *geometric_mean* of 90%. Of all the algorithms, KangasIP uses the least number of features to detect a fall. Adding more features to the detection algorithm as in KangasSIP and KangasSVIP raises the number of correctly discarded events (thus specificity) but makes the algorithms less sensitive to detecting real fall events thus lowering the overall algorithm performance.

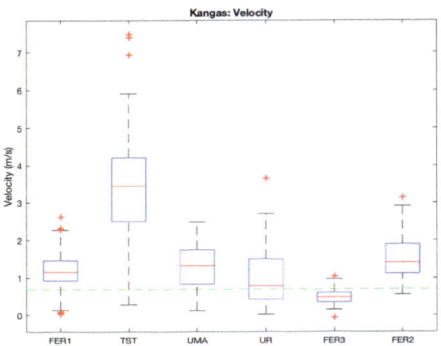

Fig. 2. Boxplot of KV feature values for falls in different datasets. Maximum whisker length is specified as 1 times the interquartile range. Horizontal line (green) represents the threshold value used on the feature

The obtained values of fall features suggest that a heterogeneity exists between the measurement contained in distinct datasets. This heterogeneity makes it difficult to set fixed threshold values in algorithms so that they could perform well on different datasets. An algorithm with threshold values set according to one dataset may not perform well on another one. The evaluation of the three selected algorithms with thresholds set to the original reported values showed that for the most datasets the values where not optimal and resulted in either poor sensitivity (not detecting all falls) or poor specificity (not being able to distinguish falls from ADL). This leads to the conclusion that more standardisation is needed in the recording process of fall detection datasets which would in turn enable a more objective performance evaluation of fall detection algorithms.

5   Conclusion

In this work six distinct fall datasets were used. Fall features were calculated and mutually compared. Three fall detection algorithms were evaluated with data from different datasets. Results showed that a heterogeneity exists among datasets and suggest that more standardisation is needed in the dataset recording process.

6   Conflict of Interest

The authors declare that they have no conflict of interest.

Acknowledgment. A part of this research is based on the Memorandum of Understanding between the University of Zagreb Faculty of Electrical Engineering and Computing, Zagreb, Croatia, and the Chung Yuan Christian University, Taoyuan City, Taiwan.

References

1. Rajagopalan, R., et al.: Fall prediction and prevention systems: recent trends, challenges, and future research directions. Sensors (2017)
2. Pannurat, N., et al.: Automatic fall monitoring: a review. Sensors (2014)
3. Patel, S., et al.: A review of wearable sensors and systems with application in rehabilitation. J. Neuroeng. Rehabil. **9**(1), 21–38 (2012)
4. Klenk, J., et al.: The FARSEEING real-world fall repository: a large-scale collaborative database to collect and share sensor signals from real-world falls. Eur. Rev. Aging Phys. Act. **13**, 8 (2016)
5. Casilari, E., et al.: Analysis of public datasets for wearable fall detection systems. Sensors (2017)
6. Gasparrini, S., et al.: Proposal and experimental evaluation of fall detection solution based on wearable and depth data fusion. In: ICT Innovations 2015. Springer (2016)
7. Casilari, E., et al.: Analysis of a smartphone-based architecture with multiple mobility sensors for fall detection. PLoS ONE **11**(12) (2016)
8. Kwolek, B., et al.: Human fall detection on embedded platform using depth maps and wireless accelerometer. Comput. Methods Programs Biomed. **117**(3), 489–501 (2014)
9. Seketa, G., et al.: Optimal threshold selection for acceleration-based fall detection. ICBHI Thessaloniki, 2017
10. Seketa, G., et al.: Real-time evaluation of repetitive physical exercise using orientation estimation from inertial and magnetic sensors. In: ENCY 2015, Budapest, May 2015
11. Kangas, M., et al.: Determination of simple thresholds for accelerometry-based parameters for fall detection. In: Proceedings of the 29th Annual International Conference of the IEEE EMBS, Lyon, 23–26 August 2007

Handling Missing Data in CGM Records

Sara Zulj[1]([✉]), Paulo Carvalho[2], Rogerio Ribeiro[3],
and Ratko Magjarevic[1]

[1] Faculty of Electrical Engineering and Computing, University of Zagreb,
Unska 3, Zagreb, Croatia
sara.zulj@fer.hr
[2] Departamento de Engenharia Informática, Universidade de Coimbra,
Coimbra, Portugal
[3] Associação Protectora dos Diabéticos de Portugal, Lisbon, Portugal

Abstract. Continuous glucose monitor (CGM) is a wearable body sensor device that automatically measures glucose at regular intervals. CGM records can be used to analyze data after the collection or for predicting certain trends in the records in real-time. Nevertheless, missing values are common in CGM records. In this paper we discuss possible methods to replace the missing values in short-length gaps, in both real-time and after the collection use.

Keywords: Missing data · Data reconstruction · CGM ·
Continuous glucose monitoring

1 Introduction

Continuous glucose monitor (CGM) is a wearable body sensor device that automatically and repeatedly measures glucose at regular intervals (ranging from every 5 to 15 min). The device usually consists of three components: a wearable sensor, a transmitter that wirelessly sends readings and a receiver nearby that displays such readings to the user [1].

Unlike regular glucose meters for self-monitoring of blood glucose (SMBG), which measure glucose from blood plasma, CMGs measure glucose in interstitial fluid. Algorithms are used to extrapolate blood glucose levels from interstitial fluid glucose [2]. Glucose in interstitial fluid can lag 5–15 min behind the blood glucose, especially when the blood glucose levels are changing rapidly [1]. There is research suggesting that this delay is a patient dependent delay [3]. Nevertheless, current CGM systems show similar overall accuracy as measured by mean absolute relative difference between CGM and laboratory reference values [4].

There is also reported efficacy of CGM use in individuals with type 1 diabetes and insulin-treated type 2 diabetes regardless of the insulin delivery method used. Some benefits include reductions in A1C and glycemic variability, increased time in target glycemic range, decreased time in hypoglycemic range, fewer hypoglycemic events in people with well-managed and poorly managed diabetes and, importantly, among those with problematic hypoglycemia [4].

© Springer Nature Switzerland AG 2020
K.-P. Lin et al. (Eds.): ICBHI 2019, IFMBE Proceedings 74, pp. 420–427, 2020.
https://doi.org/10.1007/978-3-030-30636-6_57

Proven benefits for the patient and better diagnostic dataset for the physicians contribute to increase of use of the CGMs as a daily management tool.

Danne et al. [5] report one of the key findings in visualization, analysis, and documentation of key CGM metrics: to generate a report that enables optimal analysis and decision-making, the minimum of 14 consecutive days of data with approximately 70% of possible CGM readings over those 14 days should be available. Standard reporting and visualization of CGM data are found to be important.

CGM devices and downloaded CGM records lose some of the data during monitoring, resulting in CGM records with some missing segments in the data.

In this paper we present some approaches to identify and replace missing segments in CGM records with two purposes: real-time analysis of patient's glucose trends at the moment of monitoring disruption, and post-analysis of the records after complete monitoring.

2 Materials

The data used in this experiment is obtained from the APDP (Associação Protectora dos Diabéticos de Portugal). The data was recorded using CGM iPro2 Recorder (Medtronic, Medtronic, Northridge, CA, USA) with one sample each 5 min. Dataset comprises of 67 continuous glucose monitoring records acquired from 35 different patients each during approximately 1-week-long monitoring. Baseline characteristics of the patients participating in the monitoring is given in Table 1. Some CGM records include medication and meal marks, self-reported from the patient or obtained automatically from management software.

Table 1. Baseline characteristics of participants

Diabetes type	Gender	Number of participants	Average age (years)	StdDev age (years)	Average DM duration (years)	StdDev DM duration (years)
T1DM	F	12	32.25	8.99	18.75	6.74
	M	10	30.40	12.96	19.50	9.06
T1DM Total		**22**	**31.41**	**10.73**	**19.09**	**7.69**
T2DM	F	6	71.83	4.58	13.36	11.39
	M	6	74.50	10.77	15.33	8.52
T2DM Total		**12**	**73.17**	**8.01**	**14.35**	**9.65**
without DM	M	1	38.00			
Total		**35**	**45.91**	**22.18**	**16.92**	**8.97**

3   Methods

Methods for replacing missing values in CGM records depend on when the reconstruction of the data needs to take place and the length of the missing segment. If the data needs to be replaced for offline analysis after the collection of CGM records, we considered methods that use samples before and after the missing segment to reconstruct the values of the missing segment. Whereas when simulating methods for real-time analysis of the trend, we only used samples prior to the disruption in the record.

On the used dataset we identified and evaluated missing segments considering the length and frequency of occurrence, focusing further on the short-length missing segments (less than 30 min).

3.1   Replacing Data for Analysis After Collection

As we focused this experiment on short-length gaps (less than 30 min), with known data prior and after the gap, we replaced the missing values using piecewise cubic spline interpolation (spline) and shape-preserving piecewise cubic interpolation (pchip). Both spline and pchip are using cubic polynomial to fit to the data. The advantage of spline is that it produces a smoother result, and pchip that it has no overshoots and it oscillates less if the data is not smooth. In both cases, we used the data from one hour (12 samples) before the start of the gap, and the data from one hour after the gap.

3.2   Replacing Data for Real-Time Analysis of Trends

In this experiment we focused on simple methods to estimate values of missing segments for real-time application. The important factor in glucose management is knowing to react to rate of change (RoC) of sensor glucose data. The research suggests incorporating RoC trend arrows into clinical recommendations but with addressing awareness of the limitations of incorporating ROC trend arrows in patients' daily use for decision-making [6]. An example of RoC trend arrows for FreeStyle Libre flash monitor is shown in Table 2 [7]. This system quantifies the RoC of glucose based on five trend arrow orientations. RoC is important factor in assessing the risk of hypoglycemia.

Table 2. RoC trend

Rate and direction of glucose change	Anticipated change from current reading in	
	15 min	30 min
Rising rapidly > 1.8 mg/dL/min	>+27.0 mg/dL	>+54.0 mg/dL
Rising 1.08–1.8 mg/dL/min	+16.2 to 27.0 mg/dL	+32.4 to 54.0 mg/dL
Changing slowly < 1.08 mg/dL/min	<±16.2 mg/dL	<±32.4 mg/dL
Falling 1.08–1.8 mg/dL/min	−16.2 to −27.0 mg/dL	−32.4 to −54.0 mg/dL
Falling rapidly > 1.8 mg/dL/min	>−27.0 mg/dL	>−54.0 mg/dL

We computed ROC for each record as

$$RoC(n) = CGM(n) - CGM(n-1) \tag{1}$$

where CGM is CGM records, n is the number of the sample in the record, in order to calculate anticipated change in glucose level.

Another attempt to replace the missing segment, using only previous data, is based on the similarity search and combining values from the known segments. We considered all records as the database from which similar segments can be extracted. To find similar segments, we used 1-hour window (12 samples) of observed CGM record and then computed similarity [8] search in all the other records from our database. Similarity search in this experiment is based on calculating Euclidean distance between two CGM segments (observed segment and potential similar match from other records):

$$ED = \sqrt{\sum_{i=1}^{n} \left(CGM_{obsseg}(n) - CGM_{pot}(n) \right)^2} \tag{2}$$

where n is length of the observed segment in samples, CGM_{obsseg} is observed sample, and CGM_{pot} is potential match. Potential match is extracted from all the records, excluding the records from which the observed segment is taken, using sliding window to find N best matches.

Then, to assess the values in the missing segment, we used k values following the best matched segments, where k is the length of the missing segment. Proposed values of the missing segments are given as the mean values in each position of N best matches.

3.3   Analysis of the Performance

For the evaluation of method performance, we used mean absolute error (MAE) [9]:

$$MAE = \frac{\sum_{i=1}^{n} |E_i - O_i|}{n} \tag{3}$$

where n is the length of the missing segment, E is estimate of the missing segment and O is observed segment (i.e. known real CGM data).

To simulate the possibility of data disruption at any given time, we constructed 100 random pairs of variables (*record_id*, *sample_id*). *record_id* is the identifier of the CGM record, and *sample_id* is the position in the CGM record at which we consider possible disruption. We used only those segments in records where the extracted data did not have any missing values.

4   Results

4.1   Identified Gaps

In our analysis we identified 23 total gaps in 14 out of 67 CGM records. The gap shortest in duration was 20 min and it occurred in 11 out of 23 gaps (47.83%) and longest was 23 h and 55 min which occurred once. 13 gaps were shorter than one hour (60.87%), 7 were in range of <1, 8] hours (30.43%), and 2 were longer than 8 h (8.70%). We focused our experiment to gaps shorter than one hour.

4.2   Replacing the Data

The gap we introduced to data was 20-minute-long (4 samples) which proved to be the most common length of the gap in the dataset. For the computations we used 1-hour window (12 samples) prior to the gap.

In our experiment we identified rate of change (RoC) as amount of change in the CGM record data for two consecutive samples. For each observed CGM record (Fig. 1a) we computed RoC (Fig. 1b), and defined maximal and minimal values, denoted by square marker on the figure. We used maximal and minimal RoC in the CGM record prior to the missing segment to estimate values in the missing segment. The example of replacing missing data with maximal RoC is shown in Fig. 2. This was to assess if during the gap there is any possibility to enter hypoglycemia, and the estimate was not used to truly replace missing data.

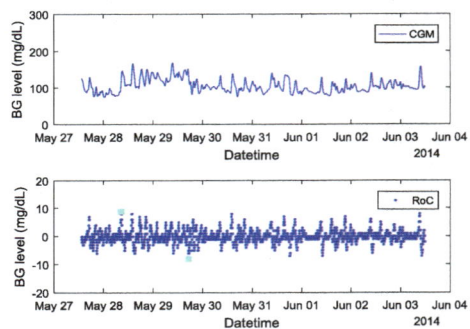

Fig. 1.   (a) CGM record; (b) RoC

Figure 3 is showing the CGM record segment from which the missing segment is excluded (gap), along with 5 best matches found in other records using the Euclidean distance. Similarity was assessed in the complete database in order to maximize the chance to find similar dynamics. Calculated Euclidean distance (ED) is shown in the legend. Replacement of the values during the gap using averaged values of matched segments is shown in Fig. 4.

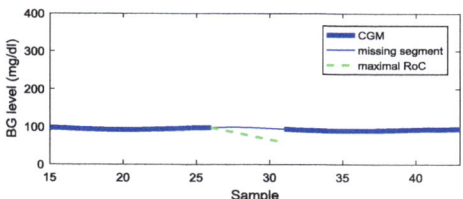

Fig. 2. Replacing with maximal RoC

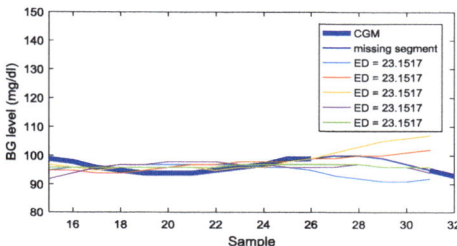

Fig. 3. CGM segment with the gap and 5 most similar matches

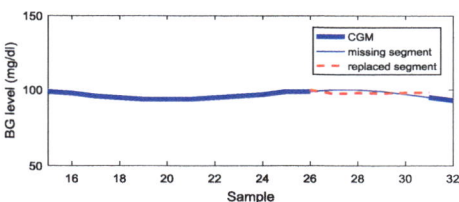

Fig. 4. Gap replacement with 5 most similar matches

For gap replacement using spline and pchip we selected 1-hour window (12 samples) prior to the gap, 20-minute gap (4 samples) and 1-hour window after the gap (12 samples). Gap replacement using spline and pchip is shown in Fig. 5.

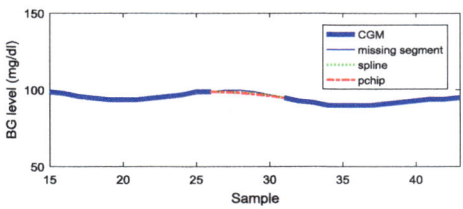

Fig. 5. Gap replacement using spline and pchip

We computed MAE for 100 randomly chosen segments, and average MAE across all 100 estimations was computed for three different methods: using averaged matched segments (AMS), using spline and using pchip. The results are shown in Table 3.

Table 3. MAE mean and standard deviation using different methods

	AMS	SPLINE	PCHIP
Mean	22.01	0.54	0.89
Standard deviation	25.83	0.32	0.87

5   Conclusions

We computed several methods to replace missing values in the short-length gaps in CGM records. We identified most gaps were 20 min. Replacing missing values in 20-minute-long gaps for offline analysis with spline and pchip showed promising result with mean error of (0.54 ± 0.32) mg/dL and (0.89 ± 0.87) mg/dL respectively. Replacing missing values for the real-time application using averaged matched segments resulted in mean error of (22.01 ± 25.83) mg/dL.

This research is valuable for development of robust and timely alert mechanisms for early warning of patients using CGM systems in case there is no data received and there is a threat of entering hypoglycemia.

Conflict of Interest. The authors declare that they have no conflict of interest.

References

1. Klonoff, D.C., Ahn, D., Drincic, A.: Continuous glucose monitoring: a review of the technology and clinical use. Diabetes Res. Clin. Pract. **133**, 178–192 (2017). https://doi.org/10.1016/j.diabres.2017.08.005
2. Mariani, H.S., Layden, B.T., Aleppo, G.: Continuous glucose monitoring: a perspective on its past, present, and future applications for diabetes management. Clin. Diabetes **35**(1), 60–65 (2017). https://doi.org/10.2337/cd16-0008
3. Schmelzeisen-Redeker, G., Schoemaker, M., Kirchsteiger, H., Freckmann, G., Heinemann, L., del Re, L.: Time delay of CGM sensors. J. Diabetes Sci. Technol. **9**(5), 1006–1015 (2015). https://doi.org/10.1177/1932296815590154
4. Kruger, D.F., Edelman, S.V., Hinnen, D.A., Parkin, C.G.: Reference guide for integrating continuous glucose monitoring into clinical practice. Diab. Educ. (2018). https://doi.org/10.1177/0145721718818066
5. Danne, T., et al.: International consensus on use of continuous glucose monitoring. Diabetes. Care **40**(12), 1631–1640 (2017). https://doi.org/10.2337/dc17-1600
6. Fantasia, K., Modzelewski, K., Steenkamp, D: Predictive glucose trends from continuous glucose monitoring: friend or foe in clinical decision making? J. Diabetes Sci. Technol. (2019). https://doi.org/10.1177/1932296818823538

7. Ajjan, R.A., Cummings, M.H., Jennings, P., Leelarathna, L., Rayman, G., Wilmot, E.G.: Optimising use of rate-of-change trend arrows for insulin dosing decisions using the FreeStyle Libre flash glucose monitoring system. Diab. Vasc. Dis. Res. (2018). https://doi.org/10.1177/1479164118795252

8. Serrà, J., Arcos, J.L.: An empirical evaluation of similarity measures for time series classification. Knowl. Based Syst. **67**, 305–314 (2014). https://doi.org/10.1016/j.knosys.2014.04.035

9. Willmott, C., Matsuura, K.: Advantages of the mean absolute error (MAE) over the root mean square error (RMSE) in assessing average model performance. Climate Res. **30**, 79–82 (2005). https://doi.org/10.3354/cr030079

Based on DICOM RT Structure and Multiple Loss Function Deep Learning Algorithm in Organ Segmentation of Head and Neck Image

Ya-Ju Hsieh[1(✉)], Hsien-Chun Tseng[2], Chiun-Li Chin[1],
Yu-Hsiang Shao[1], and Ting-Yu Tsai[1]

[1] Department of Medical Informatics, Chung Shan Medical University,
No. 110, Section 1, Jianguo North Road, Taichung, Taiwan
ii860731@gmail.com
[2] Department of Radiation Oncology, School of Medicine,
Chung Shan Medical University Hospital, Taichung, Taiwan

Abstract. Delineating organs for a long time may cause exhaustion to radiologist's eyes and mental health, it could lead to results that show different sizes of organs with therapeutic target volume. In this work, we expand on the idea of automatically delineating the organs in Computed Tomography (CT) images of head and neck through the generative adversarial network, which is a deep learning algorithm. In image preprocessing, we generate a bitmap (BMP) image by the combination of CT image and RT structure (RS) file and input it to generator network, which will improve the color and texture quality, last generate a fake Radiation Therapy (RT) image. Finally, the discriminator network takes the fake RT image as an example to compare with the original RT image. To build the predictive model, we continuously train this model to let it learn the rules of delineating organs in CT image, generating more and more images that are similar to the original samples. The approach that proposed in this paper is actually well applied in medicine, and the results of testing are similar to the selected organs or therapeutic targets' volume that was delineated by the radiologist. We can see that it not only effectively reduces the false positive rate but also promises in applying to other related images.

Keywords: Organ segmentation · Generative adversarial network ·
Deep learning · DICOM RT structure · Medical imaging

1 Introduction

The department of radiation oncology in hospital mainly treat tumors with radiation and chemotherapy. The radiologist first needs to form a DICOM Radiation Therapy (RT) image [1], which includes therapeutic target volume and important organs delineated from Computed Tomography (CT) images to assist the physician in diagnosing and determining the amount of radiation. However, repeatedly doing these actions every day causes exhaustion to radiologist's eyes and mental health, thus it could lead to

© Springer Nature Switzerland AG 2020
K.-P. Lin et al. (Eds.): ICBHI 2019, IFMBE Proceedings 74, pp. 428–435, 2020.
https://doi.org/10.1007/978-3-030-30636-6_58

results that show different sizes of organs with therapeutic target volume. In recent years, J. Pipitone et al. think whether there are effective methods to assist in the judgment of medical images [2]. Furthermore, there are more and more works had applied with deep learning algorithm in medical image segmentation [3–6]. Due to the fact that generative adversarial network (GAN) shows better results in image processing, many works have proposed to use the GAN algorithm to train and compare networks and models with little data to achieve good results [7, 8]. Dwarikanath et al. [9] trained GAN into two competitive neural networks: one is the generator network and the other is the discriminator network, performing image segmentation. The generator network will generate a fake RT image that looks like the original sample, and the discriminator network examines the truth [10, 11]. Seeliger et al. [12] point out that to build the best predictive model needed to continuously train the model, generating more images that are similar to the original samples. As a result, we expand on the idea of using GAN algorithm on automatically delineating organs in CT images of head and neck through deep learning method and use multiple loss functions to calculate the error between original sample images and generated images in this paper. This paper presents the contributions:

1. Delineating organs in medical images through GAN algorithm.
2. Carry out backward error correction through multiple loss functions and adjusts the parameters.
3. Evaluate the similarity by comparing the generated image with the original image.

The rest of the paper is organized as follows: In Sect. 2, we describe the overview of our generative adversarial network and introduce the proposed method in detail. In Sect. 3, we introduce the experimental results. Conclusions will be given in Sect. 4.

2   Materials and Methods

In this paper, we use GAN algorithm to automatically delineate the organs of head and neck in CT image. As shown in Fig. 1, the proposed organ segmentation framework includes three parts: convert the module of the CT image, automatically delineate organs or target volume and create new RT Structure (RS) file. Firstly, each patient will receive the number of DICOM image around 90 from tomography and convert it into a bitmap (BMP) file. Next, aligning images in the arrangement with z-axis from head to neck and reading required RS file information for the system, such as the pixel value of the outline and color. Last, we export the BMP file into GAN and get a trained RT image, combining it with the patient's CT image information to generate a new RS file. We will introduce the GAN algorithm we proposed in Sect. 2.1 and define the multiple loss functions detailed in Sect. 2.2.

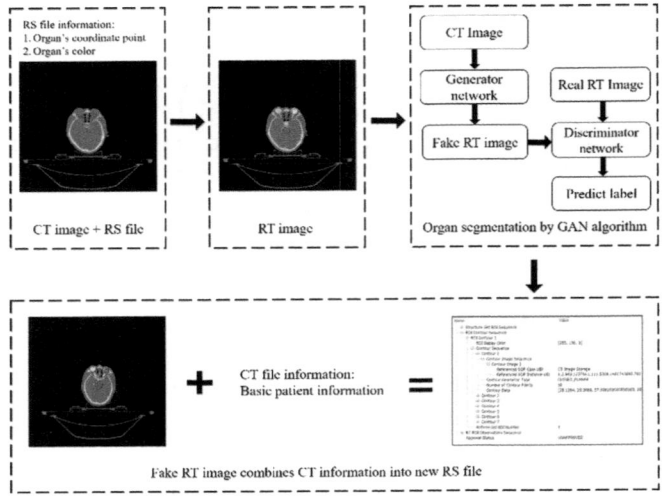

Fig. 1. The framework of our organ segmentation method

2.1 Organ Segmentation by Our Proposed GAN Algorithm

The generator network contains 11 convolutional layers, each combines a batch normalization. Except for the last layer in the generator network is applied to the sigmoid activation function to the outputs, all layers in the generator network are followed by a ReLu activation function.

The discriminator network consists of 5 convolutional layers with leaky ReLu activation function, 4 batch normalizations and 1 fully-connected layer to compare structural similarity (SSIM) and the peak signal to noise ratio (PSNR) [10] with the RT image sample that was delineated by radiologists. After several times of comparison, the trained RT image that was generated by the generator network will be very similar to the original RT.

2.2 Multiple Loss Functions

To achieve a better approach to image segmentation, we build loss function under the assumption in three major parts: color, texture and content quality [13], combining them into a total loss function with different weight.

2.2.1 Color Loss Function

In color loss, we use Gaussian blur to de-noise, and be used to build a convolution matrix which is applied to the original image then calculate the loss by Mean Square Error (MSE) function. The Gaussian blur operator is written as:

$$G(m, n) = A \, exp\left(-\frac{(m - \mu_x)^2}{2\sigma_x} - \frac{(n - \mu_y)^2}{2\sigma_y}\right) \tag{1}$$

where we defined A = 0.1, $\mu_{x,y} = 0$, $\sigma_{x,y} = 5$, and the color loss used in this paper is defined as:

$$L_{color}(X, Y) = \|X_b - Y_b\| \tag{2}$$

where X_b and Y_b are the blurred images of X and Y, resp.:

$$X_b(i, j) = \sum_{m,n} X(i + m, j + n) \cdot G(m, n) \tag{3}$$

2.2.2   Texture Loss Function

In texture loss, we build GAN to directly learn the appropriate metrics for measuring texture quality and compare the probability distribution of texture between generator and discriminator network through maximum likelihood estimation (MLE). The image generated by the generator network will be placed into the discriminator network and compare the fake(improved) image with an original sample image to meet the goal of predicting whether the input image is real or not. The degree of similarity generated by the discriminator is 0 to 1, and the value is taken as a log to calculate the error correction for texture partition. The texture loss is defined as:

$$L_{texture} = -\sum_{m} logD(F_w(I_s), I_t) \tag{4}$$

where F_w and D denote the generator and discriminator networks; $F_w(I_s)$ stands for the enhanced image that was generated by the generator network.

2.2.3   Content Loss Function

In content loss, we extract features from the activation map, which are the images that were generated by the generator network and the original sample images input to the ReLU_5_4 layer of the VGG-19 network. It will compare the error of the image content in the feature map. The content loss is defined as:

$$L_{content} = \frac{1}{C_i H_i W_i} \|\varphi_i(F_w(I_s)) - \varphi_i(I_t)\| \tag{5}$$

where C_i, H_i and W_i stands for the number, height and width of the feature maps, and φ_i is the feature map that was obtained after the i-th convolutional layer of VGG-19.

2.2.4   Total Loss Function

Our total loss is defined as a weighted sum of color, texture and content loss:

$$L_{total} = 0.5 \cdot L_{color} + 1 \cdot L_{texture} + 10 \cdot L_{content} \tag{6}$$

3   Results

In this section, we first describe some details about our experimental settings. Then, we give the experimental results on our model formulations which compare multiple loss functions. We also show results for delineating different organs in CT images.

3.1   Experimental Environment and Parameters Setting

In this paper, we totally collect 11593 head and neck CT images from 150 patients to train the model. The CT images in the dataset were preprocessed in a standard way, i.e., the organs in the images are detected and aligned then cropped and normalized to 150×150. For all the following experiments, we use TensorFlow, which is an open-source software library that provides deep learning models and makes our work easy to produce. The network was trained on an operating system of Windows with 16 GB RAM, i7-8750HQ 2.2 GHz CPU and NVIDIA GeForce GTX 1060 GPU using a batch size of 20. It was optimized using stochastic gradient descent with a learning rate of 5e–4, and training stops at 35000 iterations. We found that all the networks converge well under these settings, so we use the same parameters to train model to make fair comparisons between the original image and the image present by our experimental.

3.2   Experimental Results

The experimental results of this paper will be divided into two parts to discuss: one is the comparison of multiple loss functions with the result, and the other is the quality measurements.

3.2.1   Comparison Between Loss Function and Test Accuracy

During the training process, we carry out backward error correction by three different loss functions, which are content, color and texture. Loss value implies how well or poorly a certain model behaves after each iteration. Ideally, we expect the reduction of loss after each or several iterations. We calculate the total weight loss of returning error values to make corrections in every 1000 iterations. Figure 2 shows three different loss value step by step, in general, after 35000 iterations the three loss values will tend to be close to 0.

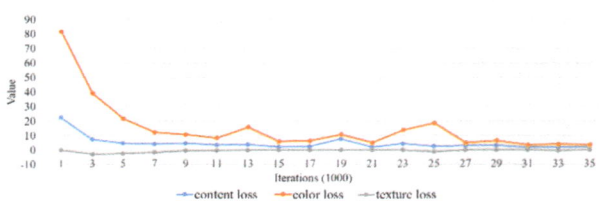

Fig. 2. The line chart shows the value of three loss functions

The training and testing accuracy are shown in Table 1, comparing with Fig. 2 that the smaller the value is, the higher testing accuracy will be.

Table 1. The training and testing accuracy show in different iterations

Training step	Training accuracy (%)	Testing accuracy (%)
7000 iterations	84.2	81.2
14000 iterations	96.5	86.9
21000 iterations	97.1	91.2
28000 iterations	97.3	95.6
35000 iterations	99.8	98.8

3.2.2 Quality Measurements

To strengthen our claim, we used two metrics to evaluate our proposed method. One is the peak signal to noise ratio (PSNR), which captures the difference in the pixel values between two images, and the other is structural similarity (SSIM), which estimates the holistic similarity between two images. Both values present by PSNR and SSIM are higher the better. In this paper, we compared the PSNR and SSIM between the original CT image that radiologist delineated the organs and the image shows in our results in every 1000 iterations, and the comparison result is shown in Table 2.

Table 2. The training and testing accuracy show in different iterations

Training step	SSIM	PSNR
7000 iterations	0.88	23.15
14000 iterations	0.91	23.58
21000 iterations	0.93	24.39
28000 iterations	0.93	24.42
35000 iterations	0.94	24.48

From Table 2, we can see that the SSIM is 0.94 and PSNR is 24.48 in the final result. As shown in Fig. 3, the comparison of the original CT image that organs were delineated by radiologists and the output responses of the discriminator network based on GAN algorithm.

There are big differences between the images produced in 7000 iterations and 35000 iterations. Moreover, the result shows in 35000 iterations is almost the same as the original CT image that organs were delineated by radiologist. From Table 1 and Fig. 3, we refer that it is possible to delineate the organs by using the approach proposed in this paper is effective and fast.

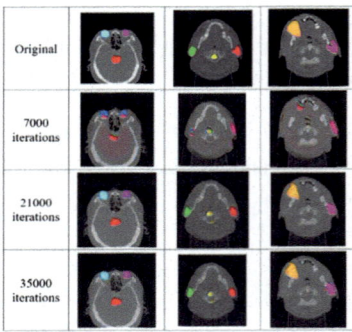

Fig. 3. Several results of our method using GAN algorithm

4 Conclusions

To reduce the working pressure from the radiologist and hope that computer-aided medicine can decrease the error that was made during delineating organs or target volume by using the GAN algorithm. We convert the image to generate training dataset for GAN algorithm to delineate the organs and target volume. The approach present in this paper is actually well applied in medicine, by using GAN algorithm to delineate organs in CT image. The comparison between the results of testing and the delineate organs or therapeutic targets' volume by the radiologist shows that SSIM and PSNR stand for 0.94 and 24.48. Infer from this result, we know that it can effectively reduce the false positive rate and apply to other medical images. In the future, we will extend the method to recognize whether the organ has lesion or the dose calculation on specific treatment, making a breakthrough in diagnosing the health condition.

Conflict of Interest. The authors declare that they have no conflict of interest.

References

1. Law, M.Y.Y., Liu, B., Chan, L.W.: DICOM-RT–based electronic patient record information system for radiation therapy. RadioGraphics **29**, 912–922 (2009)
2. Pipitone, J., Park, M.T., Winterburn, J., et al.: Multi-atlas segmentation of the whole hippocampus and subfields using multiple automatically generated templates. NeuroImage **101**, 494–512 (2014)
3. Ibragimov, B., Xing, L.: Segmentation of organs-at-risks in head and neck CT images using convolutional neural networks. Medical Physics **44**(2), 547–557 (2017)
4. Fausto, M., Seyed-Ahmad, A., Christine, K., et al.: Hough-CNN: deep learning for segmentation of deep brain regions in MRI and ultrasound. Comput. Vis. Image Underst. **164**, 92–102 (2017)
5. Lei, B., Jinman, K., Euijoon, A., et al.: Step-wise integration of deep class-specific learning for dermoscopic image segmentation. Pattern Recogn. **85**, 78–89 (2018)

6. Holger, R., Hirohisa, O., Xiangrong, Z., et al.: An application of cascaded 3D fully convolutional networks for medical image segmentation. Comput. Med. Imaging Graph. **66**, 90–99 (2018)
7. Libin, J., Hao, W., Haodi, W., et al.: Multi-scale semantic image inpainting with residual learning and GAN, NEUCOM 2018. Neurocomputing **331**, 199–212 (2018)
8. Samik, B., Sukhendu, D.: LR-GAN for degraded face recognition. Pattern Recogn. Lett. **116**, 246–253 (2018)
9. Dwarikanath, M., Behzad, B., Rahil, G.: Image super-resolution using progressive generative adversarial networks for medical image analysis. Comput. Med. Imaging Graph. **71**, 30–39 (2018)
10. Qiang, Z., Honglun, L., Baode, F., et al.: Integrating support vector machine and graph cuts for medical image segmentation. J. Vis. Commun. Image Represent. **55**, 157–165 (2018)
11. Maayan, F., Idit, D., Eyal, K., et al.: GAN-based synthetic medical image augmentation for increased CNN performance in liver lesion classification. Neurocomputing **321**, 321–331 (2018)
12. Seeliger, K., Güçlü, U., Ambrogioni, L., et al.: Generative adversarial networks for reconstructing natural images from brain activity. NeuroImage **181**, 775–785 (2018)
13. Andrey, I., Nikolay, K., Radu, T., et al.: DSLR-quality photos on mobile devices with deep convolutional networks. In: IEEE International Conference on Computer Vision, ICCV, Venice, vol. 16, pp. 3297–3305 (2017)

Author Index

A

Aramrussameekul, Worapol, 243
Arredondo, Maria Teresa, 174

B

Bocanegra, Francisco Calderón, 396
Boonjun, Sasithorn, 235
Boonpratatong, Amaraporn, 235, 243, 252
Byrne, Helen, 275

C

Canevari, Silvana, 174
Cárdenas, Jhonathan Sora, 396
Carvalho, Paulo, 320, 420
Castaldo, Rossana, 275, 288
Castro, Gustavo, 405
Chang, Cheng-Pe, 312
Chang, Cheng-Yuan, 342
Chang, Chia-Hao, 108
Chang, Ming-Kai, 15
Chang, Po-Hsuan, 15
Chang, Po-Hung, 183, 191
Chang, Yuan-Hsiang, 42
Chao, Wei-cheng, 227
Chappell, Micheal, 275
Cheimariotis, Grigorios-Aris, 389
Chen, Cheng-Hsueh, 1
Chen, Chih-Chia, 80
Chen, Jeng-Wen, 100
Chen, Ko-Chiang, 219
Chen, Kuan-Chun, 304
Chen, Kuo-Ti, 268
Chen, Mei-Fen, 115
Chen, Meng-Chi, 1
Chen, Mu-Hsiung, 1

Chen, Pei-Ying, 115
Chen, Pin-Chuan, 122
Chen, Sung-wei, 227
Chen, Wei-Hao, 91
Chen, Weikun, 335
Chen, Wen-Chien, 371
Chen, Xingguang, 335
Chen, Yu-You, 86
Cheng, Chean-Yeh, 148
Cheng, Cheanyeh, 63
Cheng, Han-Chien, 296
Cheng, Ren-Wei, 15
Cheng, Tsu-Chi, 138
Chiang, Hsiao-Ling, 312
Chiang, Hui-Hua Kenny, 91, 122, 166
Chilleri, Camilla, 328
Chin, Chiun-Li, 304, 428
Chiu, Nan-Tsing, 138
Chiu, Po-Chuan, 296
Chou, Yu-Sheng, 363
Chu, Mu-tao, 227
Chuang, Chiung-Cheng, 72
Chuang, Keh-Shih, 108
Chung, Chi-Yu, 42
Chung, Ni-Chuan, 304
Chung, Wen-Yaw, 15, 63, 148, 156
Cifrek, Mario, 335
Couceiro, Ricardo, 320
Cruz, Jennifer Dela, 148
Čuljak, Ivana, 335

D

Díaz, Martha Zequera, 396
Du, Ernie, 227
Du, Min, 335
Džaja, Dominik, 413

E
Egawa, Kana, 260

F
Fang, Yu-Hua, 33, 80, 138
Fico, Giuseppe, 174
Friebe, Michael, 9
Fu, Tieh-Cheng, 183, 191

G
Gao, Yueming, 335
García-Vázquez, Mireya Sarai, 349

H
Han, Ji-Yan, 219
He, Hsin-Yen, 281
Hemthanon, Chomkansak, 212
Hsiao, Tzu-Chien, 26, 198
Hsieh, Ya-Ju, 428
Hsu, Chian-Yun, 86
Hsu, Ching-Chi, 50, 57, 86
Hsu, Chin-Luen, 304
Hsu, Wei-Chun, 50
Hu, Wei-Chih, 9
Huang, Bo-Yu, 381
Huang, Chih-Chung, 100
Huang, Kuan-Ting, 57
Huang, Wen-Sheng, 312
Hughes, Stephen, 275
Hung, G., 281

I
Iadanza, Ernesto, 328
Illanes, Alfredo, 9
Innominato, Pasquale, 275

J
Janjarasjitt, Suparerk, 212, 356
Jesus, Diogo, 320
Jhang, De-Fu, 72
Jhang, Sin-Hua, 219
Jhou, Shu-Yu, 50
Ji, Hong-Ming, 26, 198
Juang, Chi-Long, 312

K
Kao, Szu-Ying, 72
Katsaggelos, Aggelos, 389
Kitiratchai, Pattranit, 252
Konno, Noriko, 260
Kulkarni, Vishwesh, 275
Kuo, Sen M., 342

L
Lacković, Igor, 413
Lai, Jheng-Siang, 15
Lai, Ying-Hui, 219
Lee, Kuan-Ting, 72
Leu, Jyh-Shyan, 312
Li, Kuan-Hua, 148
Li, Pin-Lu, 204
Liang, Hsin-Chin, 143
Licitra, Lisa, 174
Lin, Chia-Yu, 108
Lin, Chi-Lun, 381
Lin, Jui-Teng, 268
Lin, Kang-Ping, 115, 183, 191, 204
Lin, Wen-Chen, 115
Lin, Yin-Chih, 91
Liu, Hsia-Wei, 268
Liu, Wenzhu, 335
Liu, Xiu-Wei, 342
Lopez-Perez, Laura, 174
Lopez-Rodríguez, Mario, 349
Lu, Shao-Hung, 183, 191, 204
Lu, Wei-Cheng, 183

M
Magjarević, Ratko, 413, 420
Maglaveras, Nikolaos, 389
Manlises, Cyrel Ontimare, 100
Miyaho, Noriharu, 260
Mongkholhatthi, Waranya, 252
Montesinos, Luis, 275, 288
Muehlsteff, Jens, 320
Murase, Kotaro, 260

N
Ni, Yu-Ching, 108, 143
Nograles, Abdul Hadi, 148

O
Ou, Jin-Hao, 371

P
Paglinawan, Arnold C., 15, 156
Panganiban, Edward B., 15, 156
Pavlaković, Lovro, 413
Pecchia, Leandro, 174, 275, 288
Prati, Marta, 275

R
Ramezani, Roozbeh Falah, 148
Ramírez-Acosta, Alejandro, 349
Ribeiro, Rogerio, 420
Riga, Maria, 389

S

Sakunwitunthai, Supanat, 243
Sassananan, Setta, 235
Šeketa, Goran, 413
Shao, Yu-Hsiang, 428
Shih, Kao-Shang, 57, 86
Shimada, Takamasa, 260
Singh, Yashbir, 9
Su, Li-chi, 227
Su, Shih-Po, 166
Su, Ting-Yu, 33
Su, Xuan-Hao, 281
Su, Yi-Sheng, 129

T

Tai, Wei-Chieh, 15
Ting, Chien-Hsin, 312
Ting, Hao-Jen, 115
Toloza, Daissy Carola, 405
Tousoulis, Dimitris, 389
Toutouzas, Konstantinos, 389
Tsai, Cheng-Lun, 183, 191, 204
Tsai, Ting-Yu, 428
Tsai, Vincent, 63, 148
Tseng, Fan-Pin, 108
Tseng, Hsien-Chun, 428
Tseng, Sheng-Pin, 108
Tseng, Wei-Kung, 281
Twu, Shih-Hsiung, 129

V

Vasić, Željka Lučev, 335

W

Wang, Chih-Hao, 122
Wang, Jia-Jung, 281
Wang, Jia-Yin, 363
Watai, Kosuke, 260
Wongbuangam, Sugunya, 252
Woradit, Kampol, 235
Wu, Hsiang-Ning, 143

Y

Yang, Bang-Hung, 312
Yang, Chia-Wei, 91
Yang, Chi-chin, 227
Yang, Fan-pei Gloria, 227
Yang, Ming-Hao, 371
Yang, Yi-Fang, 363
Yao, Shu-Nung, 296
Yen, Lin-Chen, 63
Yokoi, Atsuya, 260
Yu, Ming-Hsien, 371

Z

Zamudio-Fuentes, Luis Miguel, 349
Zeng, Jing-Xiang, 122
Zequera, Martha, 405
Zhang, Wei-Ting, 91
Zheng, Haibo, 335
Žulj, Sara, 413, 420